THE EYE-OPENING BOOK THAT HAS HELPED SPUR A CONGRESSIONAL INVESTIGATION INTO DRUG PRICING, CAUSED MANY PHYSICIANS TO ALTER THEIR PRESCRIPTION PRACTICES, AND SAVED COUNTLESS PEOPLE AMAZING AMOUNTS OF MONEY

"Dr. Richard Burack has made an important contribution to the health and welfare of all Americans. His valuable new book will go a long way toward helping the consumer obtain proper and less expensive drugs. THE NEW HANDBOOK OF PRESCRIPTION DRUGS should be required reading for doctors and patients alike."

—U.S. Senator Gaylord Nelson

"I don't know what your relationship to your doctor is but this is mine: I want to know exactly what's wrong with me and I want to know exactly what he's doing about it and why. . . . Next time he says he's going to prescribe something for me I am going to raise the question of prescription prices before he writes out the name of a particular brand. He will have the HANDBOOK on his desk because I'm going to send him a copy... and if he has some reason for prescribing a high-priced brand instead of low-priced generic, I will want to know about it. We will discuss it until I am satisfied he is doing the right thing."

—Clarence Peterson,
in the *Chicago Tribune*

The New Handbook of Prescription Drugs

Updated and Expanded

Richard Burack, M.D., F.A.C.P.
with
Fred J. Fox, M.D.

BALLANTINE BOOKS • NEW YORK

Library of Congress Catalog Card Number 75-38117

ISBN 0-345-27584-5

This edition published by arrangement with Pantheon Books, a division of Random House, Inc., New York

Manufactured in the United States of America

First Ballantine Books Edition: September 1970

Revised Editions:
First Printing: September 1975
Eighth Printing: March 1979

First Canadian Printing: October 1975
Fourth Canadian Printing: January 1977

Dedication
and
Acknowledgments

This volume is dedicated primarily to Miss Helen Elizabeth Nute of New Hampshire, a wise and cultured person. It is an honor to have her as a kind, compassionate, and fiercely loyal friend. Helen Nute awakened a temporarily dormant social conscience with large doses of Upton Sinclair, and restored my appreciation for beauty with baskets of mayflowers. While she urged me to begin to write again, she patiently tolerated my procrastination. I am very, very grateful.

Once again I owe special thanks to my wife, Mary, and to our children: Ruth, Richard, Jr., Jim, Tom, and Anna. I love each of them. They were so patient when I was reading and thinking and when it may have appeared that I should have been spending more time with each of them in the beautiful mountainous out-of-doors in New England.

It will never be possible to express enough gratitude to Mrs. Charles "Betsy" Mehaffey, whose unflagging fidelity, common sense, and hard work kept my practice and me together while both of us struggled to assuage the tempers and unexpected perversities of a large and demanding number of patients. Patients demand diagnoses, but it was and always will be difficult to persuade most of them that it is far more important for the doctor to know what is *not* wrong with them. A good friend, the late and loved Dean John Fox of the Harvard School of Business Administration, understood it well. He likened the

situation to that of the captain of a Maine coastal
steamer who made no pretense of knowing "where
every single dangerous rock lurks close to the surface." "Just know where they ain't," the captain would
assure his passengers.

While Mrs. Mehaffey worked nearly four years,
using secretarial and managerial talent to keep my
office organized, Mrs. James "Mary" Haine proceeded
with tireless good humor to send bills to patients I
had served, a necessary task I wanted nothing of.
The financial transaction that occurs between doctor
and patient has always been a difficult one for me—
totally out of keeping with the concept of professional physician or surgeon who has dedicated himself to helping fellow human beings who are sick
or who imagine that they are. But since the country
has not yet recognized the practical and ethical bene-
fits to be derived from salaried doctors, the functions
performed by persons like Mary Haine are invaluable. I am fully aware that my sentiments about financial reimbursement of doctors place me very much
in the minority. In my eleven years of private practice, I always yearned for a salary and liberation
from the tyranny of overhead costs. Mine are not the
sentiments of organized medicine; they are not even
the sentiments of some of my closest doctor friends,
who have as little connection with organized medicine as I. Perhaps they will excuse what to many of
them may appear to be an eccentricity; I respect their
sentiments and merely expect them to respect the
convictions that made it impossible for me to join
the American Medical Association.*

Obviously, Senator Gaylord Nelson of Wisconsin
and Mr. Benjamin Gordon, Economist to the United
States Senate Select Committee on Small Business,

---

* Lest anyone conclude that this is meant to be a reckless
condemnation of the AMA, the record of my views about that
organization shows that while I voice strong disagreement with
many of its stands, I appreciate its fine accomplishments, past
and present. (*Competitive Problems in the Drug Industry*,
Hearings Before the Subcommittee on Monopoly, Senate Select
Committee on Small Business, 90th Congress, 1st Session [June
7, 1967], Part 1, pp. 325–326.)

remain the objects of my gratitude, for without the two of them the serious issues described in this book could never have been brought to light. Every American citizen owes a profound debt to these two public servants who have earned secure niches for themselves in American history. These two men, alone, are waging a highly successful battle to restore regulation over a vital industry grown wild as a cancer.

The scholarly volumes of hearings compiled under the direction of the late Senator Estes Kefauver of Tennessee were initially my most important source of education. Senator Kefauver's associate, Economist Irene Till, kindly introduced me to them. *In a Few Hands*, authored by the Senator with the assistance of Mrs. Till (Pantheon, 1965), has also been educational and thought-provoking. Morton Mintz's masterful *Therapeutic Nightmare*, updated as *By Prescription Only* (Houghton Mifflin, 1967), has been invaluable.

Drs. Theodore Badger, a respected senior physician, Otto Krayer, Emeritus Professor, and Paul Draskoczy, Assistant Professor of Pharmacology at Harvard Medical School, have been important mentors over the years, although none bears responsibility for any errors that may appear in the book. Rudolf Sonneborn of New York City, a bold, successful man, has been a strong, continuing source of inspiration, as have Mr. and Mrs. Shakman Katz of Baltimore. A confidant whose judgment I value highly is Giles E. Mosher, Jr., neighbor, patient, and friend.

Many thanks are due to Mrs. Paula McGuire of Pantheon Books, a helpful editor and a wise friend. A great debt is also due Donn Teal for his superb editorial advice and his fine copy editing.

For Messrs. David Currier and Owen Lock, talented editors and prudent gentlemen, I have deep respect and admiration. They were always helpful, innovative, and stimulating.

For their many overtime hours, I thank my past and present secretaries, Karen Kutrieb and Marcia Krull. Theirs were jobs of devotion and patience in typing the manuscripts.

R.B.
February 1976

To my parents; my chief, Dr. Robert
Petersdorf; my mentors, the Liscos,
Johnsons, and Bremners; and to Deb,
Steve, J. Carl, and Jude

                        F.F.
                        February 1976

Contents

Foreword   xiii

Preface: Why a Revision?   xvii

Part One: The Struggle for Rational Prescribing
  Chapter 1: Blowing the Whistle   3
  Chapter 2: The Battle Is On   39
  Chapter 3: The Reckoning Nears   87

Part Two: Basic Drug List   125

Part Three: Prescription Drug List   137

Part Four: Price Lists   329

Appendix A:
  Prescribing for Children   415

Appendix B:
  The Top 200 Drugs Prescribed in 1974   426

Appendix C:
  Some Distributors of Generic Drugs   429

Index   433

Addenda   445

About the Authors   453

Foreword

In 1966 I wrote the first edition of this book to alert doctors and patients to a serious medical, social, and economic problem: the present chaotic state of medical therapeutics. Too many, and often inferior, drugs are being prescribed, potentially toxic drugs are being prescribed for minor conditions, and drug costs to the patient are far higher than need be because doctors tend to prescribe by brand name instead of generic name. The book was purposely aimed at the public as well as at the profession for the simple reason that so much of the medical press is heavily controlled by and biased in favor of what James L. Goddard, former Commissioner of the Food and Drug Administration, has recently named "the Drug Establishment." [1]

The first *Handbook* helped catalyze some constructive action. Senator Gaylord Nelson used the occasion of its publication for a major speech in the Senate to announce that his Subcommittee on Monopoly would undertake a long-planned investigation of drug prices. The revelations of his hearings led in turn to the establishment, by former Secretary of Health, Education and Welfare John W. Gardner, of a Task Force on Prescription Drugs to consider the major scientific, clinical, legal, and administrative problems of including out-of-hospital prescription drugs as a Medicare benefit. The *Report and Recommendations* of the

[1] See his article by that name in *Esquire*, March 1969, pp. 117 *et seq.*

xiii

Task Force was published in August 1968. It substantiated the first *Handbook,* but went further. Prescribing practices, it indicated, were apparently even more chaotic, and industry control of the profession more extensive, than I had earlier realized.

So few drugs are required to treat most medical contingencies that prescribing ought to be the easiest part of office and outpatient-clinic practice. However, the practicing doctor has been confused by advertising and promotional claims into thinking that a larger number of important, superlative drugs are available than is actually the case. The *Handbook* aims to dispel some of this confusion.

Since the purpose of the *Handbook* is to be useful as well as critical, in the second, and in this, the third, edition all of the drug products most often prescribed are now included in the Prescription Drug List pages. (The first edition deliberately excluded discussion of many minor drugs and of most fixed-dosage combination drugs.) Although medical educators almost universally discourage the use of most fixed-combination drugs for a variety of reasons, the *Handbook* cannot ignore the fact that "polypharmacals" ("shotgun" concoctions, combining several drugs) are among the fastest-selling prescription items in the nation. The *Handbook* encourages the use, instead, of reliable single-entity drugs, many of them available by official, or generic, name at relatively little cost.

Like the first and second editions, this one includes a brief discussion and outline of what are called "basic drugs"; that is, drugs that could be used to treat about 90 percent of adult patients seen by the medical doctor in office, clinic, or home. Many of these drugs were once patented and expensive, but now that their seventeen-year period of patent protection has expired, they are obtainable at low cost, provided the doctor writes his prescription in a way that enables the patient to buy them by generic name. The particular attention of medical students and doctors in training is invited to this Basic Drug List.

Drug therapy is a mutual concern of the doctor *and* his patient. The patient nearly always ought to know the name of the agent that the doctor intends to prescribe, and it is at this point that the *Handbook* may have a practical, layman's use. While the Prescription Drug List cannot feasibly contain information about every minor drug on the market, it does include most drugs commonly prescribed in office practice, listed under both brand and generic names, with comments under one or the other—usually under the brand-name heading. (Since the drug industry has done such a good job of teaching brand names, the *Handbook* takes advantage of this by using those names freely for easy communication.) Often an alternative agent is suggested in the comments, if it is believed preferable because of safety, efficacy, or cost.

The Prescription Drug List pages are followed by the Price Lists, giving comparative prices for certain drugs from a variety of sources.

The appendixes conclude the *Handbook*: Prescribing for Children, compiled with the help and advice of two Boston physicians; the Top 200 Drugs Prescribed in 1974 (compiled from recently published information); and a list of names and addresses of some distributors of generic drugs. In the Index, the reader may look up a drug in three ways: by generic name, by brand name, and under the general category of illness for which it may be useful.

Preface: Why a Revision?

An updating and revision of the *Handbook* are timely if not overdue. Eight years have slipped past since the publication of the first edition in 1967 and five since its revision and updating in 1970. The latter advised the public and its doctors about many astonishing discoveries made between 1967 and 1969 by the United States Senate Subcommittee on Monopoly concerning business practices of the largest ("brand-name") pharmaceutical manufacturers.

The subcommittee's investigations have since been grinding inexorably forward, and with Senator Gaylord Nelson's re-election in November 1974 may be expected to continue. Nelson is chairman of the subcommittee. His staff's careful, brilliant research has been published in extenso and is available in every comprehensive municipal and university library.[1] Their publications have received less notice in the lay press than they deserve (and very little in the medical press), yet they have begun to have widespread effect on federal and state legislators, on cabinet officials in the Department of Health, Education and Welfare under Presidents Johnson, Nixon, and Ford, on consumer advocates, and on high-ranking officers in the Department of Defense and the Veterans Administration. The volumes of hearings presently number twenty-eight—the most comprehensive and

[1] *Competitive Problems in the Drug Industry*, Hearings Before the Subcommittee on Monopoly, Senate Select Committee on Small Business, 90th through 93rd Congresses (1967–1974), Parts 1–25.

thoroughly readable study ever published on the drug industry and the effects of its practices on the medical profession. It is time to recapitulate the high points of the volumes published since 1970, for their contents have begun to deliver a signal impact on medical practice in this nation, and in many other nations too.

A critical mass of influential people has begun to realize that the brand-name drug industry is, as has been charged, "the last of the robber barons" [2] and has begun to catalyze action to bring some order out of the disorder and chaos arising from the Organized Medicine–Drug Industry "connection." This mutually parasitic connection has enabled certain segments of the drug industry to confuse well-intentioned practicing doctors and nearly all of the public, and to corrupt certain key medical politicians and professors in the rigidly hierarchical academic medical profession. The voices of very many influential doctors who know better have been silenced, and by their silence these doctors must bear some responsibility for the lack of education of new doctors about rational therapeutics. In some cases important doctors have actively participated in a vast, expensively orchestrated industry propaganda campaign, and have thus actually "educated" a generation of doctors in how to practice *ir*rational therapeutics. The vast majority of medical doctors simply have not been vigilant: the result is that doctors of my generation are, in one key area of practice, unwittingly working against the interests of their patients without realizing that they are merely lining the pockets of some greedy profiteers who are an interested, mercenary third party to the doctor-patient relationship. This third party uses doctors as its pawns, thereby degrading a noble profession.

In response to the growing cry for reform, the drug industry has successfully sold to the politically conservative medical profession the bogey of "government interference in medical practice" and has encouraged doctors to be skeptical if not outwardly

[2] *Ibid.*, Part 1, p. 13.

hostile to the National Academy of Sciences and the
Food and Drug Administration of the Department of
HEW. I contend that the drug industry's massive
interference with medical practice—its own insidious
intrusion into the doctor–patient relationship—is
what has made government involvement necessary.

Someone has to protect the citizens. The medical
profession is not doing so. The big brand-name drug
industry is surely not going to withdraw from a position that allows it to pick with impunity the pockets
of sick people. The industry, under pressure, is de-
bating its case widely and expensively. One of the
purposes of this updated *Handbook* is to spotlight the
weakness and dishonesty of that industry's defense.

Another purpose of this revision is to encourage
the public by letting the people know that the hand-
writing is on the wall: drug-industry leaders have
begun to squabble among themselves; even a little
healthy price competition has sprouted here and there.
Many drug salesmen are afflicted today by a loss of
morale, an erosion of confidence in the future; and
among many there is a sense of guilt and shame.
They told their own families and friends never to use
certain dangerous drugs while they were promoting
the virtues and downplaying the potential adverse
side effects of these same drugs when making promotional pitches to doctors. Today also we see large
drug corporations diversifying—entering the market
for sale of medical instruments and supplies—another
healthy sign. We have even observed for the first
time in modern memory the partial loss of independence
of a giant brand-name drug corporation: Parke, Davis's
widespread promotion of a dangerous drug (Chloro-
mycetin®) and its heavy reliance on its sales, allegedly for one-third of its annual income,[3] brought it
financial trouble when the Senate made the issue public.[4]
The company is now a subsidiary of the Warner-
Lambert Drug Co.

We are at last beginning to experience the benefi-

[3] *Forbes*, January 1967, p. 158.
[4] *Competitive Problems in the Drug Industry*, Part 6, pp.
2566, 2584, 2622.

cial effects of deliberate decisions made by Drug
Efficacy Review Panels of the National Academy of
Sciences–National Research Council's study undertaken between 1966 and 1970. That study was necessary in order to comply with the Kefauver-Harris
Amendments of 1962. Sixty-three hundred drugs,
about one of every three prescription drugs on the
market, were found to lack substantial proof that
they actually have the effects claimed for them by
their manufacturers, and were therefore removed from
the market by the FDA.[5] Hundreds of highly profitable products have had to be removed from pharmacy
shelves. Wealthy and "ethical" drug corporations,
such as Squibb, Upjohn, Pfizer, Lederle, Lilly, Wyeth,
and Merck, were badly jarred by loss of revenues
from those products. They have in many cases increased the prices of their other products presumably
in order to maintain the same over-all high net profits
that have become a vested expectation for them. As
a result, the *Handbook's* Prescription Drug List and
its Price Lists were in need of revision.

The task that this need for revision posed for me
loomed overwhelming. Fortunately, Dr. Fred J. Fox
of the University of Washington Medical School in
Seattle, a former student of mine at the Harvard
Medical School, where he matriculated, a friend, and
a doctor with a keen interest in clinical pharmacology,
clinical medicine, and ethical issues in medical practice, agreed to come to the rescue. The part entitled
Prescription Drug List was drafted by him, but the burden
of editorial responsibility and especially the responsibility for any factual errors or misjudgments in that part
are mine and mine alone. It seems prudent to add that
no organization to which I belong, no one who employs
me, and no one to whom I have made an acknowledg-
ment or expressed appreciation bears any responsibility
for the contents.

The "great generic drug controversy," [6] which
raised its head first when Senator Kefauver was prob-

[5] *Ibid.*, Part 24, p. 10,648.
[6] M. Silverman and P. R. Lee, *Pills, Profits and Politics*
(University of California Press, 1974).

ing in the late 1950s and which heated up white-hot during the earlier years of the Nelson hearings, has now been settled to the satisfaction of nearly all unbiased experts.[7] It is agreed that the use of generic names in parlance . and in prescriptions, and the purchase of "generic" drugs whenever possible, are highly desirable goals.[8] This is good thinking because it will save money and allow as good if not safer medicine to be practiced.

Many fascinating discoveries and expert decisions have confirmed the first *Handbook's* plea for the use of generic drugs—information that necessitates this updated book. Also, the comprehensive discussion, in the introduction to the 1976 edition, of the generic vs. brand-name controversy will perhaps put a halt to the lingering anti-generic-drug propaganda campaign waged by the Pharmaceutical Manufacturers Association. I concluded some three years ago that the issue is kept alive by the PMA as an emotional diversionary smoke screen because it does not wish to allow time for thought and discussion of a far more basic issue, the matter of *rational* prescribing; that is, why rational prescribing is not being taught in our tax-supported medical schools, and how it is discouraged by expensive promotional schemes including control of nearly all segments of the medical press.

Any updated edition has necessarily got to provide some discussion about the serious economic position

---

[7] J. R. Crout, "FDA's Role in Drug Product Quality," speech, May 20, 1974, Boston, Mass., pp. 5 and 6. Dr. Crout is Director of the Bureau of Drugs of the FDA.

[8] *Competitive Problems in the Drug Industry*, Part 12, pp. 5085–5132. This is the lengthy, fascinating testimony by Dr. John Adriani, who was chairman of the Council on Drugs of the AMA. The punch line in his statement was: "The question, Mr. Chairman, then is not should we abolish brand names and use generic names, but when? The sooner the better. It can be done, and it will be a step forward in medicine." The astonishing disclosure that the very chairman of so prestigious and important an AMA committee advocated compulsory abolition of brand names was a startling setback to the Pharmaceutical Manufacturers Association. Little if any coverage was given this testimony in the medical press at the time or since. Not long afterward, Dr. Adriani's committee was dissolved by the trustees of the AMA.

in which individual private-practice pharmacists find themselves. These persons with good technical training have been exploited long enough by the big brand-name drug corporations, have been humiliated by far too many arrogant physicians, and are exposed daily to insult and humiliation by much of the public who have thus far been kept ignorant of the nuances of the drug company–doctor–pharmacist–patient relationship.

The naked act of forking out outrageous amounts of money for prescription medicines involves a direct confrontation of the patient with the pharmacist. By virtue of this confrontation the pharmacist has come to represent the "bad guy" in the drug-cost scandal. The revision of this book could not be complete without some words about this injustice, including suggestions as to what might be done to improve the professional image of the neighborhood pharmacist and, ultimately, the professional careers of all pharmacists. I would be intrigued to hear especially from young pharmacists and pharmacy students of their reactions to my suggestions.

It is time to remind medical students, doctors-in-training, and all of the concerned public that the aims of the drug manufacturers are different from the aims of good doctors. The manufacturers wish to maximize their profits by encouraging doctors to write as many prescriptions as possible for the most expensive drugs. Manifestly, good doctors should minimize writing prescriptions and, as purchasing agents for patients, should do all they can to keep the cost of necessary medications as low as possible. Doctors are generally in a different economic bracket from most of their patients. For many doctors, five dollars is about as important as fifty cents is to the majority of their patients; however, the doctors must learn to protect their patients' pocketbooks or they shall find themselves, one day soon, paying from their own pockets the cost difference between equivalent medicines that sell for ten or twenty times as much by brand as by generic name. The public will force their political representatives to take this step.

We can take some comfort from figures that show a recent progressive increase in the number of prescriptions written by generic or official names (often the low-cost way of doing it). *From 1966 to 1974, the number has increased by more than forty-six million. In 1974, 10.7 percent of new prescriptions were written by generic name. In 1966, the figure was only 6.4 percent.*[9] No one has noticed a national epidemic of disease or therapeutic failures in the past seven years. In fact, there is not a single documented instance of death or irreversible illness caused by a generic drug. *No such similar statement can be made for brand-name products.*

Many hours of thought were given to how best to organize the expository portion of this third edition of the *Handbook*. It was decided that the Introduction to the 1967 edition and that both the Foreword (with some alteration) and the Introduction to the 1970 edition still presented essential features of my position. Juxtaposed with the 1975 Introduction—and all three treated as "chapters" of "The Struggle for Rational Prescribing"—they provide the reader of this edition with an easy-to-read chronological unfolding of an elementary story with minimal repetition. Minor alterations have been made to the original two Introductions, and the book has a new Preface and expanded Dedication. Extensive new footnoting of the 1967 material was required to make it contemporary; the major change in the 1970 material was deletion of a brief section dealing with how the federal government has been wasting taxpayer money by paying for large numbers of second-rate pharmaceuticals under Medicaid and (by extension) under other federal programs. The Nelson hearings have now dealt with this issue nicely, and corrective action has begun. In place of the deleted section I inserted a new one describing how Dr. Charles Edwards, Assistant Secretary for Health in the Department of HEW, and formerly Commissioner of the Food and Drug Administration, testi-

[9] *Pharmacy Times,* April 1974, pp. 35–41.

fied in mid-1974 about his intention to administer a
new program proposed by then-Secretary Weinberger
of the Health, Education, and Welfare Department
that will require the use of lowest-cost (*i.e.*, generic)
drugs in all federally financed health programs.[10] This
is encouraging information.

R.B.

February 1976

It is essential for the *Handbook's* new readers to
become familiar with all the information in the introductory material, so that they may understand the
basic facts and arguments underlying the Prescription
Drug List itself. Readers familiar with earlier editions
are also urged to review this material in the light of
more recent events and to be aware of the author's
updated comments.

[10] *Competitive Problems in the Drug Industry,* Part 24, pp.
10,483–10,496.

PART ONE
The Struggle
for Rational Prescribing

1

Blowing the Whistle

(1967) *

I. *The Extent of Drug Promotion*

The U.S. has reason for looking upon its medical profession with pride, for its medical schools and teaching hospitals have succeeded well in training doctors to make correct diagnoses and to perform proper surgery. Our level of medical practice is the envy of many nations because our practicing physicians and surgeons have managed, for the most part, to stay abreast of new, important developments in diagnostic and surgical techniques. That they have been able to do so is a tribute to the profession itself, which has taken the lead in encouraging doctors' continuing education through the use of books, journals, postgraduate courses, lectures, and hospital staff conferences.

The great pity—bordering on scandal—is that too much responsibility for keeping doctors informed of developments in pharmacology has been forfeited to pharmaceutical manufacturers, who have succeeded, through advertising, in influencing practicing physicians to write prescriptions for which the patient pays a maximum price. The immensity of this advertising effort is best appreciated by considering that it costs the drug industry at least $600 million annually. Since there are approximately 200,000 prescribing doctors, the drug companies are spending more than three

* The following chapter was originally printed as the Introduction to the 1967 *Handbook*.

thousand advertising dollars each year on each doctor! These figures are taken from a prepared statement before the Subcommittee on Intergovernmental
Relations of the House Committee on Government
Operations by Dr. James L. Goddard, Commissioner
of the United States Food and Drug Administration,
May 25, 1966. Much of the advertising is misleading.
According to Dr. Goddard, in 1965 ". . . one third
of the members of the Pharmaceutical Manufacturers
Association had violated FDA agency regulations on
fraudulent or misleading advertising." * Clearly, a third
and interested commercial party has inserted itself
into the doctor–patient relationship, yet no clear warning voice has been raised against it from within the
medical profession. As Dr. Goddard said, the American doctor is "frankly under siege."

Why should doctors, among the best trained of all
professional cadres in this country, be susceptible to
misleading advertising? As medical students, were
they not provided with adequate education about
drugs? The answer is that the great majority have
been given an excellent, modern laboratory and lecture course in pharmacology, but, with few exceptions, little organized review or systematic presentation of such material after the students' second year
of medical school. The reason: those faculty members
who teach pharmacology are only rarely practicing
doctors (clinicians) as well as scientists. The scholarly, research-oriented pharmacologist has usually had
little or no experience in the actual use in humans of
the drugs that he knows so well in theory. He may
have no interest in clinical medicine, and, even if he
does, he will probably not feel qualified to play a
significant role in case discussions before members of
the clinical faculty. Unfortunately, very few of the
clinical faculty have much more than a superficial

* The PMA denied the accuracy of the charge. PMA membership numbers well over one hundred; it is very likely that
Dr. Goddard meant to direct his accusation against the twenty or
so most active, generally best-known of the PMA firms that
form the influential group known as the National Pharmaceutical Council (NPC).

interest in pharmacology as such, for tradition has taught that the cornerstone of the best medical practice is learning to diagnose. It is commonplace to hear, "Drug therapy is easy; once the diagnosis has been made, all you have to do is look up the recommended drug and prescribe it." While this may once have been a useful view, rapid developments in pharmacology (not all of them beneficial) have rendered it obsolete, and its persistence has led to an obvious result: the student ceases to continue to learn in depth about drugs, and while he receives first-rate instruction in pathological physiology, diagnosis, and surgical treatment, he frequently adopts sloppy habits with regard to the prescription of therapeutic agents.*

* Nine years after writing this, I regret that the foregoing several lines do not precisely convey my feelings. From what I have learned since 1966, I wish that I had written:

It is commonplace to hear, "Drug therapy is easy; once the diagnosis has been made, one can easily look up the recommended therapy in a proper source book and apply it." This remains by and large a useful approach to good medical therapeutic practice, provided the source book is free of any financial connection with the pharmaceutical industry. It is certainly true that many so-called "new" drugs are introduced each year, but only a handful are uniquely advantageous over older, better-known (hence, safer) drugs already on the market. Unfortunately, those beyond the second year of medical school tend to forget their *basic* pharmacology, and while they continue to receive first-rate instruction in pathological physiology, diagnosis, and surgical treatment, they begin to adopt sloppy prescribing habits. The reason is understandable: medical students are among the most impressionable and least critical of postgraduate students. They have a frightful tendency to accept at face value almost any "clinical impression" or "It has been my experience over the years to discover . . ." from nearly any imposing-looking clinician in a starched white coat who lectures to them in a crowded amphitheater. Some powerful professors are very concerned about this serious problem in medical education. An example is Professor Moran Campbell, Head of the Department of Medicine at MacMaster University Medical School in Ontario, formerly of the faculty of the British Postgraduate Medical School, Hammersmith Hospital, London, England. I have heard Professor Campbell, one of the world's foremost doctors, courageously stand up in

This unhappy state of affairs is by no means unknown to responsible members of medical school faculties, and there have been moves here and there to institute courses dealing in pharmacology during the latter two years of medical school—the so-called "clinical" years. For the practicing doctor, similarly, there is no coherent plan for periodically updating his knowledge of drugs and their use. Into the breach has stepped the pharmaceutical industry—to persuade, to cajole, and to "educate." To be sure, there is now available to all doctors and medical students a bi-weekly loose-leaf sheet called the *Medical Letter,* published by Drug and Therapeutic Information, Inc., a non-profit organization that fearlessly dispenses objective criticism of drugs old and new; but *M.L.* is not meant primarily to give comprehensive information on prices. Simply written and intelligently critical, it deserves the fuller support of the profession, however, for the struggle to control doctors' habits of therapeutic practice is a big stake and the giant pharmaceutical corporations can be expected to continue to promote, advertise, and "educate" at an increasing

---

an amphitheater crowded with several hundred young doctors to warn them about ". . . pompous asses with long white coats who'll tell you anything and you'd probably believe it." With slight exaggeration, he makes his point (I heard him in 1968) by stating: "Any one of these uncritical persons could probably stand here and tell you persuasively, 'It is my clinical impression based on my years of experience that individuals with small green spots around the anus are highly likely in later years to develop schizophrenia,' and as a result most of you for the rest of your lives would probably assiduously strip the trousers from every patient you meant to examine thoroughly and search with a torch for green spots just around the anus." Many of these "clinical impressions," including ones dealing with therapeutics, are sheer bunk tossed off by two many self-important professors. At the same time, the student has begun to have his mind assailed by the advertising and promotion boys of the pharmaceutical industry. By the time he graduates, many if not most medical students are ready for a course in clinical pharmacology and therapeutics whose major theme ought to be the *un*learning of massive amounts of misinformation.—R.B., January 1975

rate, one which even now far exceeds in cost the combined administrative and teaching budgets of all the nation's medical schools put together.[1]

What is wrong with the adoption by pharmaceutical manufacturers of the role of educator of physicians about developments in drug therapy? Let us look first at some of the unfortunate prescribing practices encouraged by the advertising and promotion policies of these manufacturers—policies disclosed during the Kefauver hearings on drugs during the years 1960–1962.

1. *Prescribing Too Many Drugs Too Often*

Many patients require no prescription, just an attentive listener, a careful examination by the doctor, and some reassurance. Too often there is a tendency to prescribe for these patients a sedative ("tranquilizer"), a vitamin capsule, thyroid or female hormones, an injection of vitamin B_{12} or penicillin, or some new drug X which the patient specifically requests. The unnecessary prescription of drugs is one of the hallmarks of second-rate medical practice, and yet when it occurs, the fault is not always entirely the doctor's. In the background there is often the fine hand of the pharmaceutical advertiser, who has made an intense effort to reach the doctor through the patient. A physician, formerly of the medical staff of one of the best-known and largest of the drug houses, testified before the Kefauver subcommittee:

It is an unfunny joke in the medical profession that the very latest information on new advances in medicine most often appears in the eminent medical journals such as *Reader's Digest, Time,* and *The Wall Street Journal*. Some of this is legitimate good reporting. However, much of what appears has in essence been placed by the

[1] P. R. Garai, "The Pill the Doctor Must Swallow," *Johns Hopkins Magazine,* Vol. XV, No. 7 (May 1964), pp. 7–9, 21–23.

public relations staffs of the pharmaceutical firms. A steady stream of magazine and newspaper articles are prepared for distribution to the lay press. These may take the form of so-called informative or background articles on conditions such as allergies or edema. Buried within the article, there is often a brief paragraph mentioning that a great drug has been discovered and manufactured by company X, and the name of the drug is given. The article does not say that the reader should rush to his physician and demand the drug, but the implication is usually clear. And, of course, there is nothing to show where the article originated.[2]

Small-town newspapers and lesser-known periodicals are especially likely to carry information prepared by public relations experts. The larger daily newspapers and the major wire services have highly skilled science reporters who weed out most of the misleading or exaggerated public relations drug claims and file them in their wastebaskets. In spite of this, much misinformation—particularly via small newspapers and some national magazines—does reach the public. One public relations executive interviewed by the Kefauver subcommittee read from a letter sent by his own organization to a large drug company that was a prospective customer: ". . . a news story on clinical results from a new drug or on the research achievements that went into this discovery automatically helps create a demand for the product." The letter, soliciting the patronage of the corporation, described what "in our opinion would have the broadest and most direct sales promotion results." This was a "feature column service providing health and medical stories built around some product for smalltown daily or weekly newspapers. Both text and illustrations are supplied in matrix form requiring no composition or

[2] United States Senate, Committee on the Judiciary, Subcommittee on Antitrust and Monoply, 86th Congress, 2nd Session, *Hearings on S. Res. 238*, Part 18, pp. 10,241 *et seq.*

engraving by the newspaper." The feature was reportedly sent to two thousand small papers, many of which could afford no wire services and welcomed the availability of this free material. In the feature mat, the name of a product was always mentioned. The public relations executive denied that his service was advertising in the strict sense and maintained, therefore, that the material need not be identified as such when published.[3]

According to another witness before the subcommittee, a physician who had previously been chief medical director of another of the pharmaceutical giants: "The patients contribute their share [to the unnecessary prescription of drugs]. Too many are unable to accept that the physician . . . is still best able to determine the proper treatment. The best doctor is not necessarily the one who gives a shot for every complaint, and the more conservative physician who does not prescribe the latest drug reported in *Coronet* may be far more competent than the one who does . . . To the pharmaceutical industry this is an open invitation to exploit both the patient and the doctor." [4]

2. *Prescribing Costly Drugs of Unproved Clinical Value*

One good example is the long-acting blood-vessel dilator, usually an organic nitrate (not nitroglycerin), which is alleged to cause improvement in angina pectoris. Evidence exists in the medical literature as convincing of the ineffectiveness of this class of compounds as to its effectiveness. When this is the case with any drug, a reasonable inference is that its usefulness is open to serious question; *effective drugs usually give obvious results.*

The so-called "tranquilizers" fall into this category

[3] United States Senate, Committee on the Judiciary, Subcommittee on Antitrust and Monopoly, 87th Congress, 2nd Session, *Hearings on S. Res. 1552,* Part 6, pp. 3212 *et seq.*

[4] Hearings on *S. Res. 238,* Part 18, p. 10,374.

too. "The simple fact that anxiety is virtually impossible to evaluate objectively and that it responds to almost any bag of asafetida[5] accounts for the market in the so-called tranquilizers," according to the same ex–chief medical director of a large drug house who has already been quoted.[6] However, these agents can certainly be effective as placebos[7] or as mild sedatives, neither more nor less effective than small doses of phenobarbital. The point the *Handbook* wishes to make, therefore, is not that the practicing doctor should never under any circumstances prescribe them, but that if he does he should know how much his patient is forced to pay for them. He needs a source to tell him how to prescribe such a drug in its least expensive dose form and by its least expensive name.

3. *Prescribing Drugs with Serious Toxic Side Effects When There Are Equally Effective Less Toxic Agents Available*

One example: though chloramphenicol is an effective drug and is the agent of choice for treatment of certain rare infections (*e.g.*, typhoid fever), its capacity to interfere with the ability of bone marrow to manufacture blood cells has been well known for years. Although this unwanted side effect most often occurs when more than the usual dose is given, there are rare persons in whom even a small dose can cause serious disease or even death. The argument that death from this cause is rare is no consolation to the families of the many persons who have been killed by unnecessary prescription of chloramphenicol. As long ago as 1952, the Food and Drug Administration re-

[5] It was a common practice in the Middle Ages to wear suspended from the neck a cloth bag filled with asafetida, a foul-smelling weed, which was believed to ward off plagues, but in fact had no such action.

[6] *Hearings on S. Res. 238*, Part 18, p. 10,374.

[7] A placebo is an inactive medication—*e.g.*, a sugar pill—whose beneficial effect on the patient is due entirely to psychological factors.

quired (upon the recommendation of the National Research Council) that chloramphenicol's package label and advertising carry the warning that it not be used indiscriminately or for minor infections. But its casual use persists. Again, this is not all the doctor's fault; the reader is referred to *Hearings on S. Res. 238,* Part 26, pp. 15,945–15,981, which contains documentary evidence showing that a manufacturer, with careful use of words, can manage to dilute the impact that a required warning label is intended to have. See also Senate Report No. 448, *Administered Prices: Drugs*, pp. 192–198. For further discussion, see below, under "The Nature of Drug Promotion."

4. *Prescribing Powerful and Potentially Toxic Drugs for Minor Conditions*

The classic example is the thalidomide tragedy, which this country was fortunately spared. Mild anxiety hardly requires treatment with drugs, and surely not in pregnancy. The lesson of the terrible thalidomide-induced defects in newborn babies seems to have been driven home to most doctors in that the prescribing of any drug at all during early pregnancy is now undertaken only after the most serious consideration by all responsible physicians. On the other hand, it remains common practice to prescribe for a simple stuffy nose a systemically taken tablet or capsule that does, indeed, help the nasal stuffiness but can at the same time cause a rise in blood pressure and a pounding or irregular heartbeat—though inexpensive, safer nose drops are known to be just as effective, though perhaps slightly less convenient.

5. *Prescribing Drugs Without Knowledge of Official Identity, Sources of Manufacture, and Cost*

It is common knowledge to pharmacologists and well-trained physicians that 90 percent or more of adult patients who are not sick enough to require hospitalization can be treated effectively with one or more of a small number of basic drugs; and the list of all such basic drugs is, in fact, a short one. Because most of these drugs are available by their official (generic) names at a cost far lower than when prescribed by unofficial (brand) names, treatment can usually be simple and inexpensive. Unfortunately, the intensive and highly effective advertising and promotion campaigns conducted by pharmaceutical manufacturers have muddied the waters and confused the well-intentioned and otherwise well-informed practicing doctor into believing that there are more essential drugs on the market than is actually the case. Furthermore, because the responsibility for publishing lists of available drugs and their sources has been forfeited by the medical profession itself to the manufacturers of brand-name drugs, the manufacturers have effectively kept practicing doctors *un*informed about the many sources of inexpensive drugs of purity, quality, and potency sold by their generic names. It is for these reasons that treatment is too often both complicated and costly.

How can a doctor care properly for the "whole person" unless he understands the impact of disease upon his patient's pocketbook? Obviously he cannot. And it is here, on the question of cost to the consumer, that the pharmaceutical company's adopted role of educator most flagrantly breaks down, for there is in it an inherent self-interest that cannot be disguised.

In summary, then, far too often a patient takes a drug when he may need none at all. Or he takes a drug with dangerous side effects when a safer drug is available. Or he takes a drug of unproved clinical value, or one which carries important risks and therefore never should be given for minor conditions. In each of these situations—and even in the happy instance when the prescription is both justified and safe—the patient is far too likely to pay much more than is necessary.

II. *Official and Unofficial Names of Drugs*

The key to an understanding of why drugs often need not cost as much as they do is a knowledge of what is meant by the terms "official" and "unofficial" with respect to drug names.

New drugs and the processes by which they are made can be protected for seventeen years under United States Patent Law. Every new drug approved for sale must be given an official (also called "generic"[8] or "non-proprietary") name, and it is by this label that it is known to pharmacologists and to the medical students whom they teach. A new drug, when developed by a drug company, is also endowed with an unofficial (also called "brand," "trade," or "proprietary") name, and this is the label by which the drug is advertised to the profession. Until only recently, these advertisements were not even required to include a prominent display of the drug's generic name,[9] but now the law says that it must be included in letters at least one half as large as those used for the brand name.

It is profoundly in the economic interest of the pharmaceutical manufacturer to "train" doctors and patients to use the brand name only, and manufacturers have succeeded mightily in doing so. More than 90 percent of prescriptions in the mid-1960s were written using brand names.[10] Brand names are frequently easier to say, spell, and remember than

[8] Technically and correctly, the term "generic" refers to classes or genera of drugs, but in common parlance it has come to be used interchangeably with "non-proprietary" and "official." To avoid confusion and pedantry, the *Handbook* adopts the popular usage.

[9] At one point during the Kefauver hearings Dr. Austin Smith, the president of the Pharmaceutical Manufacturers Association, found it impossible to locate the generic name on an advertisement until aided by a magnifying glass proffered by the subcommittee counsel.

[10] *F-D-C Reports ("The Pink Sheet")*, Washington, D.C., September 5, 1966.

generic names because it has been common for *manufacturers* to make the latter chemical tongue-twisters —which discourages their use. Besides, brand names have often been designed so as to imply what the pharmacological action of the drug is advertised to be. This is an effective merchandising technique, *e.g.,* the officially named chlordiazepoxide, a sedative, is almost universally known as "Librium®". Since 1961, generic names have been subject to approval by a committee, the United States Adopted Names Council (USAN), which includes representatives of the United States Pharmacopeial Convention, the American Pharmaceutical Association, and the American Medical Association. Why "Adopted" rather than "Official"? And can any dignified official name compete with one designed to be merchandised?

During the seventeen years for which a patent is in effect, the original developer of the drug is free to take advantage of his privileged position to recoup his investment and reap the reward of profit for his risk and enterprise. After seventeen years, anyone else is free to help himself to the process described in the patent and to manufacture and market the drug on his own, *though he may not use the original brand name; which is limited by trademark law to the use of the original coiner.*

As an illustration, we can refer to the drug dextroamphetamine, widely used for its appetite-curbing properties.* The substance was patented by Smith Kline & French Laboratories, who alone sold it in vast amounts for a seventeen-year period under the brand name Dexedrine®. The patent has long since expired, and as of now, half a hundred companies are marketing dextroamphetamine—nearly all at lower

---

* Since this was written, dextroamphetamine has generally come to be recognized as one of the most dangerous of all drugs. It became widely abused during the height of the "drug-culture" years and its danger for habituation has led to its stringent control by the federal government. Production, prescription, and dispensing of this dangerous substance are very tight now. However, its use here to illustrate an economic point remains valid.—R.B., January 1975

prices than Smith Kline & French. But the many new
producers of dextroamphetamine may not advertise
it as Dexedrine®. If Dexedrine® is the word the doctor writes on the prescription blank by force of habit,
the druggist must by law in thirty-nine states (except
within institutions) dispense Dexedrine®—and at its
brand-name price. It must be pointed out, however,
that even if the prescription reads "dextroamphetamine," the druggist is free to dispense Dexedrine®, at
the higher price; and that is exactly what many drug-
gists do, since it is not yet common-enough practice
for drugstores to keep in stock the less expensive—
but for practical purposes, identical—dextroamphetamine tablets marketed by other companies without
the trade name Dexedrine®. Such less expensive, non-
brand-name dextroamphetamine tablets are the generic equivalents of Dexedrine®.

III. The Nature of Drug Promotion

Pharmaceutical companies influence doctors in
several ways. For one thing, their salesmen, called
"detailmen," visit doctors' offices at frequent intervals to dispense samples, describe new products, remind the doctor of older ones, and sometimes to
recite certain statements that the parent company
considers of special importance and has ordered them
to commit to memory. Many of these practices provide a service that the *Handbook* has no wish to
denigrate. However, the major job of the detailman
is to sell. Many doctors by now are aware that information obtained from the detailman must be examined
critically, and that salesmen cannot be considered
authoritative sources for continuing education about
drugs. There is little chance to check on the accuracy
of what the detailman tells the doctor in the privacy
of his office, and there is plenty of opportunity for
exaggeration, dissimulation, and outright conceal-
ment.

During the course of the hearings on drugs conducted in 1960 by the Kefauver subcommittee, it was

reported that the National Research Council recommended to the FDA that a label be placed on chloramphenicol (Parke, Davis's Chloromycetin®), warning that the drug should "not be used indiscriminately or for minor infections" because serious blood disease had occasionally been found to occur with its use. The report of the hearings contains a copy of a Parke, Davis's "President's Letter" telling the firm's detailmen of the new warning label but prefacing the announcement with the statement that "Chloromycetin has been officially cleared by the FDA and the National Research Council with *no restrictions* on the number or the range of diseases for which Chloromycetin may be administered." (Emphasis in original.) Obviously, when the National Research Council recommended that chloramphenicol "not be used indiscriminately or for minor infections," it was proposing a restriction on the number and the range of diseases. The hearings report that in a "Directors' Letter" sent two months later to its detailmen, Parke, Davis included "Planned Presentation 10," which contained arguments and figures designed to enable the detailmen to allay apprehensions about the drug on the part of the physician. However, it is also reported that instructions accompanying the presentation carried this interesting admonition: "The special detail ["Planned Presentation 10"] should not be introduced unless the physician brings up the subject or unless you know that he has ceased prescribing Chloromycetin"—a position hardly in keeping with the responsibility of drug manufacturers always to keep doctors fully informed on important matters.[11]

Thus, the detailman, without realizing it himself, can transmit information to doctors that is either misleading or false; in other cases, he supplies misinformation for which the parent company cannot be blamed. As an example, a detailman recently tried to

[11] *Administered Prices: Drugs*, Senate Report No. 448, Subcommittee on Antitrust and Monopoly, Senate Committee on the Judiciary, 87th Congress, 1st Session, pp. 192–196, and documentation in *Hearings on S. Res. 238*, Part 26, pp. 15,945–15,981.

convince me that the U.S. Air Force had "three or
four years ago" been "burnt" by the purchase of
digoxin (the generic name for a commonly used heart
drug) that turned out to be "only 47 percent of
proper potency." It so happens that drugs used by
the armed services are bought by generic name through
secret bids, and that all bidders must first pass inspection by the Defense Supply Agency; no delivery
is accepted without a check on identity, quality,
purity, and potency of the material. It seemed, therefore, either that the detailman's story was incorrect
or that the Defense Supply Agency must have fallen
down on the job. When I wrote to the man's company, requesting more details, the vice-president in
charge of sales replied that the company was unaware
of the incident. This points up the importance to the
doctor of listening critically to the detailman. Drug
corporations are aware that detailmen may, by accident or design, transmit information that is not factual,
and most guard against the possible repercussions of
such practices by not supplying the men with station-
ery containing the company letterhead. Thus, misinformation is unlikely to be put in writing.

Advertisements in medical journals represent a
second method of influencing the doctor's prescribing
habits. Advertisement of drugs is entirely proper and
can undoubtedly be useful to the medical profession.
As mentioned earlier, however, advertisements are
too often characterized by misrepresentation or misleading captions, in spite of the supervision of journal
editorial boards and scrutiny by the Food and Drug
Administration. Examples would fill a book.

The Kefauver hearings contain documentary evidence of an advertisement for a steroid drug with
X-ray pictures of a large bowel showing typical
changes seen in ulcerative colitis. Although the first
picture was not labeled "Before," the second was
labeled "Barium enema following successful therapy
for ulcerative colitis." One physician wrote the company (Upjohn) to question whether the X-rays were
of the same patient. By the time correspondence between the company's advertising manager, its medical

director, and the physician had come to an end, it was clear that these X-rays were from two different patients, each with different degrees of ulcerative colitis, and that in fact neither one had ever been treated with a steroid. The company, denying intent to mislead, expressed regrets over the incident; its advertising agency refused to admit to any impropriety.[12] The prescribing of drugs is too serious and potentially dangerous to be influenced by anything less than factual, objective material. If *some* advertisements are misleading, how does the doctor know which ones to trust?

The deluge of "junk mail" that descends upon doctors daily is by now common knowledge, and most physicians are either too busy or too wise to pay it much attention. The cost of this material, however, is passed on to the consumer. And few members of the medical profession are likely to be aware that their names are obtained for mailing lists through the offices of the American Medical Association, the source from which the advertisers buy their names and addresses. This is an important source of AMA revenue: according to the general counsel to the AMA, $900,000 of income was derived from this source in 1960.[13]*

Probably the shrewdest and most effective means by which the big pharmaceutical corporations perpetuate their hold over doctor and patients is through the book *Physicians' Desk Reference (PDR)*. Although some doctors may not think of it in these terms because its format and veneer give it a cleverly noncommercial, authoritative appearance, *PDR* is in fact composed of advertising.† The 1966 rate is $115 per

---

[12] *Hearings on S. 1552*, Part 6, pp. 3084 *et seq.*, and Part 7, pp. 3301–3310.

[13] *Ibid.*, Part 1, p. 137.

* Also, the AMA receives a fee for every advertisement mailed. It is not in the financial interest of the AMA to discourage the deluge of "junk mail."—R.B., January 1975

† Since this was written, the FDA has exercised stringent supervision over the contacts of *PDR*. What a company publishes concerning its product is essentially the same as it must

column inch. With more than fifteen thousand column inches, the gross value of space in the 1966 *PDR* exceeds $1,725,000. The practitioner who habitually uses this volume to look up the names of drugs with which to treat his patients is unwittingly being influenced in his therapeutic practice by non-medical commercial interests. His very freedom of therapeutic practice is at risk. Yet many, if not most, doctors are unaware of this; here the leaders of the profession must be blamed because they have remained silent —an ironic omission for a leadership that has in recent times spent millions of dollars to fight forces they accuse of meddling in the "sacred doctor–patient relationship." It is my belief that there is no force in American life today which more directly meddles in this relationship than that segment of the pharmaceutical industry that operates through the detailman,

---

print in the drug's "package stuffer." "Package stuffers" are required by law, and they do indeed contain straightforward, honest, and comprehensive information about the drug. Unfortunately, the "package stuffer" is nearly invariably removed by the pharmacist. (He has nothing else to do with it. Surely he is not going to give it to the patient to whom he is dispensing the drug. The long list of possible adverse side effects known to be associated with use of the drug would probably scare most patients out of their wits.) Thus, doctors hardly ever get to see the "package stuffer," but they ought in 1975 to be aware that its contents are for practical purposes identical with the information published in *PDR.* Therefore, the remainder of this section dealing with *PDR* must be read in a different light. Particularly to be emphasized is that drug houses may no longer publish what they wish to publish or withhold any pertinent information from *PDR,* a practice correctly exposed in the 1967 *Handbook* and not long afterward put a stop to by the FDA. The cost of "advertising" in *PDR* remains very expensive, however, and the volume's continued use serves to perpetuate the prescription of products distributed by the richest firms—viz., brand-name drugs. Although *PDR* does give the generic name for products, its indexing is primarily by brand name. *PDR,* then, remains an industry-oriented and not a consumer-oriented volume, which serves to perpetuate the high cost of prescription drugs.—R.B., January 1975

through advertising, and, most boldly of all, through *Physicians' Desk Reference.*

The annual publication of *PDR* is an enterprise of Medical Economics, Inc., which distributes it without charge to over 200,000 practicing "doctors of medicine and doctors of osteopathy." Until recently, it was also distributed free to "pharmacies and libraries of more than 5000 hospitals," but now these institutions have been asked to purchase their copies at a nominal cost. Doubtless, most of them have done so, for of all the reference books located on hospital floors for the use of doctors and nurses, the one most often used by far is *PDR.*

PDR states that its contents have been obtained with the "cooperation" of drug manufacturers, through whose "patronage" its publication is made possible. This is euphemism. Drug houses *buy* space in *PDR* and publish what they wish to publish. Even those unethical repacking enterprises—"drug companies" owned and operated by physicians who buy up inexpensive generics, relabel them, and prescribe them under a special brand name at a higher price—are free to buy space. Since this is so, *PDR's* contents can hardly be considered authoritative. *Precisely because it is an advertising catalogue,* PDR *is incomplete; it gives prominent mention to too few generic names for widely consumed basic drugs.* The widespread use of this volume serves to conceal from practicing doctors the existence of numerous other manufacturers which very often can supply the same drugs at lower cost. There is a curious disclaimer in the foreword to *PDR* for 1960, the fourteenth annual edition: "It should be understood that in organizing the wealth of material in *PDR* the publisher is not advocating the use of any product listed by any manufacturer *nor attempting to influence the therapeutic practice of any physician.*" (My italics.) In subsequent editions the italicized portion of the sentence was dropped.

Physicians' Desk Reference has achieved its popularity not only by virtue of aggressive free distribution, but also because the profession itself offers no good alternative reference volume. I hope that the

Handbook will meet the need for a brief authoritative list of essential basic prescription drugs that can be purchased at minimum cost.

IV. The Reference Book Gap and the Role of the AMA

The *Handbook* would be incomplete without a mention of two authoritative volumes, the *Pharmacopeia of the United States of America* and the *National Formulary*. The former, usually designated as the *U.S.P.*, is published—at ten-year intervals since 1820 until very recently, when it began appearing at five-year intervals—by the private, scientific, non-profit United States Pharmacopeial Convention, Inc., which exists for the sole purpose of providing up-to-date drug standards. The convention is not dependent on drug company advertising and is, in fact, completely free of outside control or influence. Members of the board, officers, and those who serve on the Revision Committee have always been outstanding leaders in the fields of both pharmacy and medicine. With the passage in 1906 of the Pure Food and Drug Act, the *U.S.P.* was recognized by federal statute as an "official" compendium providing standards of strength, quality, and purity for the drugs it describes. Over the years, the *U.S.P.* has listed only those drugs that reflect the best practice and teaching of medicine—decisions based on creditable and firmly grounded scientific fact. Thus, the *U.S.P.* is the single most valuable and reliable authority on the composition and quality of drugs. The most prestigious thing that can happen to a manufacturer's drug is its acceptance in the *U.S.P.*, where it is listed by its official, generic name.

It is most helpful for physicians to know which drugs are contained in the *U.S.P.* However, the volume is actually of limited value as a reference to the doctor at the moment when he prescribes medications, for it has not been designed to provide information on pharmacological activity, indications for use, manufacturers, and cost of the drugs.

Because the *U.S.P.* is subject to constant revision, drugs are always being demoted from it and others promoted to it. In consequence, some drugs may be excluded or dropped from the *U.S.P.* even though they are still widely used. In order to maintain a list of those drugs that are widely used but are not acceptable to the *U.S.P.*, the American Pharmaceutical Association publishes the *National Formulary,* often referred to simply as "the *N.F.*" The *N.F.*, whose format is similar to that of the *U.S.P.*, used to contain certain drugs simply because they were widely prescribed, but now it considers therapeutic worth and toxicity before inclusion. However, the *N.F.* will include mixtures of drugs, something which the *U.S.P.* will do only rarely, since the prescription of mixtures and combinations of drugs is not generally considered the best therapeutic practice.

Because the doctor has never found it practical to use the *U.S.P.* and the *N.F.* as reference books, the AMA used to publish an inexpensive and valuable volume known as the *Epitome of the U.S.P. and N.F.,* which listed the titles of the drugs in each volume and some useful facts about them. The discontinuation of this important service about fifteen years ago is partly responsible for the gap that *PDR* has unfortunately filled.

Further responsibility for the gap lies with another decision of the AMA that discontinued publication in 1957 of an annual volume entitled *New and Nonofficial Remedies* (or *N.N.R.*). The highly prestigious AMA Council on Pharmacy and Chemistry included in *N.N.R.* descriptions of many drugs not yet official either in the *N.F.* or the *U.S.P.* but deemed of sufficient importance and worth to describe to doctors. Conversely, the council also included certain drugs which had achieved official status whenever it believed that the medical profession was not yet sufficiently well informed about them. Most reputable manufacturers used to apply to the justifiably influential council to have their new products accepted. Drugs that

were considered of little worth, or those that carried
a merchandising name or had been advertised in a
misleading fashion, were not likely to receive the
approval of the council, whose opinions were widely
accepted and served a most valuable purpose. There
is, incidentally, a "successor" to *New and Nonofficial
Remedies* entitled *New Drugs,* an uncritical compila-
tion of newly marketed agents which cannot be taken
seriously as a guide to good prescribing practice.*

* Since the pharmaceutical industry and the parasite medical
press with which it lives symbiotically could find so little in
the 1967 *Handbook* to criticize, this comment about *New
Drugs, 1966*—which was revised only once since and is no
longer in print—was viciously attacked. A giveaway sheet
called *Medical Tribune* contacted the physicians who had compiled *New Drugs, 1966* and managed to extract angry statements including wholesale denunciation of my *Handbook.*
These statements were widely distributed to nearly every doctor in the country. I would not then, and will not now, retract
my characterization of that issue of *New Drugs.* This is so
especially because in the Preface to *New Drugs* the executive
vice-president of the AMA wrote his own caveat: "Since a
monograph on a drug is included whether or not the Council's
opinion is favorable, *New Drugs* is in no sense a list of approved or accepted drugs." He also wrote, "Criticism of *New
Drugs* and comments concerning its usefulness are invited."
All I did was to take him up on it. *Medical Tribune* never saw
to it to cite these essential words of Dr. F. J. L. Blasingame's
preface.

The AMA's ex-Council on Drugs followed *New Drugs* in
1974 with *AMA Drug Evaluations.* The latter was an excellent
book that could be taken seriously as a primary guide to good
prescribing practices. The trouble is, it was too good, made
authoritative judgments on the relative values of drugs, and,
hence, raised the ire of the big pharmaceutical manufacturers.
It was consigned to the scrap heap, never to be revised or updated—a tribute to the power of the PMA in top AMA circles.
About the time that this decision was made, the AMA dissolved
its own Council on Drugs, which had been responsible for the
contents of *AMA Drug Evaluations, 1974.* It is common
knowledge that this irresponsible action was prompted by pressure from the PMA. To clarify the contents of some pages
that follow, the reader must be informed that the AMA
Council on Drugs was the successor to the Council on Pharmacy and Chemistry of the AMA.—R.B., January 1975

The overwhelming number of practicing doctors are single-mindedly concerned with giving their patients the most effective medication with the least possible chance of unwanted side effect or toxicity. Most doctors—like most people of any kind—are likely to be suspicious that a bargain may be cut-rate in quality as well as cost. There may even be a matching tendency to believe that something more expensive must also be of higher quality.

While honest skepticism is always healthy, such attitudes may be misleading. A quotation from the *Nebraska State Medical Journal,* cited in *Drug News Weekly* of January 31, 1966, asks: "Is it through no accident that cheap has come to mean inferior as well as inexpensive?" The question was asked in the context of a discussion as to the advisability of prescribing by generic name. This seemingly sensible attitude is buttressed by editorial comment in the *Journal of the American Medical Association:*[14] ". . . the physician who prescribes meprobamate [15] as such has no way of knowing that his patient will receive the drug in a form of highest quality and expected potency." The AMA did not always take this stand, however; until only recently, the AMA was on record as favoring the use of generic names in preference to brand names.[16] The preference for generic names was based on the belief that "this would avoid much needless tax on memory with its attendant confusion and errors." Dr. Austin Smith, when he was secretary of the Council on Pharmacy and Chemistry of the AMA in 1944, wrote: "One of the greatest evils of the use of protected names [*i.e.,* brand names, which are trademarked] lies in the confusion they create. The old story of methenamine being prescribed in one prescription under six different names is a standing joke in materia medica classes, and yet other examples

[14] Editorial, "Drug Names," *JAMA,* Vol. CXC, No. 6 (November 9, 1964), p. 542.

[15] Meprobamate is the generic name for a widely advertised sedative most commonly bought as Miltown® and Equanil®.

[16] American Medical Association, *New and Nonofficial Remedies, 1950,* Official Rules of the Council, Rule 4, p. xix.

just as questionable are evident in everyday practice."
Elsewhere in the same article Dr. Smith told of "a
large hospital in an eastern city [which] did away
with the expense of prescribing proprietary agents
when official counterparts were available, and unnecessarily complex mixtures and the absurd practice of
prescribing names instead of therapeutically active
agents. This pharmacy within one year effected a
saving of $50,000." [17]

To avoid the proliferation of brand names, the
Journal of the American Medical Association used to
permit only the originator of a product to advertise
under a brand name in AMA periodicals, while all
other purveyors were required to use the generic
name instead of their own brand names. Quoting the
late Senator Kefauver:

> The effect of these requirements was generally
> to curtail advertising excesses in the prescription
> field. Doctors relied heavily on the AMA *Jour-
> nal* to keep abreast of new drug products, and
> most manufacturers found it worthwhile to place
> their advertising where it counted. The Council's
> [Council on Pharmacy and Chemistry of the
> AMA] controls also tended to maintain some
> competitive balance between the large and small
> units in the industry. The Seal of Acceptance
> [indicating approval by the Council] was very
> important to small manufacturers; it was promi-
> nently displayed as proof positive to physicians
> that the product was of high quality. The fact
> that only the originator of the new product could
> use a brand name was also a marked asset; for
> the small company there was a decided prestige
> element in the recognition that it was the con-
> tributor of the development.[18]

[17] Austin Smith, "The Council on Pharmacy and Chemistry,"
Journal of the American Medical Association, Vol. CXXIV,
No. 7 (February 12, 1944), p. 435.

[18] Estes Kefauver, *In a Few Hands* (New York: Pantheon
Books, 1965), p. 74.

Sadly, the AMA attitude changed shortly there-
after; its policies were reversed in the mid-1950s after
it hired the Chicago firm of Ben Gaffin & Associates,
Inc., to research ways of improving the sale of advertising space in the *JAMA.* Whether related or not,
the facts are that the fifty-eight-year-old Council Seal
of Acceptance Program was shelved; publication of a
small volume called *Useful Drugs,* whose wide use
had the effect of "ensuring both safe and effective use
of drugs as well as limiting their number through
authoritative suggestion," [19] was discontinued; and
consideration of advertising was taken out of the ju-
risdiction of the eminent Council on Pharmacy and
Chemistry and placed in the hands of an advertising
committee. AMA advertising revenues suddenly increased dramatically, but in the words of one distinguished professor of medicine, ". . . they lost the
most valuable tool they ever had as far as being of
service to the profession, and clearly appreciated by
the public." [20] Thus it was that the Council on Pharmacy and Chemistry lost its position of authority,
contributing to the vacuum that has ever since been
filled by the pharmaceutical manufacturers.

V. The Move to Promote Generic Prescribing
—and the Reaction

Many responsible members of our government are
aware of the large savings to be made by buying
generic rather than brand-name drugs where possible, and plans are under way to introduce legislation
requiring the dispensing of generic preparations to
patients whose drugs are being paid for under tax-
supported Medicare. This comes as no surprise to
those who know that all the military medical facilities
buy and dispense only drugs that are bought by the
Defense Supply Agency of the U.S. government under

[19] Dr. Walter Modell, editorial, in *Clinical Pharmacology and
Therapeutics,* Vol. II, No. 1 (January–February 1961).
[20] Kefauver, *In a Few Hands,* pp. 76–77.

generic names from the lowest competitive bidders.
Although many of the contract winners are small and
middle-sized manufacturers (*institutional* buyers, such
as municipal hospitals, are at present their major
market), when the big corporations have entered into
sealed bidding there have been some remarkable revelations. For example, CIBA, the enormous Switzer-
land-based company, offered to sell to the U.S.
government for about 60 cents a quantity and quality
of reserpine (1000 0.25 milligram tablets) for which
the corner pharmacist must pay $39.50. The govern-
ment buys it as (generic name) "reserpine"; the corner
pharmacist buys and dispenses it as (brand name)
"Serpasil®". There are no important differences between the two; only the name—and $39. Ironically,
CIBA did not win the contract, for they were under-
bid by a company willing to sell the same drug for 51
cents.

In addition to federal government institutions, state
and municipal and many private non-profit hospitals
buy generics. Many have their own formulary, which
restricts in-hospital usage to a list of selected basic
generic drugs, the appropriate one being substituted
for the expensive brand-name item wherever the institution's own committee on drugs (consisting of its
own physicians and pharmacists) deems it appropriate
and suitable. This meets with nearly unanimous acceptance on the part of the doctors, but is anathema
to brand-name manufacturers. According to corporate thinking, the formulary restricts the doctor's
freedom of choice. Therefore, the National Pharmaceutical Council, Inc. (NPC), whose relatively few
dues-paying members are exclusively heavily advertised brand-name drug manufacturers, is, according
to its executive vice-president (who appeared before
the Kefauver subcommittee in May 1960), "particularly concerned with the practice known as substitution." He went on to say

. . . a physician, in prescribing a particular brand
of drug for a patient, may be doing so because
that brand has characteristics which the physician

wants his patient to have and which may not be present in other brands. The generic name does not indicate to the dispensing pharmacist what these characteristics are and he cannot necessarily tell from reading the prescription why the prescriber chose the brand he did. If the pharmacist is permitted to substitute the so-called generic equivalent, he *very likely* is not substituting a drug with equivalent characteristics and may be defeating the very purpose of the physician in selecting the brand of the drug he chose.[21]

The statement is nonsense. In seventeen years of clinical experience, an instance where a prescription was written for a brand-name drug because of "characteristics" other than the identity of its major ingredient has never come to my attention. Furthermore, close physician colleagues I have questioned are unaware of any such instances. The representative of the National Pharmaceutical Council ended his prepared remarks by asserting: ". . . we insist that the medical profession be left free to prescribe exactly what it sees fit and that the public be assured that it gets what the doctor prescribed." [22] Any implication that the generically named drug does not contain what the doctor prescribed is false.

The council proposed to spend $140,498 in 1960 alone to protect this "freedom" of doctors. It is difficult not to believe that the National Pharmaceutical Council is in reality prepared to spend large sums of money to perpetuate and exploit a situation which many in the medical profession (and a growing number of lay persons) find distasteful: *viz.*, the undue influence which multi-million-dollar promotion has applied to the practicing doctor and to the public. With the assistance and prodding of the National Pharmaceutical Council, the majority of the fifty individual state pharmacy boards have influenced state legislatures to adopt resolutions prohibiting a phar-

[21] *Hearings on S. Res. 238*, Part 21, pp. 11,695, 11,699.
[22] *Ibid.*, p. 11,701.

macist from substituting one brand-name drug or a
generic-name drug for another. This has taken place
quietly; doubtless, few citizens are aware of it. Of
course, the council is not entirely successful: the
Director of Drugs and Drug Stores of Michigan, Mr.
O. K. Grettenberger, testified before the Kefauver
subcommittee that an attempt by the Michigan State
Board of Pharmacy to suspend the license of a pharmacist, one E. L. Casden, for filling a prescription
for Meticorten® with another brand of prednisone
instead was not justified under law. A state court
found that "chemically and by assay the drugs were
identical." [23] Meticorten® is the Schering Corporation's form of prednisone, and is often ten times as
costly as prednisone sold by generic name or even by
other brand names.[24]

The druggist, himself the object of advertisements
and of the "educating" salesmen, in his honest desire
to be a helpful, reliable partner of the doctor passes
along to him dark rumors of generically named drug
tablets which do not dissolve in the gastrointestinal
tract (a phenomenon which must be very difficult to
document) and remarkable testimonial anecdotes of
his own as to the impotence of generic penicillin
(classically, about a patient with fever, treated with
generic penicillin G without apparent effect, who im-
proves only after the doctor switches to a brand-name
penicillin G). Doctors are human, and while they
may recognize that such stories are usually impossible
to prove and are often lacking in logic, the seeds of
doubt may be planted and take root—for after all, is it
not axiomatic that quality always costs a little more?
Did not the National Pharmaceutical Council distrib-
ute a pamphlet listing twenty-four "reasons" why brand
names should be specified on prescription blanks?
This pamphlet was even made available as a handout
in drugstores; unfortunately, a brilliant point-by-point
dissection of this fatuous document made before
Senate subcommittee hearings by Dr. Walter Modell,

[23] *Ibid.*, pp. 11,592–11,593.
[24] *Ibid.*

the distinguished Professor of Therapeutics at Cornell Medical School and the New York Hospital, goes unread.[25] The campaign to make doctors and patients ill-at-ease about prescribing and using generic drugs has been highly successful; prejudice against the use of generics is deeply instilled and will be overcome only gradually.

The big brand-name drug houses, through their executives and representatives, openly disparage products sold as generics and undoubtedly influence some doctors to adopt a similar view. For example, I received a "Dear Doctor" letter from the vice-president in charge of sales of one of the largest corporations; the letter began, "Although there is nothing unusual about substandard drugs being sold by small manufacters lacking quality-control procedures . . ."

The entire incident surrounding this letter deserves extended comment, for it is rich in revelation. The letter was in response to my request for further information regarding the allegation made by his detailman that a U.S. government agency had unwittingly bought substandard digoxin. While disowning knowledge of the allegation, the vice-president did make reference to three recorded instances in which substandard digoxin was, in fact, sold by two small companies. He enclosed a reproduction of an article from the *Brooklyn Eagle* of January 1963 describing a "Crack-Down on Heart Drug as Too Weak" and "seizure" of digoxin tablets from two Manhattan drugstores, and also enclosed a pamphlet published by the National Pharmaceutical Council. In the first place, the disparaging reference to generic manufacturers was uncalled for, since there is reason to believe, as will be shown later, that the word "big" could have been used as meaningfully as "small" in describing manufacturers who produce substandard products. Second, since digoxin is sold generically by more than fifty small companies, it makes no more sense to blackball all of them for the quality-control slips of two than it would be to blackball the vice-

[25] *Ibid.*, pp. 11,608–11,627.

president's corporation for the recorded quality-control slips of other brand-name manufacturers. The presentation of material of this nature to a physician searching for a factual report shows surprising evasion and irresponsibility.

Finally, the NPC pamphlet "Misconceptions About So-Called 'Generic Equivalent' Drugs" is worth analysis. Its general thesis is that there is no such thing as a "generic equivalent" because, in addition to the major ingredient in a tablet or capsule, there are also inert substances: bases to create bulk, adsorbents, disintegrants, and binders to hold the tablet together. The pamphlet implies that the know-how required to produce a tablet or capsule that will disintegrate properly and release the active drug is somehow unlikely to be the possession of those who manufacture generic drugs. To be sure, there are incompetent manufacturers who have marketed improperly compounded tablets that do not, for example, disintegrate as they should, but the information supplied in the *Handbook* will make it possible for doctor, patient, and pharmacist to buy generic drugs with a high degree of assurance that they meet the specifications of the *United States Pharmacopeia*. As a matter of fact, all important techniques of drug compounding are common knowledge and within the ability of any conscientious manufacturer, large or small.* Most of these techniques are among the oldest arts of medicine. The substances used as bases are milk sugar, salt, starch, and a simple sugar, mannitol. For absorbents, both milk sugar and starch will do. As a disintegrant, cornstarch is the popular choice and works well. Binders in general use are gelatine, gum acacia, gum tragacanth, molasses, dextrin, and, less commonly, cellulose. Physicians and lay persons alike will recognize all of these substances as inert materials about which there can be little

---

* Obviously, this was slightly overstated. The matter of easy solubility and its relation to ease of absorption into the blood was not well understood. The big manufacturers, the small manufacturers, the PMA and the *U.S.P.* itself were all a little slow to appreciate this too. See the *Handbook* sections dealing with chloramphenicol and digoxin.—R.B., January 1975

mystery. As for modern tablet-making machines, they are available to anyone wishing to buy them. (The interested reader can find excellent brief monographs on tablet making and tablet coating in any pharmacy library.)

The NPC pamphlet is correct in stating that there is no generic name for tablets or capsules that contain two or more active drugs. However, this is because the *United States Pharmacopeia* does not include combinations and nearly every teacher of pharmacology and clinical medicine discourages their use—and with good reason. A tablet or capsule containing a mixture of drug limits the doctor to a fixed-dosage ratio. Nevertheless, in support of such combinations the pamphlet states categorically that it is "more economical to prescribe a single preparation than to prescribe separate ingredients by generic names." This does not agree with my observations. (See "Drugs for High Blood Pressure" and "Drugs for Gastrointestinal Disorders" in the Basic Drug List.)

The council pamphlet refers, in passing, to the "minimum requirements" of the *United States Pharmacopeia,* subtly implying that *U.S.P.* standards can be exceeded or bettered, and some readers could infer from it that brand-name drugs do just that and generics do not. For example, with respect to the matter of dosage, it happens that the human body is not delicately sensitive to small variations in dosage of most drugs.[26] Therefore, in many cases the *U.S.P.* permits the weight of a tablet to vary somewhat. Thus, a tablet stated to contain 100 milligrams of a drug may in some cases contain as little as 95 or as much as 105 milligrams. Exceeding 105 milligrams can be as potentially serious as failing to provide 95 milligrams. It makes no sense to think in terms of "exceeding" the dosage requirements of the *U.S.P.*

"Why do so many physicians specify drugs by brands?" asks the council, which proceeds to answer its own query in part by saying of generic drugs:

---

[26] An illustration of this fortunate degree of tolerance is in the almost universal practice of giving adults the same dose of most drugs without respect to body weight.

"The patient taking such a drug may suffer an unexpected reaction, not experienced with the drug with
which the physician is familiar containing the same
active agent. Is the reaction due to the drug or to
some inert ingredient used by the maker as a flavoring
agent, binder, or for other purposes of dosage formula-
tion?" Now, allergic reactions can *theoretically* occur
from these substances (although I have never personally seen one), but there is no basis for believing
that a flavoring agent, base, adsorbent, disintegrant,
or binder used by a manufacturer of generic drugs is
any more likely to cause allergy than one used by
a manufacturer of brand-name drugs. Actually, allergy
to a medication is nearly always due to its *major*
ingredient, and for this reason a strong argument
can be made for referring to drugs by generic name.
In many cases the same drug has several very different-
sounding brand names: [27] if a patient had shown an
allergy to this drug under one brand name and the
physician switched him to another brand without
realizing that it was the same drug, the result would
be continuation or worsening of the allergic reaction.

Having nearly rested its case, the National Pharmaceutical Council pamphlet takes up the matter of
prescriptions written for welfare patients: "Some individuals take the position that prescriptions for welfare
patients should be written generically, on the theory
that some public funds presumably will be conserved,
and that 'generic equivalent' drugs are good enough
for the patient who cannot pay for them. Are reasons
which dictate a physician's choice of a reliable brand-
name drug for a sick patient any less valid because
the patient cannot pay for the best treatment available?
Are there in fact tremendous savings to be achieved
by relegating the welfare patient to the class of second-
rate citizen?" The council has an admirably sensitive
social conscience, but it is reminded that when the
President of the United States, a senator, a representative, or any other high government official becomes

---

[27] Syncillin®, Darcil®, Alpen®, Chemipen®, Dramcillin®,
and Maxipen® are all brand names for a particular kind of
penicillin.

ill and is hospitalized at Walter Reed Hospital or the United States Naval Hospital in Bethesda, Maryland, he is treated with drugs bought by generic name from approximately one hundred different companies of which only about twenty are large and well-known manufacturers.[28] Is there any reason why other citizens should not have access to these same medications?

VI. What About Research?

There is merit to the argument that some large pharmaceutical companies do important research and maintain facilities to provide a number of public services for which they are never adequately compensated in dollars. On the other hand, few manufacturers of generic drugs do research and none is equipped to provide an adequate supply, let us say, of rare antitoxins should need ever arise, whereas some of the big companies are in a position to do so. It has been pointed out, however, that the large corporations spend nearly four times as much for advertising and promotion as they do for research, and it has been said that much of the latter takes the form of "molecule manipulating" attempts to produce a drug that will have the same pharmacological effect as an agent already patented and marketed by a competitor. Upon discovering such a compound, the company may patent it, market it, and join in the competition even though the new drug offers no substantial advantage over the older, better-known one. It is the proliferation of such drugs, each with its own brand name, and each launched with a giant promotional campaign, that has caused much of the confusion besetting the doctor. Activity of this sort could conceivably be beneficial by giving rise to price competition. Unfortunately, this rarely happens because the major manufacturers, with a few exceptions, peg their prices at practically the same, often identical figures.

However, while one can therefore legitimately ques-

[28] *Administered Prices: Drugs*, p. 247.

tion the value of introducing "copycat" drugs, it is
not entirely fair to question the kind of research
(*viz.*, molecule manipulating) that makes them available. Anyone aware of the nature of pharmacology
knows it is impossible to predict when a small change
in molecular structure is going to cause significant
beneficial change in pharmacological effect or in toxicity. (A mere increase in potency is not beneficial,
however, for it makes little difference to the patient
whether he swallows a 10 or a 500 milligram tablet.)
There is no doubt that the pharmaceutical industry has
made many important research contributions.[29] Many
conscientious physicians undoubtedly feel that this one
factor alone justifies prescribing brand-name items
even though their patents have expired and patients
have to pay more than if generic equivalents were
prescribed. There is something to be said for this view,
*provided public money is not involved (as with welfare
or Medicare patients) and that private patients who
foot drug bills directly are agreeable. Patients (who
are "captive consumers") have a right to know for
what services they are paying.* Other equally conscientious physicians may take the view that the
responsibility of the doctor is to his patient's immediate welfare—including his pocketbook—and
may not wish to allow an ideology of sorts to influence
therapeutic practice.

VII. The Substantive and Crucial Quesion: Are Brand-Name Products Superior?

It is the contention of the *Handbook* that no one
is in a position to make ironclad guarantees for any
manufactured product, drugs included, and that there

[29] About two-thirds of the *Handbook*'s basic drugs were developed entirely or in part by the pharmaceutical industry, but
the patents by now have expired on more than half of these.
Addendum: And by 1975 at least three-fourths of the drugs
considered basic are either non-patented or so cross-licensed
that there is a broad spectrum of prices for the same item,
e.g., ampicillin, an important antibiotic.—R.B., January 1975

is no good reason to believe that brand-name drugs are necessarily more reliable than generics as to quality, purity, and potency. There is compelling evidence for this view in Table 1 (page 53), which presents details of major drug recalls [30] during the period 1966–1967. This information was supplied by the Food and Drug Administration to a congressional committee. The facts speak for themselves: *All of the recalls involved products of the largest and best-known corporations.* It is plain that a pharmaceutical manufacturer's reliability is not related either to size or to advertising budget. One wonders, even, whether physician, pharmacist, and patient have not been placing exaggerated confidence in certain well-known firms. It would be incorrect to infer that all large pharmaceutical manufacturers are not reliable in their overall production, but the evidence does point up the injustice in wholesale condemnation of all smaller drug manufacturers.

Because 90 percent of the drugs currently sold in the U.S. are produced by about two dozen of the largest brand-name drug manufacturers, it is fair to ask whether the number of their substandard products is nonetheless disproportionately smaller than would be expected. It is possible to provide a tentative answer, since the Kefauver subcommittee did its work so thoroughly. In the hearings the then Commissioner of Food and Drugs, Mr. George Larrick, testified: "We confine sampling to drugs which we have reason to believe may be misbranded or adulterated." [31] Mr. Larrick provided data showing the number of samples taken per one-million-dollar volume of business in the cases of several large and several small companies during the decade 1950–1960. In the cases of Merck, CIBA, Schering, and Carter Products (Wallace Laboratories), one sample alone was taken per $1 million of business; for Smith Kline & French, Lederle, Pfizer, and Upjohn the range was from one to less than five per $1 million. For small companies, how-

[30] The removal from the market of drugs discovered not to meet *U.S.P.* standards or of drugs which are mislabeled.
[31] *Hearings on S. 1552*, Part 22, p. 12,113.

ever, the situation was strikingly different, for here
the number of samples ranged around one hundred
per $1 million and in several instances was even more
numerous! [32] This kind of sampling, in effect, spot-
lights the violations of the small companies, upon
which the enforcement work is concentrated.

Furthermore, with respect to the activities of the
major drug companies, Dr. Barbara Moulton, formerly
an FDA staff member, testified, "Private conferences
between representatives of industry and the Food and
Drug Administration staff members are also the rule
rather than the exception with respect to regulatory
action under the law." Thus, when a large manufacturer was concerned, situations more commonly
than not were rectified by informal rather than official
agreement. This way, damaging reports of official recall actions were often avoided, for the FDA records
of such informal agreements were allegedly incomplete.[33]

Not least of the reasons forcing us to believe that
brand-name drugs are not necessarily better than
those sold by generic names is a finding made in the
spring of 1966 by the United States Food and Drug
Administration. At the direction of its new, no-
nonsense Commissioner, Dr. James Goddard, the
agency sampled 4600 drugs from 250 manufacturers.
Quoting Mr. Winton B. Rankin, Deputy Commissioner,
as he addressed the American College of Apothecaries
on October 15, 1966, in Boston, Massachusetts:
"About 2600 of the drugs were sold by their generic
name only and about 2000 by brand name. They
represented 20 of the most important groups of drugs
used in medicine—antihypertensives, oral antidiabetics,
anti-infectives, digitalis and digitalis-like preparations,
for example. Antibiotics were not included because
every lot of antibiotics for human use is checked by
FDA before sale." Deputy Commissioner Rankin then
went on to reveal to a hushed audience of pharmacists
that "7.8 percent of the generic-named drugs were

[32] *Administered Prices: Drugs*, p. 246.
[33] *Ibid.*

38 *The New Handbook of Prescription Drugs*

not of acceptable potency, 8.8 percent of the brand-
named drugs were not of acceptable potency." Later,
in reply to a question from the audience, the speaker
made it clear that the difference between the 7.8 and
8.8 percent figures is not large enough to allow one
to conclude that generic drugs are necessarily better
than those sold by brand name.

2
The Battle Is On (1970) *

I. The Scene, and What the Handbook Is About

A highly respected medical educator once wrote, "The secret of the care of the patient is in *caring* for the patient." [1] Two or three generations of American physicians, most without ever having known him, have been deeply influenced by his words. We physicians are proud of the quality of scientific medicine in the United States, but many of us recognize that all is not well in our medical-care system. [2] One gravely disturbing problem concerns the quality of prescription writing. Some of us, because we *care* for patients, are unwilling to sidestep this issue, which is "controversial" because it involves large sums of money and corporate profits.

It is a fact that owing to circumstances largely beyond his control, the prescribing habits of the independent practicing doctor are in themselves causing illness. [3] Also, enormous sums of money are being spent by patients because of faulty prescribing. [4]

* The following chapter was originally printed as the Introduction to the 1970 *Handbook*.
[1] F. W. Peabody, "Care of the Patient," *Journal of the American Medical Association*, 88:877–882 (March 1927).
[2] For an excellent discussion, see *Time*, February 21, 1969, pp. 53–58.
[3] *Competitive Problems in the Drug Industry*, Hearings Before the Subcommittee on Monopoly, Senate Select Committee on Small Business, 90th Congress, 1st and 2nd Sessions (1967–1968), Part 2, p. 565.
[4] *Ibid.*, Part 3, pp. 838, 839; Part 10, p. 4066.

Some doctors prescribe too many drugs, and potentially toxic drugs for minor conditions. They have insufficient regard for the cost of drugs and little
knowledge of how the patient can obtain them at
least expense. The nation's outstanding medical weekly,
The New England Journal of Medicine, published an
editorial commenting on these charges when they were
made in the first edition of the *Handbook,* and stated,
"[The author's] purpose is to spell out convincingly
some of the ills that we all know exist." [5] Not long
afterward, Senator Gaylord Nelson of Wisconsin
provided the first proof.

Nelson's Subcommittee on Monopoly discovered
in November 1967 that from 3,500,000 to 4,000,000
million Americans were being dosed each year with
a course of Chloromycetin®. Chloromycetin® (chloramphenicol) is a potentially dangerous drug. If physicians had limited its use to conditions where it was
truly indicated, only 10,000 persons at most would
have received it.[6] Death from aplastic anemia following administration of Chloromycetin® for trivia such
as acne, sore throat, the common cold, minor urinary
infections, even infected hangnail, has been the documented fate of many hundreds and possibly the fate
of several thousands of Americans in recent years,
many more than were injured by thalidomide in the
U.S.[7] The thalidomide incident caused more widespread indignation because the victims, though they
remained alive, were horribly disfigured for all to see,
while Chloromycetin's® victims are dead and have
been buried, out of sight. Until Nelson exposed the
scandal, Parke, Davis & Co. is reported to have
been reaping one-third of its profits from the sale
of Chloromycetin® [8] and spending tens of thousands
of dollars annually to advertise and promote it. The
drug's potential toxicity had been known to the medical

[5] Editorial, *New England Journal of Medicine,* 277:155–156
(1967).

[6] *Competitive Problems in the Drug Industry,* Part 6, p.
2566.

[7] *Ibid.,* pp. 2167–2752.

[8] *Forbes,* January 1967, p. 158.

profession since the early 1950s,[9] and that it had been overprescribed was common knowledge to most medical authorities.

Chloromycetin® is a dramatic example of the danger of bad prescribing. However, severe injury from drugs is very common. At least 1,500,000 persons in this country are admitted each year to hospitals because of adverse side effects of drugs, according to testimony before the Nelson subcommittee by Colonel Robert Moser, Chief of Medical Services at Walter Reed Hospital and one of the nation's foremost authorities on drug-induced disease. The injury that bad prescribing costs public and private treasure is incalculable.

What is responsible for this state of chaos? The root cause is economic. A couple of dozen giant pharmaceutical manufacturing corporations have all but wrested from the medical leadership responsibility for the continuing education of the busy doctor in drug prescribing, and the doctor has not been given the right kind of information to help him practice rational, economical therapeutics. Information about comparative costs and authoritative views on comparative efficacy have been drowned out by a flood of exaggerated, misleading, even false advertising claims aimed at doctors by pharmaceutical houses, which have all but filled the communications void separating true medical educators from practicing doctors. It cannot be denied that the pharmaceutical industry exerts undue influence upon the profession at every level from the student to the busy practitioner to the professor and educator. Its tools are simple: money and flattery.

Let there be no mistake about it: there is a basic conflict between the aims of the drug industry and the aims of good doctors. The industry seeks to enlarge the consumption of its products and spends $3,000

[9] Richard Burack, *The Handbook of Prescription Drugs* (New York: Pantheon Books, 1967), p. 9. Also *Competitive Problems in the Drug Industry,* Part 6, pp. 2584, 2622.

per doctor per year to this end.[10] Faced with this advertising siege, good doctors should consciously seek to minimize drug consumption—in order to optimize it. Rational prescribing must include consideration of comparative efficacy of drugs and of comparative costs.

Many members of the medical profession, though by no means all, are aware of the chaos and understand at least partly what lies behind it. Unfortunately, most doctors in influential positions have not been quick to make effective moves to correct things. Some are intimidated, like most people, by the thought of standing up to a five-billion-dollar industry; others are so heavily indebted to it for "retainer," consultation, and drug-testing fees, for research grants and fellowship support, for many small personal obligations, that they dare not speak out—or are unwilling to. Some privately express displeasure over drug corporations persuading doctors to use drugs that they might not want to prescribe if left to themselves, but only a rare few have had the courage to speak out unambiguously for the record.[11] Prominent, influential physician educators may be members of the board of giant drug corporations while masquerading under the protection of academic titles; they may also fail to make public disclosure of these financial connections when publishing industry propaganda,[12] and do deny such associations when asked. A key pharmacology professor on the Drug Efficacy Review Committee of the National Academy of Science–National Research Council, its present chairman in fact, admitted

[10] James L. Goddard, "The Drug Establishment," *Esquire*, March 1969, pp. 117 *et seq.*

[11] Some recent examples, all before the Nelson subcommittee, are: Dr. W. B. Bean, University of Iowa; Dr. J. M. Faulkner, Boston, Mass.; Dr. George Baehr, New York City; Dr. George Nichols, Jr., Boston, Mass.—all in December 1968; Dr. A. Dale Console, Princeton, N.J., in March 1969; and Dr. John Adriani, New Orleans, La., Chairman of the Council on Drugs of the American Medical Association, in May 1969.

[12] Samuel Proger, ed., *The Medicated Society* (New York: Macmillan, 1968), pp. 204–225.

in a telephone interview with a staff member of the Nelson subcommittee[13] that he is a consultant on the payrolls of three drug firms,[14] which pay him a substantial income additional to his salary from his medical school appointment. His committee's job is to give important advice to the United States Food and Drug Administration (FDA), whose decisions based on that advice could seriously affect drug manufacturers' profits. Millions of dollars lie in the balance. The public is entitled to know if that professor has ever divulged to the FDA the extent of his financial connections with the very industry his committee's recommendations will regulate. Are there other influential men in similar potential conflict-of-interest situations, who sit on public or private drug advisory committees, or who, as kingpins in a highly authoritarian profession, mold the opinions of others? These are fit questions for a level-headed congressional inquiry.

What, for instance, would the present medical leadership and the giant pharmaceutical concerns say if it were discovered that the author of this book, Dr. Richard Burack, had for years been receiving a "retainer" fee from one or several manufacturers of generic drugs, or that he "consulted" for several who paid him as much money as he receives annually from other sources, or that he was a member of the board of directors or owned shares of stock in such a company?

The drug industry is run by businessmen who have been more successful at making profits than all other businessmen on the American manufacturing scene. They make so much profit and manage to do it with so little risk that they have been called "the last of the robber barons." [15] Patients are being exploited

[13] Economist Benjamin Gordon.

[14] James Ridgway, *The Closed Corporation . . . American Universities in Crisis* (New York: Random House, 1968), p. 99.

[15] *Competitive Problems in the Drug Industry,* Part 1, p. 13. See also U.S. Department of Health, Education and Welfare, Task Force on Prescription Drugs, *Report and Recommendations* (August 30, 1968), pp. 18–19.

by some well-known corporations with astonishingly
disreputable records, including federal convictions for
criminal offenses. This is happening only because the
medical profession, the group entrusted with defending
the patients, has fallen under the spell of men who
claim to be ethical but who, like many businessmen,
are governed by marketplace morality. Former Commissioner James L. Goddard of the Food and Drug
Administration has boldly written: "If the [Drug]
Establishment insists on following its present course . . .
an awakened public will have no alternative but to
demand a system of governmental control . . . The
Drug Establishment may well find itself in the position
of explaining to Congress why it should not be made
into a public utility." [16]

What can be done? The welfare of the public
demands clear-cut separation between the pharmaceutical industry and the medical profession. This
need not mean that medicine and industry cannot
cooperate. It does mean that transactions such as con-
tracts to do drug testing should be handled by a neutral
third party to keep medicine–industry contacts at a
minimum. The financial dependence of the profession
on the drug industry is wrong. It is the patient who
pays for this. One of the best-paid professions
should pay for its own meetings, its own cocktails,
its own printed meeting programs, its own medical
journals, and its own continuing education. Hardly
any of us doctors is invulnerable to criticism on this
score. While much of the free material supplied doctors
is little more than worthless trash corresponding to
the calendars sent out by many business firms, this
is not always the case. "Little gifts," such as doctor
bags and stethoscopes, free prescription drugs, cases
of baby foods, and vitamin products, are accepted
and rationalized by impecunious medical students and
young doctors in training as unimportant though
personal; their receipt of these "little gifts" has led
ineluctably to the receipt by institutions of "big gifts,"
which are less personal but more important. Acceptance is rationalized by saying that it is an old

[16] Goddard, "The Drug Establishment," p. 154.

American tradition for questionable money to be cleaned up by its passage through the university.

The consumer-patient has a right to know about the financial ties of the industry and the profession. Doctors must know about them too, and must be persuaded to divest themselves of these connections and to prescribe rationally with economy in mind. The profession's single reason for existence, after all, is to provide the public with a service. Medical leadership—local, state, and national—must come to understand that it is in the long-term interest of the profession to avoid incurring obligations to the industry. Responsible physicians (and legislators) prefer that the impetus for reform originate in medical circles. Unless it does—soon, and without compromise or equivocation—there is a strong likelihood of federal legislation, always unpleasant compared with education and self-imposed reform.

I feel compelled to say that nearly all I have read and observed during the two years since the first *Handbook* appeared has caused me to doubt that rational prescribing practices will come about through traditional approaches to the medical profession. I fear there is too much disorganization and inertia, too many fixed habit patterns and preconceived ideas among the rank and file, and too much possible conflict of interest, authoritarianism, and self-perpetuation among the elite of the medical establishment—the men who mold the attitudes of students and of doctors in training. A very serious matter alluded to already is the communications gulf between leading educators and the doctors in the field, which drug promoters have been quick to bridge with slick, giveaway journals and sheets, so seductively easy to read. The over-all influence of this "commercial press" upon medical therapeutics is profound.

There is no more effective way of catalyzing reform than by demonstrating to the individual citizen how his pocketbook and health are affected by a problem. The pharmaceutical industry, while it has done much that is constructive, has also caused trouble in the medical profession and in the doctor–patient relationship. We in the profession would be wise to take strong corrective action without delay.

II. Rational Prescribing

Appropriate selection of a drug by the doctor includes:

1. *Using the Right Drug for the Right Patient at the Right Time in the Right Amounts*

No one disagrees with this. Admittedly, the decision is based on judgment; there can be honest differences. The shibboleth has it that "the doctor must be free to order what he wishes." The trouble is, the doctor is not as free as he thinks. He is the object of an advertising campaign designed to influence his therapeutic practices; the comments in this book's Prescription Drug List pages show what the drug industry's propaganda siege has done to him.

2. *A Consideration of Cost*

Modern industry and government decision-makers have long been used to asking themselves, "Is this desired effect worth the cost?" Doctors ought to think the same way. Admittedly, it is harder for them: they are dealing with human beings, there are emotional factors, and they have too few hard facts about relative effectiveness of different drugs promoted for the same conditions. In fact, there is evidence that brand manufacturers are reluctant to support drug testing that might supply this kind of information.[17] Even so, the doctor can begin to apply common-sense economy by always asking himself two questions:

1. Is the possible benefit to be derived from this drug worth its cost?

[17] *Competitive Problems in the Drug Industry*, Part 2, p. 461.

2. Has the benefit to be derived from new drug X been proved so much greater than that to be derived from old drug Y as to warrant the difference in cost?

About cost there can be little dispute. The wholesale cost of drugs is fixed by manufacturers, and figures are available to those who wish to plow through price catalogues. The *Handbook* supplies comparative price information about most of the drugs sold by prescription over American drugstore counters and offers some views on economy.

Choosing the best drug for the least money in prescription writing has been given short shrift in medical education. How can a discussion on economy be introduced when neither instructors nor students have any precise information on costs?

The basic pharmacology course in the second year of medical school provides no in-depth study of the economics of drug prescribing. Beyond that stage in his education, the doctor is putty in the hands of an industry propaganda machine which has every reason to avoid discussion of drug prices. At no point is he prepared to resist this advertising onslaught. There is going to have to be a big change; an informed profession ought to be in a position to guard patients from exploitation at the same time that it keeps prescriptions simple, safe, and effective. Since the doctor is a purchasing agent for his patient, one can justifiably ask whether he is acting within the bounds of propriety if he makes drug-prescribing decisions without a knowledge of comparative costs. One can also justifiably question whether any professional person should be "educated" by advertisements.

III. Generic Drugs Have Brand-Name Equivalents That Cost More

When a manufacturer has come up with a new drug and has received FDA permission to sell it, it becomes known to doctors by two names. One is its official (also "established" or "generic") name. The other is the brand (or "trade" or "proprietary") name. The brand name is nearly always easier to say, spell, and remember. Unlike the generic name, it usually has a "merchandizing" quality too, often suggesting what the pharmacological action of the drug is claimed to be. For example, the sedative officially known as chlordiazepoxide hydrochloride is much better known by the brand name Librium®. On the prescription blank the doctor can, at the present time, legally write either name. Naturally, he tends to write "Librium®".

For the seventeen years of patent monopoly on a new drug, it makes no difference to the patient whether the doctor writes the brand or the generic name on the prescription blank, because usually only one company's product is available by either name (although a patented drug *can* be licensed to other distributors). However, it does make a great difference to the drug company if the doctor gets into the habit of writing the brand name. Once he is "trained" to do this, he is likely to continue in the habit after the seventeen-year protection period has come to an end—and that is exactly what the manufacturer wants. Why? Because at the expiration of a patent other manufacturers can start marketing the same drug, usually at a much lower price, *but they may not market it with the original brand name because brand names are protected nearly indefinitely by trademark law, though not by patent law.*

The brand-name manufacturers have shrewdly arranged to take advantage of the busy doctor's fixed habit patterns. During the 1950s, a number of the biggest and best-known drug sellers financed a group that traveled the length and breadth of the nation and "advised" individual state pharmacy boards on how to lobby for passage of an "antisubstitution" statute by their state legislature wherever they were not empowered to achieve the same end by "regulations." Thanks to the "advisory" group's successful work, at least forty-four of the fifty states now have these antisubstitution statutes or regulations.

See what happens: Abbott Laboratories originally marketed a good sleeping medication, officially named pentobarbital but much better known to doctors and the public as Nembutal®, its brand name. The patent on pentobarbital expired years ago, and scores of other firms have been selling it since, at very low cost. The biggest and best teaching hospitals know all about this and have been buying their pentobarbital at great savings, but the average physician either does not know of the availability of generic drugs, or if he does, has been led to believe that they might be inferior. So he goes on writing "Nembutal®". *But even in case the* PATIENT *should be wise to what is going on and wish to shop around for the less costly generic, the antisubstitution law has him fixed.* The law in forty-four states says that the pharmacist *must*, under threat of severe penalty, dispense the brand-name article if that is the name written on the prescription—and of course, this article commands the brand-name price. The manufacturer thus manages to perpetuate his product monopoly long after the patent has expired.

The main reason for writing the *Handbook* was that I was particularly incensed over this system in which industry uses propaganda to prejudice doctors against prescribing drugs by their official names and then uses antisubstitution laws to wring maximum prices from captive consumers.[18] (A famous pharmacologist has recently referred to brand names as "phony" names and has pointed out that their use makes possible all kinds of serious as well as ludicrous mistakes.[19]) It was necessary to argue in the first edition that "brands" are not better than "generics." However, the present edition need not dwell at length on the question of generic equivalency, since it has been settled for us by the Task Force on Prescription Drugs of the United States Department of Health, Education and Welfare (HEW). Results of their fourteen-month study, conducted with the help of two hundred consultant experts, were made public in

---

[18] The late Senator Estes Kefauver once defined the patient as a "captive consumer": "He who buys does not order."

[19] *Competitive Problems in the Drug Industry,* Part 1, p. 285. Statement by Dr. Walter Modell, Director of Clinical Pharmacology of Cornell University Medical College.

September 1968. HEW had this to say: "We have reached the conclusion that—except in rare instances—drugs which are chemically equivalent, and which meet all official standards, can be expected to produce essentially the same biological or clinical effects." [20] HEW testimony on the Task Force Report is unequivocal: "It is evident that the issue of chemical equivalency and clinical equivalency has been clouded by articles, publications, press statements, and promotional claims which seem designed to make the issue appear much larger." And: ". . . lack of clinical equivalency among chemical equivalents meeting all official standards has been grossly exaggerated as a major hazard to the public health." [21]

Dr. Philip R. Lee of HEW testified on the Task Force findings on September 25 and dealt with a publication circulated some six weeks before by the Pharmaceutical Manufacturers Association (PMA). An accompanying PMA news release had referred to "the astonishing myth" that drugs which cost less by generic name might be as good as the same drug sold at a high price by a brand name. According to Dr. Lee, "At the most, Task Force staff and our consultants agree, there were only two or three [generic drugs] which demonstrated statistically significant lack of biological equivalency, and in one case, the differences were described as being without any practical clinical importance." [22] Benjamin Gordon, Staff Economist of the Nelson subcommittee, asked, "Are there two or three? Which is it?" and the answer he received from the Task Force director was, "There are two. One of them, as you have probably surmised, is chloramphenicol." As for the second, the scientists "pointed out quite clearly that although differences were detected, these were not of any clinical importance." Not one of the *Handbook*'s "basic

[20] *Ibid.*, Part 9, p. 3718. Testimony of Dr. Philip R. Lee, Assistant Secretary for Health of the Office of Health and Scientific Affairs, U.S. Department of Health, Education and Welfare.

[21] *Ibid.*, p. 3726.

[22] *Ibid.*, pp. 3726–3729.

drugs" was called clinically substandard in generic form.

The chloramphenicol matter was quickly straightened out and, as far as is known, caused no harm. There is at present no known reason to suspect any given generic drug of being less effective than its expensive brand counterpart. In other words, doctors are now justified in discarding any prejudice they may still have against prescribing drugs by their generic names; they can write a generic name on a prescription blank with as much assurance of quality as when writing a brand name. There is no longer any excuse for depriving patients (and taxpayers) of the savings to be had by shopping for low-cost drugs. There is a lot of money to be saved by buying drugs by their official name, and, as will become clear from the Prescription Drug List, even more can be saved by doctors prescribing *therapeutic* equivalents—*i.e.,* equally safe (often safer) drugs that provide the same clinical effect at lower cost—and most often by their prescribing no drug at all.

IV. *The Use of Generic Drugs When Possible Makes Prescribing Safer*

The HEW Task Force Report establishing the effectiveness of generic drugs failed to emphasize an obvious point: that the doctor who makes it a practice to use generic drugs where indicated will practice safer medicine. The reason is not that "generic" manufacturers are necessarily more reliable than brand-name manufacturers, but that drugs which are widely sold as generics have stood the test of time. After seventeen years or more of use, the medical profession has found that they are effective and relatively safe. Drugs still under patent protection and available only by brand name are newer. Less is known of their short-term and long-term toxicity, which is why outstanding medical educators constantly warn against the casual use of new drugs.

It is even possible to take issue with the often-made statement that "generic" manufacturers are not *necessarily* more reliable than brand-name manufacturers. Table 1 below demonstrates that major FDA recalls of violative and substandard drugs during fiscal year 1966–1967 were all the responsibility of big brand-name corporations.[23] Also in fiscal year 1966–1967, 32.5 percent of PMA manufacturers (generally the well-advertised brand-name manufacturers) had according to FDA, marketed "violative" products, as compared with only 15.5 percent of non-PMA manufacturers.[24]

V. How U.S. Taxpayers Soon May Save Large Sums in Federal Health Programs

The 1970 *Handbook* included in this place a brief section entitled "How Medicare and Medicaid Money Is Being Wasted." To illustrate the point, there was an analysis of an advertisement aimed at pharmacists by one of the largest manufacturers. The advertisement listed eighty-eight of its products under the heading "Handy Reference . . . Products Now Covered for Reimbursement Under Medicare" (which included Medicaid in many states). It was shown by the *Handbook* that fewer than one-third of the products (twenty-eight) were acceptable either to the *U.S.P.* or to the *N.F.* Of the twenty-eight, 43 percent (twelve) provided a pharmacological effect that could be provided by equally effective and safe, but less costly, drugs. Of the remaining 57 percent (sixteen), one-third (six) could be prescribed and bought by generic name at very large savings. The aim of the breakdown was to highlight the waste of millions of dollars of taxpayer money on trivial, duplicative products of questionable quality; expensive, unnecessary dosage forms; and outrageously high-priced brand names

[23] *Ibid.*, Part 2, p. 789.
[24] *Ibid.*, p. 787. Statement of Dr. James L. Goddard, Commissioner of the Food and Drug Administration, U.S. Department of Health, Education and Welfare.

Table 1. Major Drug Recalls, Fiscal Year 1966–1967

Company	Drug	Quantity	Hazard	Depth	% Recovered	Reason
AYERST (Am. Home Prods.)	progesterone (Lingusords®)	15,045,092 tablets	moderate	doctor	30%	cross contamination penicillin
SQUIBB	nystatin (Mycostatin®)	18,500,000 tablets	moderate	branch warehouse	10%	subpotent
ABBOTT	sterile water solutions	3,500,000 bottles	serious	doctor	10%	nonsterile
ROCHE	chlordiazepoxide (Librax®)	570,374,450 tablets	serious (injury)	doctor	17.9%	adulterated
PFIZER	meclizine HCl (Bonine®)	6,905,408 tablets	moderate (injury)	retail	40%	not given
CIBA	aminoglutethimide (Elipten®) NDA	41,600,000 tablets	serious (injury)	doctor	20%	not given
PFIZER	physician's samples	40,000,000 tablets	serious	doctor	not given	label mixup
RICHARDSON-MERRELL	bacitracin (Bacimycin®)	656,700 ½ oz tubes 810 100 g jars 10,450 ⅛ tubes*	serious	wholesale	not given	subpotent
BURROUGHS WELLCOME	polymixin B sulfate (Aerosporin®)	1,258,533 10 cc	moderate	retail	4%	subpotent

* There is assumed to be an omission of a word in the record; probably this should read "⅛ g tubes."

53

rather than official names. The *Handbook* maintained
that tax money should properly be limited to payment
for drugs and drug dosage forms necessary to promote
health and maintain life.

The wheels of democratic government grind slowly,
haltingly, but surely. On December 19, 1973, a member of the President's Cabinet addressed a special
Senate Health Subcommittee of the Senate Labor and
Public Welfare Committee. Caspar Weinberger, Secretary of HEW, paid tribute to the HEW Task Force
on Prescription Drugs which had been ordered into
action by President Lyndon Johnson eight years earlier,
just after the Nelson hearings began to unearth its
findings. Secretary of HEW at that time was John W.
Gardner, who assigned the organizational work to
Dr. Philip R. Lee,[25] then Assistant Secretary for
Health in the HEW structure.

[25] Dr. Lee, a well-trained, experienced doctor as well as a
good administrator, is no longer in government. In 1969 he
became Chancellor of the University of California and in 1972
became Director of the University of California in San Francisco's Health Policy Program—richly deserved rewards. His
major associate in searching out and analyzing data for the
Task Force was Dr. Milton Silverman, an accomplished
chemist, pharmacologist, and a distinguished medical author
who had been a recipient of the Lasker Award for outstanding
medical reporting. Dr. Silverman joined Dr. Lee in California
in 1969, where he is now on the pharmacology and pharmacy
faculties. Drs. Silverman and Lee are co-authors of an important and erudite book based largely on the findings of the
Nelson hearings and their experiences while directing the Task
Force, whose final report was in 1969. Their book, entitled
Pills, Profits and Politics, was published in 1974 by the University of California Press. Readers of the *Handbook* will have
observed that I have had occasion to make frequent reference
to it. Its value to me lay partly in helping to confirm what I
had myself learned about pills, profits, and politics from other
sources, in providing choice morsels of information about
which I did not know, and in serving as an important check
on reference sources. Although Dr. Silverman and I might
hold some honest differences of opinion about where the professional future of pharmacy students should, and probably
will eventually, lie, his and Dr. Lee's book is a substantially
accurate account of the opinion of most unbiased authorities

Secretary Weinberger, an appointee of a President from another political party than Lyndon Johnson's, demonstrated bipartisan respect for the assemblage of data, conclusions, and recommendations of the Task Force by referring to them as "landmarks in the consideration of prescription drug issues." He made reference to a committee of outside experts in politics and economics which had reviewed the Task Force conclusions, and gave them his imprimatur. Although he remarked that instances of biological inequivalency could happen, he stated that, "All the evidence to date indicates that clinically significant differences in bioavailability are not frequent." (The reader who reads the section entitled "The Digoxin Incident" in Chapter 3, "The Reckoning Nears," may more fully appreciate the significance of Secretary Weinberger's statement; he will note that the digoxin problem, real-

---

in government, medicine, pharmacy, consumerism, and even of some of the more farsighted pharmaceutical executives. I recommend *Pills, Profits and Politics* enthusiastically as an easily readable, comprehensive, meticulously documented source book. The best signal that Silverman and Lee struck the roots of the issues they discuss is the contemptuous review their book received in the giveaway sheet called *Medical Tribune.* Supported nearly exclusively by drug advertising, *Medical Tribune* is very widely circulated to all practicing doctors who like its easy-to-read though superficial style. A disturbing side of this publication lies in its self-serving editorials, which are well and convincingly written. They carry an authoritative ring and many doctors are profoundly influenced by them. Somehow these doctors fail to perceive that those who provide this giveaway reading matter have a big financial stake in the doctor–pharmacist–patient relationship. When Secretary Weinberger's policy will have been implemented and when state legislatures throughout the country will have repealed antisubstitution statutes, the pharmaceutical industry will switch its advertising money to those publications whose major audience is pharmacists rather than doctors. *Pills, Profits and Politics,* because of its cogency and the deep respect that its co-authors enjoy, will undoubtedly help to catalyze implementation of the Weinberger policy reform proposal. If politics is "who gets what and how much," *Medical Tribune*'s antipathy to Drs. Silverman and Lee's fine book is understandable.

ized by the FDA as a potentially serious one in 1970, had been solved by late 1973 through the coordinated efforts of the *U.S.P.* and FDA to raise biopharmaceutical standards and police them.[26] In fact, the FDA set forth the new program assuring solution of the digoxin problem in the *Federal Register* on January 22, 1974.)

Mr. Weinberger must have been privy to all of the progress and confidence before then, because as he spoke before members of the Senate Health Subcommittee on that now famous December 19, 1973, he announced that HEW intended to publish regulations limiting the amount of money that it would disburse in payment for any drug to "the lowest cost at which the drug is generally available, unless there is a demonstrated difference in the therapeutic effect." [27] There was no equivocation; the Administration, through the Secretary of HEW, had informed itself of the issues and had come down hard on the side of paying only for generic drugs in federally financed health programs. The secretary was quick to append words, however, conveying the intention of the gov-

[26] *Competitive Problems in the Drug Industry*, Part 24, p. 9955. The present Commissioner of the FDA was so well satisfied that the problem was solved that on February 20, 1974, testifying before the Subcommittee on Monopoly, he answered a direct question from Senator Nelson by stating: ". . . we believe the new program will give every assurance that the digoxin being marketed will meet the new standards." His deputy, Dr. J. R. Crout, Director of the Bureau of Drugs in the FDA, commented: ". . . we assume that as the bioavailability data come in and as manufacturers demonstrate repeatedly that they can make a good batch, they will drop out of this certification program. So we view this certification program as a transient and not a permanent phenomenon on the digoxin scene" (*ibid.*, p. 9956). On February 21, 1974, Dr. Daniel Banes, Director of the Drug Standards Division of the *United States Pharmacopeia*, referred to the coordinated actions of the *U.S.P.* and FDA; he said: ". . . in my opinion, given these two quick reactions, with a strict U.S.P. dissolution standard and FDA's program, there should be no problem in the future with digoxin" (*ibid.*, p. 10,237).

[27] Transcript of Hearings Before the Senate Health Subcommittee, December 19, 1973.

ernment not to interfere with doctors' prescribing practices. Should a doctor wish to continue to prescribe by brand names and insist that his Medicare and Medicaid patients receive the branded items, he would still be free to do it; he would have only one problem: the government would not pay for them.

There were the expected cries of outrage from the PMA's chief executive, C. Joseph Stetler. He sounded the standard stale anthem that is critically examined, stanza by stanza, in the following section, entitled "The Profits of the Brand-Name Manufacturers."

As if to underscore the serious intention of HEW to proceed with the Weinberger cost-cutting policy, responsibility for weaving the details of its implementation was entrusted to the reliable, sensible Dr. Charles C. Edwards. Dr. Edwards, a political conservative who had once had close ties to the AMA, had been appointed Commissioner of the FDA during President Richard Nixon's first term in office. Many, who mistakenly believe that the prescription price issue is the cause of liberals only, feared that this man would reverse the trend set by his most important predecessor in recent years, Dr. James L. Goddard. The liberals soon discovered that they had nothing to fear in Dr. Edwards's appointment; and they, as well as most of the people who have been closely following the issues that this *Handbook* describes, believe that Dr. Edwards has been the most effective and intelligent Commissioner of the FDA in modern memory.

Dr. Edwards's accomplishments as Commissioner of the FDA led to his promotion to Assistant Secretary for Health in HEW, the highest medical office in our government. On March 6, 1974,[28] he presented an official statement at a hearing of the Subcommittee on Monopoly and summarized his efforts to date to implement the HEW policy to limit drug reimburse-

[28] *Competitive Problems in the Drug Industry*, Part 24, pp. 10,483–10,496.

ment "to the lowest cost at which the drug is generally available." Dr. Edwards put himself on the line: "We believe this policy could result in savings of 5 to 8 percent in the overall HEW reimbursements for prescription drugs and have a beneficial impact on drug pricing throughout the country. I would like to take this opportunity to reaffirm the Department's commitment to this policy and assure this committee that regulations to implement this policy are being developed." He stated that the issues that faced him in this task were complex, because they affected so many interested parties. He outlined seven major issues besetting him, and how he and his staff had tentatively decided to meet each one. Briefly, they were:

1. ". . . this policy will in no way adversely affect the quality of drugs. As you know, the Department's firm position in this regard is that in terms of quality and therapeutic equivalence, with few exceptions, no significant difference between chemically equivalent drugs has been shown. We, therefore, do not believe that allegations of inequivalency can or should stand in the way of this drug reimbursement policy."

2. ". . . we must insure that the policy in no way restricts the availability of needed drugs to a recipient."

It was evident that he was having some trouble understanding how to establish "the lowest cost at which the drug is 'generally available'" and had decided to skirt the issue by declaring, "It has never been the Department's position that the reimbursement level should be established at the *absolutely* [my emphasis] lowest cost." He was worried: "The regulations must insure that at the established reimbursement level a continuing supply of the drug will be available to all pharmacies." Thirty-five states presently providing out-of-hospital drugs under the program require pharmacists to dispense by use of the dispensing, or service-fee, method. No usual and customary markup is allowed. The pharmacist is allowed to add a "service fee," usually upward of $2 to the cost of the medication. It would be reasonable for HEW to mandate extension of these regulations to the remaining fifteen states, establishing a uniform national policy with regard to both Medicaid and Medicare if and when Medicare or any other HEW health program should, one day soon, begin to provide out-of-hospital prescription drugs.

Establishing a reasonable figure for the lowest cost "generally available" ("lowest cost" has more recently come to be named "maximum allowable cost," or "MAC") has been touted as a very difficult and complicated project. On the contrary, determining maximum allowable cost is no Manhattan Project. The task can be assigned confidently to a small staff of clerks who perfunctorily peruse catalogues of well-known reliable manufacturers and distributors of generic drugs who ship their products to any part of the country with remarkable promptness. Smaller, regional manufacturers of generic drugs would merely be expected to meet the same wholesale cost levels.

3. "At a later time we would hope to perhaps extend this policy to other drugs." It was necessary to decide how extensive the initial MAC program should be, and wisely Dr. Edwards recognized that it would be impractical to establish a maximum reimbursement level for *all drugs,* or even for most. As a solid start, he proposed concentrating on the two hundred most prescribed drugs, the same two hundred covered in the Prescription Drug List pages of this *Handbook*.

Dr. Edwards was not about to bite off more than he could for the moment chew with his mouth closed. Critics of Dr. Edwards's intention to keep his program simple might point to the "Top 200 Drugs Prescribed" list (Appendix B) and correctly show that most of the products are still patent-protected; and that no government agency is likely to be able to establish a maximum allowable cost on these patented items; and that prescriptions containing the generic name cannot save a customer money if only one manufacturer sells it at its own high price. These criticisms are correct, but fail to take into account the rapidity with which patents are expiring on presently well-known products. Also, doctors (especially the new breed), increasingly conscious of their role as responsible purchasing agents, recognize so-called "new" drugs as duplicative and unnecessary and turn more and more away from commercial sources for information about drug therapy. All the while, the FDA may be expected to maintain its high standards in overseeing test results claiming safety and efficacy. By continuing responsible action, the FDA will continue to put the damper on the introduction of "me too" "new" drugs, products which have no uniquely new attributes. Without the senseless proliferation of products, there will be little to ballyhoo and the large pharmaceutical manufacturers will find it increasingly difficult to introduce senseless but expensive products into the "Top 200" to displace products whose patents are close to expiration. The game of artificially induced obsolescence will become ever harder to play successfully. Dr. Edwards's disarmingly modest first move can be expected to have a very important impact on the cost of most prescription medicines—sooner than is generally recognized.

4. The "source"—the company—to be used to determine maximum available cost was briefly discussed as a problem by Dr. Edwards. This was touched upon under point 2 above; the *Handbook's* suggestion is not far from Dr. Edwards's own expressed ideas.

5. While this is, for the record, an important issue to raise, in practical terms there will be no difficulty in Dr. Edwards's problem of determining "availability of the drug, disparity of prices among equivalent products, demand for the product, *and ability of the manufacturer to produce quality drugs.*" (Emphasis is mine.) The italicized statement is a joke. Senator Nelson placed in the record of his hearings the following information which may surprise many readers: [29]

. . . Squibb, Pfizer and Wyeth have recently joined SKF [Smith Kline & French], Robins and Parke, Davis as purchasers of antibiotics and other generic dosage forms from Mylan, a pri-

[29] *Ibid.,* p. 10,165.

vate formula manufacturer in Morgantown, West Virginia. Mylan's private formula sales to major drug manufacturers jumped to $4,800,000 in fiscal year 1973 ending March 31 from $2,200,000 a year earlier.

Emerging as Mylan's top major pharmaceutical marketing customer in fiscal year 1973, Squibb purchased $1.3 million erythromycin in the first year it bought anything from the Morgantown private formula manufacturer. Mylan is the sole supplier for Squibb's erythromycin, introduced in 1972.

A Squibb spokesman said the company decided to use Mylan rather than processing erythromycin itself because of the "difficult technology involved." Mylan is one of the few companies capable of making the product, the Squibb spokesman said.

So the Pharmaceutical Manufacturers Association, to which all but one of the best-known ("reputable," "ethical") high-price drug manufacturers belong, disparages the purchase of generic drugs,[30] while its member firms are quietly buying inexpensively from small "generic" manufacturers, pasting their own labels on the bottles, and selling the products at high prices under brand names!

6. Dr. Edwards made it clear that *two* elements determine the cost of any drug product: the wholesale cost of the item and the pharmacists' profit. MAC will have to deal with both elements—another of the problems with which policy will have to deal.

7. A final important issue: Dr. Edwards addressed himself to those problem situations in which a doctor might stubbornly insist that a Medicaid or Medicare

---

[30] C. Joseph Stetler, head of the PMA, had reacted to HEW's announced policy favoring purchase of generic drugs in government programs as "radical, a gamble, a disservice to the American public." He warned that the policy would "relegate Medicare and Medicaid beneficiaries to second-class medical care" (Silverman and Lee, *Pills, Profits and Politics*, p. 169).

patient receive the expensive brand equivalent to an
available inexpensive generic drug. In response to a
question from Senator Nelson, Dr. Edwards stated
that the physician would be required to state on an
appropriate form the reason why it is necessary for
the patient to receive the expensive item. This seems
an eminently fair requirement from which no doctor
should shy away. The argument of most physicians
has been that the practicing doctor knows better than
anyone what medications to choose for his patient.
The cost of out-of-hospital prescription drugs may
well become an explosive voter issue in 1976.

VI. The Profits of the Brand-Name Manufacturers

Independent economists (Dr. William S. Comanor,
Professor of Economics, Harvard University; Dr. Wil-
lard F. Mueller, Chief Economist and Director, Bureau of Economics, Federal Trade Commission; Dr.
Leonard G. Schifrin, Chairman, Department of Economics, College of William and Mary; Dr. Henry B.
Steele, Associate Professor of Economics, University
of Houston [31]) have made it amply clear to Senator
Nelson and his subcommittee that the few drug firms
controlling 90 percent of the retail prescription market do not function in a truly free and price-competi-
tive marketplace—*i.e.,* one free of monopoly, restraint
of trade, and price fixing—and that they make unusu-
ally high profits.

[31] These are to be distinguished from certain other economists paid by the drug industry to appear before the subcommittee to "make a case" in return for exorbitant fees—up to
$1200 a day. Admitting that their fees were higher than usual,
one rationalized that there was a risk to his professional reputation in appearing. "You should see the stream of [uncom-
plimentary] letters I've got from my testimony," he is quoted
as saying (*National Observer,* March 18, 1968, p. 45). Another
allegedly said, "None of us made any pretense whatsoever that
we were going down as completely objective professionals"
(*ibid.*).

Table 2. Profit as a Percentage of Total Sales, Pharmaceutical Manufacturers Versus American Industry

Company	Fiscal Year											
	'62	'63	'64	'65	'66	'67	'68	'69	'70	'71	'72	'73
Abbott	10.3	11.1	10.7	10.4	10.1	9.3	9.0	8.0	5.1	8.7	7.6	7.4
Am. Cyanamid	9.1	9.3	10.5	10.8	9.9	7.5	8.4	8.3	7.3	7.9	8.0	7.7
Am. Home Prods.	10.6	10.6	10.1	10.2	10.3	10.6	10.3	10.3	11.2	10.5	11.1	11.2
Bristol-Myers	8.1	8.2	8.7	8.5	8.4	7.1	6.9	7.3	7.1	7.6	7.0	7.5
Carter-Wallace	13.6	12.7	13.9	13.7	12.2	11.6	—	8.4	8.3	14.6	9.0	6.4
Lilly	11.9	10.6	12.0	13.2	13.6	13.1	14.7	15.5	13.3	15.9	4.7	16.0
Merck	12.2	13.5	15.6	18.0	18.1	17.0	15.9	15.6	15.3	15.2	15.4	16.0
Olin Mathieson	4.6	4.7	5.1	5.8	6.0	7.0*	5.7	6.6	7.6	6.9	7.8	9.2
Parke, Davis	10.5	11.7	12.9	14.6	13.3	8.8	7.4	7.6	(bought by Warner-Lambert)			
Pfizer	9.5	9.7	9.3	9.8	9.9	9.2	8.9	8.9	9.5	9.3	9.4	9.4
Richardson-Merrell	10.7	10.3	9.9	9.6	9.7	9.6	8.2	8.3	7.3	8.4	8.2	8.2
Robins, A. H.	15.6	10.7	12.6	14.2	14.1	12.0	—	12.3	12.6	11.9	13.7	13.2
Schering	11.7	11.4	11.6	12.2	12.8	12.6	12.9	12.8	13.5	12.9	15.3	17.3
Searle	24.4	26.0	28.0	26.1	20.1	20.1	18.5	17.4	15.9	15.8	15.4	12.7
Smith Kline & French	16.9	16.8	17.8	17.3	16.4	16.2	15.0	12.8	12.6	12.6	12.2	11.9
Sterling Drug	10.4	10.4	11.2	11.1	9.7	9.8	9.6	9.5	9.7	9.6	9.6	9.5
Syntex	7.1	23.0	32.0	29.2	33.5	28.6	—	—	—	—	—	—
Upjohn	13.4	13.4	14.2	15.3	14.1	11.0	10.3	10.1	9.1	9.5	9.1	10.6
Warner-Lambert	9.4	10.1	10.1	10.0	9.6	7.9	8.4	8.9	8.0	7.8	8.2	8.3
Pharm. Mfrs.	11.6	12.3	13.5	13.7	13.3	12.1	10.6	10.5	10.2	10.9	10.1	10.7
All U.S. Mfrs. (500)	4.2	4.4	5.0	5.5	5.6	5.0	4.8	4.6	3.8	3.9	4.1	4.5

* Now Squibb Beech-Nut, Inc.

The 19 corporations above supply most of the expensive brand-name drugs and drug products cited in the Prescription Drug List and the Appendixes. The 15 whose profits are shown in Table 3 (as a percentage of invested capital) are included here, too. (Source: Standard and Poor's individual annual reports, and *Fortune*, October 1956 to 1973.)

Table 3. Profit as a Percentage of Invested Capital

Company	'62	'63	'64	'65	'66	'67	'68	'69	'70	'71	'72	'73
Abbott	13.1	14.4	14.9	15.2	14.9	14.4	14.7	13.9	15.5	8.7	13.4	14.1
Am. Cyanamid	12.3	13.1	15.0	15.6	14.8	10.7	12.5	13.0	12.5	11.1	12.1	12.7
Am. Home Prods.	27.2	26.5	26.4	25.9	24.5	25.1	25.4	26.2	25.8	26.7	26.3	28.2
Bristol-Myers	19.0	20.0	21.5	23.3	25.0	20.1	19.5	21.1	19.7	17.8	17.4	12.4
Lilly	13.5	13.3	15.5	18.5	20.5	19.2	21.1	21.1	20.7	18.7	7.1	21.3
Merck	14.4	16.6	19.5	23.7	27.1	25.4	24.3	23.9	24.1	24.4	24.3	25.7
Olin Mathieson	8.2	8.4	8.9	10.0	11.9	13.5*	12.9	8.2	0.1	4.1	—	11.0
Parke, Davis	11.9	13.2	14.8	17.4	16.0	10.2	8.9	9.7	(bought by Warner Lambert)			
Pfizer	14.9	14.7	14.8	15.8	16.3	13.9	13.9	14.6	15.1	15.1	15.0	15.9
Richardson-Merrell	14.5	14.1	13.2	13.7	14.7	14.1	13.4	13.4	14.2	12.3	13.7	13.9
Schering	13.9	13.8	16.3	17.6	20.1	20.0	21.1	22.1	21.3	21.5	23.2	25.6
Smith Kline & French	31.2	30.9	31.0	31.6	28.7	26.9	24.9	23.1	22.7	21.5	20.9	20.9
Sterling Drug	20.4	19.6	20.7	21.6	21.1	20.6	19.8	19.5	19.2	18.8	18.3	18.1
Upjohn	14.7	15.3	16.1	18.5	16.8	15.4	13.6	14.1	13.5	12.5	14.7	19.0
Warner-Lambert	18.4	18.9	20.1	21.1	21.1	16.8	17.9	18.7	14.4	14.5	15.0	15.3
Average	16.5	16.8	17.9	19.3	19.6	16.3	17.6	17.4	17.0	16.3	15.8	18.2
500 U.S. Mfrs.	8.9	9.1	10.5	11.8	12.7	11.3	11.7	11.3	6.5	9.1	10.3	12.4
Pharm. Profit × 100 / All Mfring. Profit	187	185	169	163	154	144	150	154	262	179	153	147

* E. R. Squibb separated from Olin Mathieson in 1967. The figure given is for a new corporation, Squibb Beech-Nut, Inc. The 15 corporations above supply most of the drugs cited in the Prescription Drug List. They are also among the 500 largest manufacturing industries in the United States. Data are taken from annual issues of *Fortune* in the years 1962–1973, and from annual reports of individual corporations.

Four other important drug manufacturers are not large enough to be included in *Fortune*'s 500, but figures for their profits as a percentage of sales are shown in Table 2.

Table 4. Rates of Return of Drug Manufacturers and All Manufacturing Industries, 1956–1973

| Year | Profits after taxes as a percent of stockholders' equity | | Profit rank of the drug industry among all manufacturing industries* |
	All drug manufacturers	All manufacturers	
1956	17.6	12.3	2
1957	18.6	11.0	1
1958	17.7	8.6	1
1959	17.8	10.4	1
1960	16.8	9.2	1
1961	16.7	8.8	1
1962	16.8	9.8	1
1963	16.8	10.3	1
1964	18.2	11.6	1
1965	20.3	13.0	1
1966	20.3	13.5	2
1967	18.0	11.3	1
1968	17.9	11.7	1
1969	19.1	11.3	1
1970	15.5	9.5	2
1971	15.1	9.1	2
1972	15.3	10.3	2
1973	18.1	12.4	1

* Rank among the 26 industries for which profits are reported separately in the Quarterly Financial Reports.

The source of these data is the Quarterly Financial Reports of the Federal Trade Commission and the Securities and Exchange Commission for the years 1956–1965. The source of the data for the years 1966–1973 is the *Fortune Directory of the 500 Largest U.S. Industrial Corporations.*

There is no question about how big their profits are; tables 2 to 5 provide this information. The data come from Standard and Poor, in part from annual issues of *Fortune* magazine, from corporation annual reports, and from government data. The corporations listed in the tables are the biggest and/or best-known American firms which sell drugs largely by brand name.

Peruse Tables 2 and 3 and notice the following:

1. Profit as a percentage of the sales dollar is consistently more than twice that of all the rest of the 500 most profitable native manufacturing enterprises.

2. Profit as a percentage of invested capital [32] consistently runs at least 50 percent higher, occasionally

[32] "Invested capital" = "net worth," the sum of capital stock, surplus, and retained earnings at the year's end.

Table 5. Profit (Net) for Major Pharmaceutical Manufacturers, in Millions of Dollars[8]

Fiscal Year	'56	'57	'58	'59	'60	'61	'62	'63	'64	'65	'66	'67	"Excess Millions of Dollars" potentially available for research in 1967.‡ (See text.)
Abbott	10.9	12.7	12.9	13.0	12.4	12.0	14.8	19.5	22.6	24.7	26.7	28.1	12
Am. Cyanamid	44.3	51.3	43.8	52.3	46.8	49.4	59.3	66.3	81.6	93.1	94.4	70.3	41
Am. Home Prods.	31.3	38.6	42.4	46.7	48.6	50.2	53.4	56.9	69.1	76.5	93.8	104.1	43
Bristol-Myers	5.6	6.4	7.2	8.9	10.8	13.0	16.1	19.1	23.1	33.4	39.4	52.0	13
Carter-Wallace	2.0	4.5	5.6	7.0	8.9	7.5	8.8	9.1	11.4	11.2	10.6	9.9	5.7
Lilly	30.1	32.3	23.7	23.5	18.8	23.1	25.5	25.8	31.7	41.8	46.4	53.7	27.4
Merck	20.2	23.1	27.7	30.0	27.8	27.2	29.2	35.8	44.9	59.6	75.9	89.3	52.4
Olin Mathieson (incl. E. R. Squibb)	44.8	36.4	9.4	37.4	34.7	32.1	34.1	37.0	41.3	50.5	66.7	40.1†	4.5
Parke, Davis	17.6	27.9	28.0	31.0	30.5	22.3	19.1	22.2	26.2	32.8	31.8	21.0	28.4
Pfizer	18.3	22.9	24.0	24.9	26.1	31.4	36.5	40.3	44.7	53.1	61.6	58.3	26.9
Richardson-Merrell	7.0	7.9	10.1	12.2	14.4	17.0	17.3	17.5	17.8	20.4	24.2	25.1	10.2
Robins, A. H.	—	—	2.0	2.7	2.8	3.2	4.6	5.5	7.4	9.5	10.4	12.0	6.3
Schering	10.6	15.4	12.5	11.9	9.9	10.0	10.2	10.5	12.0	14.3	16.8	19.0	9.4
Searle	6.6	6.9	7.0	7.3	7.5	9.9	13.8	18.5	24.2	23.2	22.9	26.6	15.5
Smith Kline & French	18.1	20.6	20.8	25.0	24.4	27.1	30.5	34.0	38.7	42.2	41.3	42.1	27.2
Sterling Drug	16.9	17.8	19.1	21.0	22.2	23.4	24.8	26.4	29.2	33.6	40.4	44.2	17.2
Syntex	—	0.6	0.05	0.6*	0.3	0.4	0.8	3.8	8.4	10.5	19.0	19.2	15.8
Upjohn	15.2	17.4	20.0	23.2	22.8	22.8	23.3	25.8	29.6	37.2	36.4	30.1	22.0
Warner-Lambert	11.4	15.0	15.0	16.4	16.5	17.4	28.6	30.2	34.0	39.1	43.2	51.6	18.1

* Loss.
† Squibb is no longer a subsidiary of Olin Mathieson. It is now Squibb Beech-Nut, Inc.
‡ A gross underestimate, since the savings incurred through increased tax-deductible income is not considered. Far more "excess millions available for research" could have been had in every case if less had been spent for advertising and promotion. These data have been expressed above as percentages with respect to invested capital (Table 3) and to total income from sales (Table 2).

twice as high. (Economists prefer to use Table 3 data as an indication of profit making. Profit as a percentage of net worth is a more significant expression of corporate success than profit as a percentage of sales.)

Faced with the statistics in Tables 2 and 3, apologists for the drug industry take several predictable tacks. One is: "It's a high-risk industry, one based on innovation and invention. Hence, higher profits than usual are justified." The answer: Brand-name manufacturers are, on the contrary, in a very *low*-risk industry. Every year but five since 1956 (when figures became available), the drug industry has been first in the nation in profit rank among all manufacturing industries. Table 4 shows this. Were corporations failing or making a poor profit, the industry's average profit figures and profit rank could not regularly be as high as they are. As a matter of fact, no major drug manufacturer has suffered a business decline* in fifteen years.[33] Contrary to what the apologists claim, the economic strength of the industry is largely *due* to the remarkable ease with which their chemists can, by molecular manipulation, innovate and invent drugs that duplicate the pharmacological action of agents already patented by competitors. Although these can be patented and marketed as "new," they rarely have significant advantages over the older drugs of which they are copies. This is not to say that molecule manipulation is a bad research approach, for occasionally it gives birth to important new drugs. But most of the time, it predictably provides "me-too" drugs, marketed (successfully) with exaggerated claims *without introducing price competition.* For the doctor, this practice brings confusion; and what confuses doctors is not good for patients.

Faced with Table 4 data, industry apologists might claim that profit rank is not a good index of "risk."

* This "chapter" was written before Parke, Davis's takeover by Warner-Lambert.—R.B., January 1975

[33] *Competitive Problems in the Drug Industry,* Part 5, p. 1578. George Squibb's testimony.

The answer: There is no better index of risk than the probability of incurring a loss.[34]

It is usually at this point that one hears, "Well, no matter what you say, it is a fact that while the cost of everything else is rising, the cost of drugs is declining," and reference is made to the imposingly named "Consumer Price Index of the United States Bureau of Labor Statistics." What is not pointed out is that for drugs the BLS figures provide no index of the actual amount being spent, since the newest, most expensive drugs that sweep medical practice like fads are unrepresented among the short list of prescription drugs it monitors. The best way to make this clear is to quote the Honorable Arthur M. Ross, former Commissioner of the Bureau of Labor Statistics: "Although prices for identical prescriptions over a period of time have been declining, the newer drugs that appear on the market are generally more expensive than those available over the years. As a result, the cost of an average prescription has been rising." [35] The number of prescriptions written in 1967 was 1.1 billion; the average one cost $3.43 (by one estimate), about 50 percent more than fourteen years ago.

Industry apologists and propagandists then play their trump: "The high profits are necessary for research." The answer: Not true. Not true for the following reasons:

1. Money for research comes out of gross revenues, not net profit.[36] Research is written off as a tax-de-

---

[34] *Ibid.*, p. 1818.
[35] *Ibid.*, Part 1, p. 184.
[36] Table 5 was set up to show that even if research funds did come from net profit, each of the major corporations would have millions more available for research if only it were willing to accept the same level of net profit as all the rest of manufacturers in the U.S. 1966 is taken as a typical year. The column on the far right shows that the "Excess" available would have ranged from 52 millions in the case of Merck and Co. down to 4.5 millions in the case of Olin Mathieson (which at the time was E. R. Squibb's parent company). No board of directors in their right minds would take money for research out of net profit; it would be too disadvantageous tax-wise.

ductible expense like advertising and administration. (Therefore, the taxpayer and/or the patient subsidizes 50 percent of it.) On the average, research outlay uses less than 10 cents on the sales dollar. Outlay for advertising uses around 25 cents on the sales dollar, probably more.[37]

2. According to the report of the HEW Task Force on Prescription Drugs on August 30, 1968, much of industry research is wastefully directed toward making duplicative drugs and combination drug products which "have been found generally unnecessary by leading clinical pharmacologists."

3. If and when a drug company does devise an important, unique drug, it is provided with many years of patent monopoly in which to recoup its investment and reap a profit. (The architects of patent law reasoned that limited-life patent monopoly provides incentive *while encouraging disclosure of socially important inventions,* but that perpetual monopoly discourages inventiveness.)

4. Suppose, for the sake of argument, that points 1 to 3 do not exist. Suppose that research is dependent on high profit. A social and political issue then arises. The burden of paying for prescription drugs does not fall evenly on the populace. According to the HEW Task Force report, less than 10 percent of people, the elderly (usually not the wealthiest people), buy nearly 25 percent of the drugs. One must question if it is appropriate to expect the elderly sick and the poor to bear the brunt of research costs so that the pharmaceutical industry can come up with more duplicative, high-cost, highly profitable, patent-protected drugs to be sold back to the same elderly sick and poor people.

In summary: brand-drug manufacturers are the most successful in the nation. Their profits are the highest, their risk is low. The cost of the average prescription and the number of prescriptions are steadily rising. The high net profit is not necessary to

[37] *Administered Prices: Drugs,* Senate Report No. 448, Subcommittee on Antitrust and Monopoly, Senate Committee on the Judiciary, 87th Congress, 1st Session.

fund research programs, but even if it were, it would
be socially unjust.

VII. The United States Needs
a National Drug-Label Law

"Label" means here the placing on any drug con-
tainer (bottle, cardboard box, etc.) of the official (or
generic) name of the drug as well as directions for
its use. The most important reason for insisting on
label is that it is essential for public health—so essential that it should be mandatory and automatic
unless the doctor specifically requests its omission.

Dr. Helen Taussig of Johns Hopkins, one of the
nation's most outstanding doctors, outlined the situation well enough in 1963 in the *New England Journal
of Medicine* in an article [38] where she described a
side of the thalidomide disaster that is not well known
to doctors and legislators. That the U.S. was largely
spared the tragedy of children born without limbs,
thanks to the good work of a single public servant in
the FDA, does not detract from the lesson Dr. Taussig intended to teach. She pointed out that tablets
and capsules containing thalidomide were marketed
throughout the world under at least fifty, and possibly
as many as a hundred, different brand names. Usually
the brand name gave no indication to doctors or to
the public about the active ingredient of the tablets or
capsules, and it was therefore impossible for doctors
to warn their patients or for government authorities
to broadcast clear-cut warnings to their populations.
An alert Brazilian reporter had a suspicion that thalidomide was being sold in pharmacies in his own large
city, São Paulo, because he had suddenly become
aware of numbers of limbless newborns. Upon inquiry,
however, he was told by authorities that thalidomide
was not being sold in São Paulo. He persisted in his

[38] Helen B. Taussig, "The Evils of Camouflage as Illustrated
by Thalidomide," *New England Journal of Medicine*, 269:92–
94 (July 11, 1963).

questioning, and discovered that thalidomide was indeed being widely sold but that it was known to the public and the "authorities" only by its brand names: Slip®, Ondasil®, Verdil®, Sedin®, and Seralis®. When this was made known, 2.5 million tablets containing thalidomide in pharmacies and pharmaceutical factories in São Paulo were confiscated by officials. Countless children and their parents must always be grateful to that inquisitive reporter.

The *Handbook* warns that in spite of all the FDA's fine work in screening new drug applications, and in spite of the important 1962 Kefauver-Harris Amendment to the Pure Food and Drug Act (which somewhat tightened the clinical testing requirements on new drugs), tragedy is likely to strike again as a result of unexpected drug toxicity. A tragedy could become a cataclysm if medical and government authorities were unable to act surely and swiftly to check it. Avenues of communication will have to be kept wide open. Delay or confusion due to any future misunderstanding of what words mean cannot be tolerated. It is imperative that medical and government leaders take every step now to encourage a "one drug–one name" habit of mind on the part of doctors and lay persons. The best way would be to pass legislation making it mandatory that all medications dispensed by pharmacists be labeled with the generic name of the active drug or drugs within. The possibility of disaster is too great to justify opposition based on anyone's wish to be "free from compulsion." The public has a right to be protected.

What kind of mishap can be visualized? We have already had a taste of what could happen in the form of death from brain hemorrhage in patients taking certain drugs for mental depression. Patients taking this class of drugs (the best known is Parnate®) were unexpectedly found to be intolerant of certain cheeses and a number of other foods rich in a potentially toxic substance called tyramine. Tyramine is ordinarily easily destroyed by the body, but the mechanism for doing this is paralyzed by the drugs, and ingestion of tyramine can cause sudden sky-high rises in blood pressure—enough to cause death from rupture of major arteries in the brain. More recently, pharmacologists have become aware that many commonly used drugs can grossly modify the rate of breakdown of anticoagulation drugs.[39] Failure to recognize this "drug–drug interaction" has led to poor control of treatment with anticoagulation drugs—a dangerous situation. Sulfonamide drugs, by markedly potentiating the effect of some oral blood-sugar-lowering agents, have precipitated life-threatening coma. Many more examples could be cited, and the list is growing longer as our already overmedicated society increases its exposure to ever more combinations of drugs.

A mandatory label law would be a great boon to the everyday practice of medicine, as well as to patient safety.[40] Busy doctors are forced to waste too much time trying to discover the identity of tablets and capsules being taken by their new patients, who often show up with a paper bag filled with unlabeled bottles. The pharmaceutical manufacturers must be very well aware of this, as they have taken to publishing color photographs of their largest-selling tablets and capsules in a special glossy section in the middle of a commonly used advertising catalogue known as *Physicians' Desk Reference* (*PDR*). Physicians are forced to waste valuable time, frequently in vain, trying to match patients' medications with the pictures —time which could be better spent if only the bottles had been labeled in the first place. In the absence of sure identification of medication, no physician can be certain that he understands the basis of his patient's symptoms.

There is no adequate justification for opposing or delaying passage of a national drug-label law, but ingenious reasons have been invented by those who fear its possible secondary economic effect: that doctors and patients will become educated about the

[39] *Clin-Alert,* No. 103, May 8, 1968.

[40] Senator Nelson recently introduced a bill to provide for mandatory labeling, but as of this writing (December 1968) it has not yet been acted on.

generic names of brands, and price competition will
ensue. It has also been claimed that labeled bottles
in bathroom cabinets and bureau drawers will encourage self-medication, and that patients themselves will
defeat the purpose of the legislation by mixing different tablets and capsules in a single bottle. I can only
emphasize that it is in the patient's interest to ask his
doctor to write the word "Label" on any prescription
blank and to see to it that the order is carried out by
the pharmacist.

VIII. Drug Testing—Some Problems and Suggestions for Improvement

Before a corporation can market a new drug, it
must be approved by the FDA, which bases its decision on reports by doctors who have tested the drug.
New drugs, then, must be tested, and the doctors
who do the testing ought to be paid for their services.
At present, any "qualified" person can make his hospital, laboratory, or private practice facilities available
to the industry; and for many doctors, drug testing
has become a major source of income.

As a result, we are faced with several sticky administrative and ethical problems. It is not our intention here to dwell upon the sick spectacle of those
rare physicians who have been grossly dishonest—
who have contrived and criminally submitted false
reports to companies which have, probably unwittingly,
used the data to seek FDA approval of a product. No
one condones this, and once found out, these physicians have been disbarred by the FDA from further
testing. It is more important to ponder the relationship that most physician drug testers and most drug
makers presently enjoy.

Drug testing as a tedious, demanding job if it is to
be done well. Objectivity and honesty are essential.
However, objectivity is not encouraged by the present
practice, which (1) leaves the choice of investigators
up to the drug companies; (2) all too often results
in raw data being given to statisticians in the employ

of industry (the possibility of bias is too great a risk); and (3) leaves the payment of the investigator or of his medical school department to the industry. This makeshift arrangement leaves room for conflict of interest: the independent practitioner who tests drugs can become dependent upon the industry for a significant part of his annual earnings. Will he, in every case, be coldly objective and forthright in his evaluations, to the extent of providing industry time after time with unpromising reports? Or will he soften or modify what he writes for medical journals because industry executives are his "friends," who pay him, wine and dine him, fly him to meetings, flatter him? Is there a possibility that he might be struck off a company's list of drug testers if he should persist in being "uncooperative"? The dangers are clear.

Similarly the professor who undertakes to test drugs in return for a drug corporation's grant of funds to his department through his university is in a dangerous game. From the public's point of view, his involvement could be even more sinister than that of the individual private practitioner. The academician's publications carry more weight within the profession, and his opinions are likely to carry more weight with the FDA. Whether money is earmarked for "research funds" or personal income matters little. Money is what nourishes medical academic life, and personal or department or university obligation is a natural enemy of objectivity.[41]

[41] In an address given at the 50th Annual Meeting of the American Association of University Professors, in St. Louis, April 10, 1964, the Walker Professor of Economics and International Finance at Princeton University, Dr. Fritz Machlup, had the following to say:

"One incident during my term of office has, more than anything else, reinforced my belief in the importance of tenure. It had to do with a young medical researcher in the last year of his probationary period who had discovered toxic qualities of a drug distributed by a company which was supporting his university with generous research grants. Should he publish the report of his findings? Would he risk non-renewals of his appointment if his publication angered the donor and the chairman of his department? As it was, or as I am told, the

The following selections are from letters by some doctors who tested Indocin® (indomethacin) for Merck, a giant drug manufacturer. The letters were in the FDA files, became available to the United States Senate, and are reported in the Nelson hearings. Nothing in them is illegal, but their tone and contents are disturbing. Physician investigators' names and other identifying information have been omitted. Italics are added.

On the letterhead of a medical center, the following was sent by a drug-testing doctor to Dr. Nelson H. Reavey Cantwell of the Merck, Sharp & Dohme Research Laboratories. The date is May 11, 1964.

Dear Nelson,

The enclosed letter is from a very fine patient. I thought you would be interested in her very vivid and articulate description of the adverse symptoms she encountered with Indomethacin.

I would emphasize that these do not alarm me nor indicate any evidence of organic damage but *I am afraid they will offer some practical problems in marketing this drug.*

Needless to say, I am very grateful for all of your kind efforts in regard to my trip to Japan.

I'll look forward to seeing you on my return. I think *we must get together* and plan on publishing some of the data which we have collected. Best regards always.[42]

---

young man decided to publish and he lost his post. I discouraged him from filing a complaint with the AAUP because it would be impossible to prove that his chairman's decision not to renew the contract was influenced by his decision to publish the embarrassing findings of his research. Just think how easy it would have been for this scientist to postpone publication by just one year; and what consequences for the health, perhaps the lives, of many could be entailed by postponement of such publications by as little as a month."

(Louis Joughin, ed., *Academic Freedom and Tenure*, A Handbook of the American Association of University Professors [University of Wisconsin Press, 1967].)

[42] *Competitive Problems in the Drug Industry*, Part 8, p. 3453.

It is not an investigator's business to be concerned about "problems in marketing" a drug. An investigator has no business taking favors from a drug house (whatever "all of your kind efforts in regard to my trip to Japan" means). A drug tester who requires assistance interpreting his data ought to be provided with disinterested expert help outside of industry.

Another letter addressed to Dr. Cantwell that was reported in the hearings reads, in part:

> I also contacted Dr. —— [department head], to ask if funds of the sort you proposed were permitted by the department. He was entirely agreeable and felt that such uncommitted funds offered greater latitude in opportunity to work and visit in other laboratories, *as well as provide enjoyable contact with the commercial firm.*[43]

One can be reasonably certain that this particular investigator and department head would not consciously allow obligation to the industry to affect experimental results or publications. One gets the feeling, however, that an initial reluctance to accept drug company funds has been rationalized. The rationalization usually goes: "I'm sure enough of myself to know that I'll not be anything but objective, and if *they're* willing to give me *that* much money, enough to pay the better part of another technician's salary,[44] merely to make some informal clinical observations on a certain drug, why shouldn't I take it?" The motives of the industry are rarely given thorough consideration. The industry knows what is going on in the mind of the rationalizer but is willing to pay well for even a few informal reports about its drug's usefulness from an academician in a famous medical school. Whether any company would readily undertake to fund a "double-blind study" (see page 80) in

[43] *Ibid.,* p. 3460.
[44] To be put to work on some other research project that the investigator finds more interesting.

which its drug was compared for efficacy and safety with another drug already on the market is doubtful.[45]

An excerpt follows from another letter reported in the hearings:

Dear Dr. Cantwell:

I received your letter this morning and *want to thank you for suggesting a grant* for the rheumatalogy section at the University of——— [a large state university].

Since you were here we have started a number of new patients on indomethacin (the LX capsules). At least three of the patients complained of severe epigastric distress within 30 minutes after taking the capsule. Therefore, in the next few subjects we started them out on 1 capsule twice a day increasing 1 capsule daily until they reached the maximum 6 capsules and *believe it or not we encountered no distress.* This is the method we will follow for the time being, *with our fingers crossed.*[46]

This tester, with the fingers of one hand crossed and the fingers of the other clutching a grant, sounds a little biased.

Obviously, some drug testers have unwittingly left themselves wide open to criticism through their financial relationship with industry. Many do not even recognize their vulnerable position. They are not above the taint of suspicion. As Dr. William Bean, Professor and Chairman of Medicine at the University of Iowa, has recently written, "The physician who is in the pay of pharmaceutical manufacturers is in no position to keep public confidence in his objectivity." [47]

Financial ties are not the only ones that disturb

[45] *Competitive Problems in the Drug Industry,* Part 2, p. 461.
[46] *Ibid.,* Part 8, p. 3452.
[47] "The Medical Profession and the Drug Industry," *Ethical Issues in Medicine* (Boston: Little, Brown and Company, 1968), pp. 227–248. Quoted in *Competitive Problems in the Drug Industry,* Part 10, p. 3962.

critics of drug testing. Here is a statement to the Senate Subcommittee on Monopoly by Dr. A. Dale Console, now a practicing physician in New Jersey:*

> The relationship that exists between the medical profession and the drug industry is an unhealthy one and in many ways a corrupt one. It is important to remember, however, that it is not only money that has the power to corrupt. Having spent more than six years in the business of influencing doctors and investigators, and some five years as a member of Fellowships and Grants Committee [of E. R. Squibb], I can assure you that while large grants and other monetary rewards play an important role, that role is minor relative to other inducements and techniques that can be used to destroy objectivity. An incident that will always remain fresh in my memory will perhaps illustrate the point I wish to make.
>
> Sometime in 1956, when I was still a Medical Director [for E. R. Squibb], the lagging sales of one of our products led management to decide that the product needed a boost. The boost took the form of obtaining an endorsement from a physician who was a prominent authority in the field. We knew that the particular physician was being subsidized by another drug company and so management decided that it would be simple for me as Medical Director to "buy" him. I objected since I felt that the doctor was incorruptible and because I felt the product did not deserve endorsement. My business colleagues overruled me and I was left with a blank check to win his favor. I was free to offer him a large grant to support any research of his choice

---

* Dr. Console has since died of a heart attack. The big professor he "gulled" lives on, but the Senate Subcommittee on Monopoly and the author of this book have made a pledge not to reveal his famous name. This was Dr. Console's wish; his intelligence and talent were accompanied by compassion.— R.B., January 1975

"without strings" or to retain him as a consultant with generous annual compensation. I was quite certain that the doctor would throw me out of his office if I approached him with any of the techniques suggested by my colleagues. They all had the obvious odor of a bribe. I decided, therefore, to use a stratagem that was more likely to be effective and that I thought (at the time) would be easier on my conscience.

I took the doctor to lunch, and after the usual two Martinis, I told him exactly what had been going on and of my disagreement with my colleagues. In this manner we established a physician-to-physican relationship in which we were both deploring the questionable tactics used by the drug industry. Conversation gradually shifted to the product and, to make a long story short, we got our endorsement almost as a personal favor. My travel expenses and the price of the lunch made up the entire cost to the company.

I recall this out of a hundred similar incidents only because the doctor was, and still is, a highly respected authority. My attitude toward him still is one of profound respect and admiration, since I must confess that the device that gulled him would have fooled me had I been in his place.

We are still human in spite of being physicians. As humans, we are vulnerable to all forms of flattery, cajolery, and blandishments, subtle or otherwise. The drug industry has learned to manipulate this vulnerability with techniques whose sophistication approaches perfection . . . Any employee of a drug firm who is worth his salt has an expert's appreciation of their power, a gourmet's taste for their subtleties, and the deft delicate touch that leads the doctor to hang himself. These techniques are used not only by physicians employed by a drug company but also by more experienced detailmen.

I know of no effective way to deal with this type of hanky-panky that goes on every day between the medical profession and the drug industry. It seems impossible to convince my medical brethren that drug company executives and detailmen are either shrewd businessmen or shrewd salesmen, never philanthropists. They make investments, not gifts.[48]

It is essential for drug testers to remain at arm's length from those who hire and pay them. One system that might help them do this is outlined below:

The profession and the public could support moves to establish a drug-testing center through which all industry requests for clinical drug testing would be funneled. This center might be located at the National Institutes of Health. Details would need to be worked out, but, as envisioned, those who were qualified and wished to test drugs would apply for and be granted permission to participate. Drug testers would be provided with drugs, placebos (dummy "drugs" of identical appearance), and where possible with identical-appearing tablets of another drug with the same or similar pharmacological effects. All tablets, capsules, etc., would be coded. No investigator would be told what corporation's product he was testing, nor would any corporation be allowed to know which groups of investigators were testing its product. This is the well-known "double-blind study." The drug makers would pay the testers via the center.[49] The advantages of such a system can be enumerated:

1. The public could be assured that the FDA was being provided with objective data to help it decide whether a drug warranted marketing.

2. Drug testers would be free of pressures from industry. Manipulation of unwitting investigators would be difficult (perhaps illegal).

3. Drug testing would cost the industry less money. Everyone in the industry and outside it knows that

[48] *Competitive Problems in the Drug Industry,* Part 11, p. 4480.

[49] Senator Nelson has meanwhile introduced legislation to accomplish these ends, but no action has yet been taken on it (August 1969).

drug-testing bills can at present be padded; this would be hard to do with a national drug-testing center in operation.

IX. Manipulating More Than Molecules

The medical profession can take no pride or comfort in knowing that a rare physician will *consciously* allow himself to be manipulated in connection with promotional schemes on the part of the drug industry. Antisocial behavior of this sort cannot be condoned. It must be exposed and it should be made illegal. The following is an illustrative case:

In the course of a private suit over injuries suffered from taking the drug MER-29, a considerable number of internal documents of the William S. Merrell Co. (a division of Richardson-Merrell, Inc.) were made available to the plaintiff's attorneys. Among these documents was a letter [50] headed by the statement: "To be given to ———, M.D., as suggested letter to *Medical World News.*" This was followed by the typewritten name R. H. McMaster, M.D., a Merrell corporation executive. The letter is addressed to William H. White of *Medical World News,* a widely distributed commercial journal supported by medical advertising. (No reason exists to suggest that Mr. White was aware of the existence of this document.) The letter begins, "As one of the participants in the Symposium of Hypocholesteremic Drugs at the American Medical Association Meeting, Miami Beach, I was quite surprised and concerned about your article, 'Breakthrough on Cholesterol,' in the June 17 issue . . ." and continues, "As stated by the M.W.N. reporter, I definitely did not agree with the remarks attributed to Dr. ——— concerning MER-29." (This doctor had brought to the attention of the audience that MER-29 was a probable liver toxin, and he has been proved correct.) Three paragraphs follow, ex-

---

[50] Exhibit 63 in the case of *Ostopowitz* vs. *Wiliam S. Merrell Co.*

tolling MER-29 for its relative non-toxicity (with emphasis on its lack of toxicity to the liver), citing "our own experience" and the reported experience of others who had been testing the drug for the corporation.

Among the letters to the editor in the July 15, 1960, issue of *Medical World News* is one attributed to the doctor to whom the letter described above was sent.[51] The sentence with the "definitely did not agree" in it has been omitted and a fourth paragraph appears to have been added in which a cholesterol-lowering drug marketed by another firm is depreciated as "noneffective." Aside from this, the *MWN* letter is identical with the portion of the "suggested letter" in the Senate files.

According to a "Brief for the Plaintiff" argued before the New York Supreme Court in August 1968 (*Ostopowitz vs. William S. Merrell Co.*), the Richardson-Merrell organization then "had the audacity" to send the *MWN* letter to the FDA as testimonial evidence supporting their application to have the drug released for sale. The brief charges that, in a previous lower-court trial, the corporation president defended the practice by arguing that it was analogous to President Johnson's use of speechwriters.

Anticipating that many practicing doctors might have read about MER-29's possible liver toxicity in *Medical World News,* the corporation supplied its detailmen with a copy of the letter in the form of a bulletin with selling tips.[52] The bulletin's cover contains only the words "An Answer to Medical World News," and on the first page the letter is introduced with the caption "Doctor ———— Speaks Up."

The Richardson-Merrell case is not the only available example of physicians or prominent medical educators putting their signatures to industry propaganda. Doctors and medical educators have no business being cats'-paws to industry. Their primary

[51] *Competitive Problems in the Drug Industry*, Part 10, pp. 3971–3972.
[52] *Ibid.*, p. 3971.

obligation is to the public, who must not be viewed as an abstraction.

X. Drug Houses as Sources of Support for Medical Schools

Medical school administrators, understandably preoccupied with raising money to support research programs and professorships, are likely to believe that "gifts" from the pharmaceutical industry are necessary and acceptable, that the need for dollars is a fact of life and the origin of the dollars a secondary consideration. A well-intentioned tendency to categorize drug-house money as too important to turn down is likely to be revaluated by some in view of a survey by the Association of American Medical Colleges published in the November 25, 1968, issue of the *Journal of the American Medical Association*.

The data therein show that funds expended in 1966–1967 for sponsored research in all U.S. medical schools came from six sources:

Federal grants and contracts	$344,480,141
Non-federal divisions of government	12,732,011
Foundations	16,926,247
Voluntary health agencies	16,823,251
Individuals and others	9,777,507
Industry	9,001,266
Total	$420,231,581

For the sake of argument, let us assume that "Industry" means "Drug industry." Industry's $9 million represents a little more than 2 percent of the total expenditure for sponsored research and 1 percent of what the drug corporations spend annually for advertising and promotion. Since this is so, it is hard to understand why medical school administrators deem drug-industry contributions essential.

Part of the reason seems to be that the drug industry restricts its gifts to prominent, show-window examples—not without an eye to soft-sell promotional advantage. A professional chair named after the drug house which has established it causes the prestige of an institution of higher learning to rub off onto the drug house. An idealist dreams that philanthropic industrialists in other than drug-manufacturing enterprises will come to the rescue and get the profession off the hook by replacing these few restricted funds. One can imagine an Eastern Airlines, Union Tank Car, Polaroid, or Prudential Chair of Pharmacology, but the application of a drug manufacturer's name is inappropriate. If some medical students have deemed it wise to return drug company "gifts," [53] could not medical school administrators do the same, especially if provided with an alternative source of funds?

XI. Some Problems to Ponder

There are grave ethical implications, possible conflicts of interest, and reason to revaluate the role of professional responsibility in the following situations:

1. When a doctor, acting as purchasing agent for a consumer, prescribes a drug without adequate knowledge of its cost relative to that of another drug with the same clinical effect.

2. When many physicians base their prescribing practices to a large extent on information supplied them by industry salesmen ("detailmen") and other commercial sources. This is unprofessional.

3. When many physicians prescribe dangerous drugs for non-indicated purposes.

4. When doctors lend their names for articles and letters written or solicited by members of the pharmaceutical industry.

5. When doctors own shares of stock in drug com-

[53] *New York Times* (Late City Edition), February 1, 1969, p. 27.

panies whose products they are evaluating and/or prescribing.

6. When doctors are paid directly by a drug firm to evaluate its products.

7. When influential doctors or medical educators, particularly in high academic positions, are large stockholders and/or serve as policy-setting members of boards of drug corporations. These men are in a position to mold the attitudes of other doctors and of the public and to make policy decisions in key medical and pharmaceutical organizations—a possible conflict-of-interest situation. The implications are particularly serious when doctors, especially educators, fail to disclose fully their industry affiliations.[54]

8. When prominent professors receive regular "retainer" or "consultation" fees from drug firms while simultaneously advising government or private agencies on matters of policy that çan severely affect sales of drug firms' products.

9. When medical organization and publications are largely or wholly dependent on income derived from drug advertising.

10. When so-called "independent" giveaway medical magazines (which subsist nearly exclusively on drug advertising) are becoming a factor of some importance in the physician's "education" and, through editorial and news policies, are in a position to influence doctors' attitudes on social, economic, and political issues in which the magazine might have a financial interest.

11. When many medical students accept "gifts" of doctor bags and instruments, cocktail and dinners, and "free" weekend trips from the drug industry;

---

[54] The courts have developed standards for deciding issues relating to the performance of a director's duty to the corporation and its stockholders, and these are generally applicable in state and federal courts. The basis of the duty may be expressed in Justice Benjamin Cardozo's phrase, a "duty of constant and unqualified fidelity" (*Competitive Problems in the Drug Industry,* Part 10, p. 3973). It is naïve, if not illegal, for a medical educator to serve as a drug-corporation director in the belief that he can be a "consumer advocate."

when physicians accept fellowships or research support from the drug industry; and when medical schools accept endowments for professional "chairs" from the drug industry.

3

The Reckoning Nears [1]
(1975) *

I. The Character of the Onslaught Against Us

In the raging controversy over whether so-called generic drugs are the therapeutic equivalent of their expensive brand-name counterparts, the Pharmaceutical Manufacturers Association (PMA), whose principal members are twenty-one corporations each with assets exceeding $100 million,[2] has been actively confusing both the medical profession and the public. The important PMA members are the corporations that generally charge exorbitant prices for drugs sold by brand name.

While it is impossible to provide any comprehensive examination of the attempts by the PMA to justify its members' pricing and promotional policies, it is reasonable to remark that any expert who has followed closely the public statements and the testimony by such experts[3] as the Honorable Charles C.

* The following chapter is, in effect, the Introduction to the 1975 *Handbook*.

[1] M. Silverman and P. R. Lee, *Pills, Profits and Politics* (University of California Press, 1974). (Taken from the title to Chapter 6.)

[2] *Competitive Problems in the Drug Industry*, Hearings Before the Subcommittee on Monopoly, Senate Select Committee on Small Business, 90th through 93rd Congresses (1967–1974), Part 24, p. 10,224.

[3] *Ibid.*, pp. 9948–9977, 10,163–10,183, 10,217–10,223, 10,230–10,247, 10,423–10,428, 10,483–10,496.

Edwards, M.D., Assistant Secretary for Health in the Department of HEW; the Honorable Alexander M. Schmidt, M.D., Commissioner, Food and Drug Administration; Dr. William S. Apple, Executive Director, American Pharmaceutical Association (APhA); Dr. Edward G. Feldmann, Associate Executive Director for Scientific Affairs, APhA; Dr. Daniel Banes, Director, Drug Standards Division, *United States Pharmacopeia;* Dr. Henry E. Simmons and Dr. J. R. Crout, past and present Directors of the Bureau of Drugs of the FDA, respectively—will conclude that although the PMA has spent a lot of money justifying its members' policies, it has shown a surprisingly poor ability to debate controversial issues on the facts and a striking propensity to counterattack and defend its members against public criticism with nothing more than half-truthful, misleading statements that amount, simply, to propaganda.

Yet the PMA has managed to confuse sincere doctors with outdated information. Some doctors have unwittingly used this information in "Letters to the Editor" of important newspapers in efforts to block impending progressive legislation at state levels.[4]

The PMA has bought expensive, full-page advertisements whose purpose is to imply that only the biggest and wealthiest corporations have a reputation for integrity. One such advertisement was actually accepted by the editor of *Clinical Pharmacology and Therapeutics,* one of the nation's most distinguished journals.[5] In the center of the page was a large medicine bottle labeled "Reputation." Beneath was the bold statement, "There is no generic equivalent," and the claim that the advertisement was being placed as a "courtesy" to the medical profession.

Such an advertisement failed to cite the recorded instances where the PMA's member firms had either withheld important laboratory information from the

[4] J. Argue, "Letter to the Editor," *Manchester Union Leader,* March 1, 1973.

[5] *Journal of Experimental Therapeutics,* January–February 1969, facing p. 1.

FDA (see Addenda) or had deliberately falsified laboratory data submitted to the FDA; had been found guilty in federal courts of violating criminal statutes; had been found by FDA to have placed false and/or misleading advertisements in medical journals; had persuaded influential medical figures into rendering endorsements for inferior products that were not selling well, by techniques that included outright bribery as well as subtle flattery; had allegedly conspired to monopolize and had allegedly actually monopolized to fix prices on important pharmaceuticals; had allegedly lied to the United States Patent Office; and had failed[6] and openly refused[7] to place the same warnings about serious adverse side effects in advertisements and claims for drugs sold overseas, when they were well aware of the danger and were forced to advertise the danger to doctors in this country. It did not mention the fact that PMA members are influencing medical students and doctors by holding "educational symposia."[8] And,

---

[6] *Competitive Problems in the Drug Industry*, Part 6.

[7] *Annual Meeting of the Stockholders of the Warner-Lambert Co. 1972.* Ninety-seven percent of the stockholder vote was "No" to a resolution that the corporation change its policy by divulging to foreign doctors what U.S. law now demands that it tell U.S. doctors about the toxicity of its Chloromycetin®, a product of its Parke, Davis division. I attended the meeting as a proxy voter.

[8] One such symposium dealing with the treatment of high blood pressure was held under the noses of the Dean and professors at Dartmouth Medical School about three years ago. Since I am licensed to practice medicine in that state, I received an invitation to attend. Rather than doing so, I sent a letter to the sponsoring corporation in order to express my resentment at any attempt by an interested third party to influence doctors in the selection of drugs to treat high blood pressure and added that if every doctor *truly* knew the ins-and-outs of pharmacology and therapeutics, the corporation might have a hard time staying in business. I received an animated letter in response that recited how much volunteer work the corporation's members were doing in their communities to fight drug abuse and admitted that the corporation was deeply committed to educational activities within the medical profession.

of course, the "Reputation" advertisement failed to mention that millions of persons are made very ill, permanently maimed, and killed by drugs sold by its member firms—and especially that about 1,500,000 persons are admitted to hospitals each year from adverse reactions to drugs and that from 18 to 30 percent of all persons admitted to hospitals have been reliably estimated to have their hospital stays prolonged because of adverse reactions to drugs.[9] In a recent study of six cooperating hospitals, the alarming estimate was made that 130,000 or more *medical* (*i.e.*, not surgical, obstetrical, pediatric, etc.) patients die of adverse reactions to drugs given them while hospitalized.[10] Nor did the PMA's advertisement make the point that an estimated one-seventh of all hospital days is devoted to the care of drug toxicity at an estimated yearly cost of $3 billion![11] Nor did the PMA advertise its obvious implications in this situation, since it openly boasts that its member firms sell 95 percent of the prescription medicines used in the U.S.[12] Those are not generic drugs.

II. "Derogatory Euphemism"

Some brand-name manufacturers have gone so far, in the opinion of Dr. William Apple, Executive Director of the American Pharmaceutical Association, as to utilize "derogatory euphemism" to denigrate smaller manufacturers of generic drugs. An interesting exchange took place during one of Senator Nelson's subcommittee hearings on February 21, 1974.[13] The

[9] K. L. Melmon, "Preventable Drug Reactions—Causes and Cures," *New England Journal of Medicine*, 284:1361–1368 (June 17, 1971).

[10] S. Shapiro, et al., "Fatal Drug Reactions Among Medical Inpatients," *Journal of the American Medical Association*, 216:467–468 (April 19, 1971).

[11] Melmon, "Preventable Drug Reactions."

[12] *Competitive Problems in the Drug Industry*, Part 24, p. 10,224.

[13] *Ibid.*, pp. 10,177–10,178.

subcommittee had just heard the following testimony from Dr. Edward Feldmann, Associate Director for Scientific Affairs of the APhA: "In recent years we have heard a number of disquieting speeches, and we have read a number of disturbing articles—all emanating from DPSC [Defense Personnel Support Center] spokesmen—which *in toto* [Dr. Feldmann's emphasis] have served to cast doubts and suspicion on various unnamed drug manufacturers. These speeches and articles have suggested that problems pertaining to unreliable drugs produced under shoddy conditions of manufacture are widely prevalent on the American drug market."

He was suddenly interrupted by Benjamin Gordon, Economist for the subcommittee, who asked, "What is a 'schlock' manufacturer? This word 'schlock' is used especially by the big firms."

He was answered by Dr. Apple: ". . . it is certainly a derogatory euphemism,[14] frequently employed by industry propagandists to describe a small firm which concentrates on producing drug products which are in the public domain . . . I suppose the inference is that such a firm cuts corners . . . That is, that these firms, schlock manufacturers, cut corners on quality; they cut corners on legal standards; *and that they are in business to make a fast buck* [*sic!*]. I don't know of any."

Senator Nelson interrupted immediately. "Any such manufacturers?"

Dr. Apple: "Mr. Chairman, I cannot identify any particular manufacturer that meets this description." [15]

---

[14] "Schlock" is neither a euphemism nor a neologism.

[15] Dr. Apple was being charitable. He might have mentioned how a prominent laboratory's intravenous fluids were bottled in containers whose caps were contaminated by sewer organisms. An epidemic of bloodstream poisoning (septicemias) and several deaths resulted from the use of these fluids. He might have cited other instances where brand-name corporations have put out substandard drugs. One such corporation was forced by the FDA to close down a plant for a lengthy period. An FDA inspector had termed the plant "a disgrace." (See Addenda.)

Mr. Gordon interjected, "Actually, that word is also onomatopoeic.[16] In [this] sense it is an invidious word. It is supposed to engender hostility toward a person who can be identified by that word."

Dr. Apple proceeded to say, "I agree with you that the term is frequently used, especially in speeches in pharmacy meetings. It is used frequently in discussions. It has crept into the literature. I regret that it has even crept into some of the comments by eminent scientists in our field who tend to use this euphemism without identifying anyone."

Mr. Gordon then asked, "Well, is it possible for you to send a letter . . . [to those who use it] to find out exactly what evidence they have on this particular subject, and perhaps submit it . . . for our records?"

Dr. Apple's responsive letter[17] dated August 13, 1974, advised Mr. Gordon that the question was put to the "Academy of Pharmaceutical Sciences, which has been most verbal in challenging the Association's [*i.e.*, American Pharmaceutical Association's] opinion that the quality of the nation's drug supply is very high, to have their members identify firms which they individually regard as warranting the characterization 'schlock manufacturers.' " Dr. Apple's letter continued: "This is to advise you that the Academy of Pharmaceutical Sciences leadership has declined to query its membership . . . I personally have met with the leadership of the APS [APhS] on numerous occasions, during which generalized disparaging comments were made about the ability of some manufacturers to produce quality products. When I have asked them to name names, they have refused . . . We feel that your inquiry has served a useful purpose, namely to put everyone on notice that your Subcommittee expects those who question the quality of the nation's drug supply and FDA enforcement of the laws assuring that quality to come up with hard facts if they wish to have their charges seriously considered."

[16] *Ibid.*, Part 24, p. 10,177.
[17] *Ibid.*, p. 10,758.

III. The Peculiar Case of Max Feinberg

As a result of the Nelson hearings, two HEW Task Force Reports on Prescription Drugs, and other in-depth studies, state legislatures throughout the country have for several years attempted to pass consumer protection bills enabling citizens to obtain low-cost generic drugs. It should be no surprise that the Pharmaceutical Manufacturers Association and many state pharmacy boards have in each case lobbied against the passage of these progressive acts. What was a surprise was the frequent appearance of a mysterious Max Feinberg, who invariably and persuasively argued against the enactments.

Feinberg, the legislatures were told, was Chief Inspector for the Medical Division of the Department of Defense, and his was the final word as to the suitability of a prospective manufacturer of drugs to sell to the Armed Forces. The impression was given that Mr. Feinberg's years of service made him uniquely able to ferret out weaknesses in the manufacturing practices and products of corporations large and small, even where FDA inspectors were unable to do so; Feinberg argued that the FDA had approved places that simply would not pass *his* inspection and that as a result the American people were being dosed with drugs which the Department of Defense would not touch with a barge pole. His major contentions were two:

1. "The rejection rate on the Department of Defense plant inspections is 45% and the rejection rate on pre-contract award inspections is 42%."

2. "Based on my experience of drug plants, it is my firm conviction that the primary problem lies in the fact that many producers in the business today are in gross violation of FDA's Good Manufacturing Practices Regulations. Those same firms are manufacturing drugs on a daily basis." [18]

Senator Nelson has said that, Mr. Feinberg for

[18] *Ibid.*, pp. 10,424–10,425.

several years made public statements which, if true, should frighten the American people, and that he had decided to go to the heart of the matter by asking the Department of Defense for the specific data on which Mr. Feinberg based his charges. He was especially interested in the 45 percent plant and 42 percent product rejection rates.[19] This is what Senator Nelson found out: Mr. Feinberg, in fact, had been surveying only 10 percent of the Department of Defense's prospective contractors as a result of a conscious selection process. He pre-decided that the other 90 percent of the firms were fully capable. Thus, the rejection rate was not 45 percent of all prospective contractors; it was, at most, 4.5 percent.[20] And of the 4.5 percent, how serious were the allegations and how well had Mr. Feinberg made his inspections? The Commissioner of the Food and Drug Administration stated that ". . . many of the statements are unsupported totally by any evidence . . . that he has provided to us." [21] Dr. J. R. Crout, the new Director of the FDA's Bureau of Drugs, and successor to Dr. Simmons, in that role said, ". . . it is quite clear that most of the violations . . . are relatively trivial and unrelated to the quality of the drug." [22] Mr. Feinberg had supplied twelve examples of "gross violations." [23] On breakdown, one firm is listed twice so that the total number of plants involved was really eleven. Five of the eleven plants were operated by members of the Pharmaceutical Manufacturers Association.[24]

The Department of Defense (for which Mr. Feinberg was making the decisions) admitted to Senator Nelson that only 5 percent of drug products that they obtain on contract are, in fact, subjected to laboratory testing. The remaining 95 percent are prejudged as satisfactory. "In other words, the rejection

[19] *Ibid.*, p. 10,425.
[20] *Ibid.*
[21] *Ibid.*, p. 9966.
[22] *Ibid.*, p. 9967.
[23] *Ibid.*, p. 10,426
[24] *Ibid.*

rate is less than 2.5 percent of the drugs to be bought, not 42 percent." [25] As for the identity of the rejected drugs, they were *"not on production runs of drugs, but on special runs of drugs done by a new company wishing to make the drug . . . never having made it before."* [26] (Emphasis is mine.)

Senator Nelson remarked that ". . . even the president of the Pharmaceutical Manufacturers Association and his counsel, Mr. Cutler, were taken in by Mr. Feinberg." [27] It cannot be underestimated what considerable damage Mr. Feinberg's deceptive and misleading speeches and articles have done by confusing doctors, legislators, and consumer groups and by casting doubt on the integrity of the Food and Drug Administration.[28] Senator Nelson apologized to the witness before him at the time, Major General George J. Hayes, Medical Corp, U.S. Army, and Principal Deputy Assistant to the Secretary of Defense, for the length of his introductory remarks about Mr. Feinberg and asked if the general had any comments on the matter.[29] General Hayes answered, "Mr. Chairman, I would say that your statement is like a breath of fresh air coming into a crowded room . . . I agree with everything you said in the statement." [30]

IV. Chloromycetin® vs. Chloramphenicol:
An Instructive Story

The PMA was desperate for an example of a generic drug that, having met all of the posted requirements for manufacture of the *U.S.P.* or the *N.F.*, performed

[25] *Ibid.*

[26] *Ibid.*

[27] *Ibid.*

[28] I was present when Mr. Feinberg addressed a New Hampshire state legislative committee in a public hearing on January 15, 1973. Mr. Feinberg did make claims similar to those cited by Senator Nelson.

[29] *Competitive Problems in the Drug Industry*, Part 24, p. 10,428.

[30] *Ibid.*

differently from its brand-name counterpart. After
months of questioning by Senator Nelson and his staff,
they were unable to supply an example. But one day
their luck changed (temporarily).

1966 was the year when the patent on Parke,
Davis's Chloromycetin® (generic name: chloramphenicol) expired (see also Chapter 2, "The Battle
Is On"). Other firms set about manufacturing and
selling chloramphenicol at lower prices. A fish breeder
in California had been in the habit of emptying the
contents of Chloromycetin® capsules on the surface
of the water in his fish tanks, presumably to diminish
bacterial contamination. When he did so, the powdered
material would rapidly go into solution in the water
and, of course, become as invisible as the sugar that
goes into solution when added to tea. This fish breeder,
aware of the availability of less expensive generic
chloramphenicol, bought and tried some. To his
surprise he found that several of these newer products
formed a fine film on the surface of the water and
only very gradually went into solution. One day in
1967 he informed Parke, Davis of his observation and
they were able to confirm what they had not known
themselves.[31] Here, then, was precisely what the PMA
and its member firms were looking for; namely, a
generic drug product which had met the *then* current
official requirements of the *U.S. Pharmacopeia,* had
been "certified" by the Food and Drug Administration,
and was nonetheless *presumably* inferior to that of
a comparable, expensive "brand."

Parke, Davis gave normal human volunteers doses
of their own Chloromycetin® and of several of the
generic chloramphenicols. They demonstrated beyond
question that, after ingestion of their own product,
the active drug could be detected in the bloodstream
sooner, reached a higher peak concentration, and then
more rapidly disappeared from the blood. Several of
the competitive products made their appearance in
the blood a little later, reached lower peak concentrations, but remained circulating in the blood for a

[31] Silverman and Lee, *Pills, Profits and Politics,* p. 150.

significantly lengthier period.[32] The PMA and Parke, Davis claimed "better biological availability." The reliability of the standards of the *U.S.P.* and *N.F.* were questioned, and it was implied that large and well-known manufacturers and distributers were naturally the only ones to trust, because they are the "reputable" companies. Doctors sat up and listened; they were impressed.

When the chloramphenicol matter had been thoroughly investigated by scientists, the reason for the variation in "biological availability" was discovered very simply to be that the drug is, by its very nature, hard to dissolve in water and that solubility is enhanced by using active ingredients with very small crystal (or particle) size.[33] Under these conditions the powder presents more surface area relative to mass and solubilization in water is enhanced. It was a simple matter for the generic manufacturers to make the necessary adjustment in the physical properties of their active ingredient, and the matter was quickly corrected. Although the corrective action took place more than five years ago, one still frequently hears about the Chloromycetin® episode, particularly from doctors who are biased against the use of generic drugs. The reader is referred to pages 40–41 for what happened to Parke, Davis's profits as a result of the affair.

From this important observation with chloramphenicol, it became immediately apparent to all concerned that any important drug with low water

[32] There is only one human disease, typhoid fever, for which chloramphenicol may be a therapeutic agent of choice. Neither Parke, Davis nor the PMA nor anyone else has demonstrated that short-lived, high-peak blood concentrations of chloramphenicol are more effective in treating typhoid fever than lower-level sustained concentrations. My intuition as a clinician and pharmacologist is that the product with the sustained level (in pharmacological terms, "longer circulating half-life") might be expected to be more effective because successive doses would accumulate and an around-the-clock better-sustained high or higher blood level of drug would result.

[33] Chloramphenicol can be obtained either as a pure, amorphous powder or as a finely crystalline material.

solubility might be able to be shown to be deficient in "biological availability." In order for absorption of a drug to occur from intestine to bloodstream, the drug must first be in solution in the intestinal fluid, which is mainly water. Thus, immediately after the chloramphenicol episode was understood, the *U.S.P.* and *N.F.* added to their official specifications for all types of relatively water-insoluble drugs a new, important, mandatory "dissolution specification." This means that tablets or capsules with a relatively insoluble active ingredient must be shown to be able to deliver up the drug in solution in a simple laboratory bench test. The solution rates were shown to parallel "biological availability" (that is to say, blood levels) when the same products are swallowed. As a double check for a handful of important drugs, the tablets or capsules must actually be swallowed by human volunteers and the drug must be shown by chemical measurement to be in the bloodstream. It is noteworthy that no complaints of clinical inefficacy for "generic chloramphenicol" were ever filed by practicing doctors.[34] The chloramphenicol affair, while it provided temporary propaganda grist for the PMA, led to certain stringent new controls by the Food and Drug Administration and new official requirements by the *United States Pharmacopeia* which strengthened the case for the use of generic drugs and weakened the case for "brands." It took the digoxin episode (see page 100) to nail down more solidly the case for using generic drugs.

V. "The Astonishing Myth"

The PMA, encouraged by the chloramphenicol incident, tried to move heavily over to the offensive. The association published a *Bibliography on Biopharmaceutics* (Washington, D.C.: Pharmaceutical Manufacturers Association, 1968). The PMA had been smarting from the conclusions of the HEW Task

[34] Silverman and Lee, *Pills, Profits and Politics*, p. 150.

Force on Prescription Drugs conducted in 1967 and 1968, and particularly hateful to the PMA was the conclusion that the "lack of equivalency among chemical equivalents meeting all official standards has been grossly exaggerated as a major hazard to the public health." [35]

The PMA's publication has been described by Silverman and Lee (p. 154) as "supposedly a bombshell that would demolish the Task Force conclusions." The president of the PMA, aware that the *Bibliography* contained 501 references to articles in the scientific literature, disseminated a broadside saying, "This unique publication refutes the astonishing myth that there are not significant differences among dosage forms of the same drug." It was a hollow statement. Responsible scientists knew that such might be the case; the crucial question was, and remains: How often do they actually occur and what threat do they pose to patients? Once again, Senator Nelson entered the picture by asking technical consultants to the Task Force to review the PMA "bombshell" and evaluate it. Here is the summary of their review, taken verbatim from Silverman and Lee's *Pills, Profits and Politics* (p. 155):

Of the 501 studies only 221 were actually conducted in human subjects. Of the 221 only 76 were—by PMA's own evaluation—"adequately designed or controlled experiments." Of the 76, only 12 represented comparison between what might seem to be different brands of the same chemical equivalent. And of these final 12, most compared different dosage forms (such as tablets vs effervescent solutions), or different salts (such as sodium derivatives vs potassium derivatives), or different coatings (such as delayed release products vs rapid release products). Some of these

[35] *Competitive Problems in the Drug Industry*, Part 9, p. 3726. Testimony of Dr. Philip R. Lee, Assistant Secretary for Health of the Office of Health and Scientific Affairs, U.S. Department of Health, Education and Welfare.

final products failed to meet existing USP or NF standards and thus would be illegally on the market.

At the most, Task Force staff and consultants agree, there were only two or three [36] which demonstrated statistically significant lack of biological equivalency, and in one case the differences were described as being without any practical clinical importance.

One drug company public relations official is quoted as having later quipped, ". . . the PMA should be charged with treason in time of war. Their damn bibliography merely gave aid and comfort—and lots more ammunition—to the enemy." [37]

The Task Force never gloated, however, and by no means became arrogant or complacent. In its final report, it emphasized that even though there were so few documented cases in which generic products had met *U.S.P.* and *N.F.* standards and yet failed to perform properly in controlled human trials, ". . . others may be reported in the future . . . [and] these cannot be ignored, and the problem deserves careful consideration because of the medical and economic policies which are involved."

VI. The Digoxin Incident

In addition to the chloramphenicol incident, there has been one other which has provided fodder for the PMA's propaganda mill though its discovery has been a blessing in disguise to consumers. I refer to the well-publicized "digoxin incident," which has led to

[36] Benjamin Gordon asked, "Are there two or three? Which is it?" The answer he received from the Task Force director: "There are two. One of them, as you have probably surmised, is chloramphenicol." About the second: the scientists "pointed out quite clearly that although differences were detected, these were not of any clinical importance." (*Ibid.*, pp. 3726–3729.)

[37] Silverman and Lee, *Pills, Profits and Politics*, p. 154.

so much more rigorous strengthening of *U. S. Pharmacopeia* and FDA standards that the case for "generic equivalence" has probably been absolutely vindicated. The way is now clear for Secretary of HEW Caspar Weinberger to expedite action on his proposed policy (December 19, 1973) to exclude payment of brand-name prices wherever possible in all government programs where drugs presently are or may in future be dispensed—viz. Medicaid, Medicare, or any national health plan.

The digoxin incident involved a powerful and widely used heart drug. Almost every person in the U.S. who has heart failure (often called "cardiac decompensation") or who has a common irregular heartbeat called atrial (auricular) fibrillation receives a nearly daily dose of either digoxin or its close relation, digitoxin. (See the Prescription Drug List for a discussion of each.) More than 85 percent of all digoxin sold in this country is made by one manufacturer, Burroughs Wellcome, who sells it by the brand name Lanoxin®. Approximately forty-four other companies also manufactured digoxin in 1969 and thirty-five manufactured it in 1975. They include such well-known firms as Endo Laboratories Inc.; Lakeside Laboratories; Lederle Laboratories; Parke, Davis & Co.; Philips-Roxane Labs.; Rexall Drug Company; Wyeth Laboratories; and a considerable number of lesser-known but highly respected firms.[38]

In April 1970, the FDA inaugurated a program to systematically test marketed batches of digoxin tablets. FDA suspicion about digoxin stemmed from a *clinical* observation made by a group of doctors in New York City. Their hospital, in an economy move, made a decision to switch from Lanoxin® to a less costly product sold as digoxin. The doctors noticed that they had to increase the dosage of the new product in order to maintain the same therapeutic effectiveness. Their observation was reported to the FDA, whose laboratories found considerable tablet-to-tablet varia-

---

[38] *Competitive Problems in the Drug Industry,* Part 24, pp. 9952–9957 and 10,673–10,723.

tion in the amount of active digoxin produced by several companies. Only one corporation consistently produced tablets with a uniform quantity of digoxin: Burroughs Wellcome, whose Lanoxin® brand was among the most expensive. Ironically, Burroughs Wellcome's home division, in England, was having very serious difficulties, with both tablet content and bioavailability.

At first, the reason for observed tablet content nonuniformity was inexplicable. Attempts to uncover the cause were unsuccessful, and between April and November 1970, the FDA had to make nearly eighty recalls of digoxin tablets for reasons including both inadequate tablet uniformity and grossly too much or too little of the active drug in many tablets. (However, lest the reader be misled as to the enormity of the problem, only about 2.5 percent of all digoxin tablets were suspect.) It is intriguing to know that no clinical reports of trouble with digoxin were either published by doctors or made by them to any federal agency. Yet in October 1970, the FDA asked every manufacturer of digoxin tablets to submit samples of every batch for testing by the FDA in order to ensure that *U.S.P.* requirements were met. All manufacturers cooperated. *It was not until fourteen months after the FDA had initiated corrective measures that the problem became generally known to the medical profession:* J. Lindenbaum et al. described their experience with digoxin in the *New England Journal of Medicine* in December 1971.

In the Lindenbaum study, normal volunteers were given tablets from four commercially marketed batches. One batch which had given very low serum digoxin levels was discovered by the FDA not to meet *U.S.P.* specifications. Sufficient numbers of tablets of another batch which had provided very low blood levels could not at the time be found for analysis. It was the FDA's conclusion that the problem lay in tablet subpotency and not in "bioavailability." *Subsequently, however, sufficient tablets from the lost batch were located and chemical analysis did show that they contained the requisite amount of digoxin.* Only then did the FDA realize that they were dealing with digoxin tablets that met *U.S.P.* specifications and yet, upon being swallowed, delivered up the active drug to the bloodstream in insufficient amount. The problem facing the FDA, then, was twofold:

1. All but one U.S. manufacturer had serious trouble making tablets with a constant content of digoxin.

2. Some tablets with a proper amount of digoxin could be swallowed and yet not deliver the active ingredient to the bloodstream. (This was not, by the way, one of those rare instances where the coating on the tablet fails to dissolve and the object passes through the intestine into the feces intact. Digoxin tablets are not coated.)

In attempting to account for the first problem, it is not hard to make an educated guess as to the cause. The total weight of an average digoxin tablet is 100 milligrams. Practically all of this weight is accounted for by pharmacologically inert ingredients: binder, disintegrant and filler. A mere one-fourth of 1 milligram of *active* drug is in the tablet. Imagine that many kilograms of binder, disintegrant, filler, and active drug are carefully weighed out in exact proportions and then are mixed thoroughly together. Imagine then that many thousands of 100 milligram quantities (chemists might use the word "aliquots") are carefully measured from the mixture to be stamped into tablets. Notwithstanding how accurately the initial ingredients were measured and how proportionally correct were the measurements, the likelihood that each 100 milligram tablet of the mixture would contain exactly one-fourth of 1 milligram of digoxin seems small, indeed. Admittedly, if mixing were always homogeneously perfect, one might *theoretically* expect that each tablet would contain one-quarter of a milligram of digoxin. But the statistical likelihood that mixing is always perfect seems small. A way to ensure that a proper amount of digoxin would end up in each and every tablet would be to measure out aliquots of digoxin individually and add each to an approximately 100 milligram mixture of binder, disintegrant, and filler. As a matter of fact (from a call to Dr. Daniel Banes of the *U.S.P.*), I have found that the problem of tablet content uniformity has long been known to tablet manufacturers, who express the matter more succinctly and more scientifically by stating that wherever the excipient/active ingredient ratio is high, tablet uniformity is difficult to attain.

Thirty-five firms (of the original forty-four) continued to manufacture digoxin after October 1970 and met the new rigid standards for *U.S.P.* tablet content uniformity. The FDA knows this because it monitored and tested multiple individual tablets from each batch in its own laboratories. What was surprising to discover was that the firms accomplished their feat by *closer attention to mixing* and not, as imagined, by measuring individual aliquots of digoxin!

The explanation for problem number two, the availability problem, is more elusive. It had long been known to the *U.S.P.* that certain binders of an "earthy" composition—such as bentonite, a naturally occurring colloidal substance (hydrated aluminum silicate)—can exert as-yet-poorly-understood binding upon digoxin. Unfortunately, it was not the custom of the *U.S. Pharmacopeia* to delineate excipients. Notwithstanding our lack of uniformity in manufacture, all thirty-five firms still manufacturing digoxin for sale in the U.S. have consistently met the new blood-level guidelines set up by FDA *and also the new dissolution standard set up by the U.S.P.* Firms must now literally demonstrate that when their digoxin tablets are swallowed, the active ingredient appears in the bloodstream at therapeutic levels. The FDA monitors this closely. The tablets must also disintegrate sufficiently rapidly to allow solution of their active ingredient into a test fluid. This is monitored closely by the *U.S.P.* The *U.S.P.* requirement is that between 55 and 90 percent of the active digoxin must go into solution within one hour. It is very important to know that passage of the dissolution test parallels passage of the "bioavailability" test as shown by blood test. Addressing himself to the importance of the issues raised by the chloramphenicol and digoxin experiences, the present commissioner of the FDA, Dr. Alexander Schmidt, said, "Mr. Chairman [Senator Nelson], in my opinion the issue of bioavailability is being overdrawn. As we have learned more about nonequivalency problems, it has become clearer that they are limited in number and are manageable." [39] He continued: ". . . we believe that the impact of our quality assurance program on the drug industry has made that industry one of the most quality-control conscious industries in the country. This has resulted in a drug supply for this nation that we believe to be of the highest quality in the world." [40]

Note that the commissioner drew no distinction between generic-named drugs and their brand-name counterparts. It would have been redundant because his subordinate, Dr. J. Richard Crout, Director of the Bureau of Drugs, had delivered a speech on the FDA's role in product quality at the 28th Annual Technical Conference of the American Society for Quality Control in Boston on May 20, 1974. He described the immensity of the laboratory operation carried out at the National Center of Drug Analysis in St. Louis, where, in fiscal 1973, 89,033 assays were carried out on drug samples taken from commercial traffic. Dr. Crout also described the prodigious amount of batch-by-batch testing that goes on: approximately 30,000 batches of antibiotics and 400 batches of insulin were examined during 1973 in the FDA's Washington laboratories. He said that the total number of recalls in 1973 for defective products was only 179, well below one-tenth of 1 percent of all drugs produced. Dr. Crout began to terminate his prepared speech by saying, *"Finally, I would comment that when product deficiencies do occur, they are not necessarily more common or more severe among generic than brand-named drugs . . ."* (Emphasis is mine.) For stoppers he added these points:

[39] *Ibid.,* p. 9961.
[40] *Ibid.,* p. 9963.

Many generic drugs are, in fact, made by large manufacturers, while some of the brand-named preparations marketed by larger firms are in fact produced by smaller manufacturers.[41]

There may have been a time in the past when the "brand name/generic name" issue was linked more closely to the "big firm/small firm" issue or the "high quality/low quality" issue. But, if such a case ever existed, it is no longer true today. There is simply no convincing evidence that the systematic use of the brand name in prescribing drugs would provide greater protection of the public from those defects which do occur. [Emphasis is mine.]

VII. Upjohn and Orinase®

Notwithstanding the new *U.S.P.* and *N.F.* awareness of the potential problem of "biological availability"— caused by the chloramphenicol affair—their responsible alacrity in providing new official standards for relatively insoluble drugs, and their expressed determination to maintain increased vigilance for any other unwanted phenomena that might require further revisions of standards, the Upjohn Company of Kalamazoo (see Upjohn in Tables 2, 3, and 4, pp. 63–65) took premature advantage to exploit the fears of doctors and used the *Journal of the American Medical Association* to carry a "scientific" article to "educate" them.[42]

An individual working in an Upjohn Company laboratory, aware that the very commonly prescribed drug tolbutamide (brand name: Orinase®), which lowers blood sugar levels, is relatively insoluble, fabricated tablets meeting the not-yet-revised *U.S.P.*

[41] See Price Lists (pp. 329–412) about Mylan Laboratory's production for brand-name houses.

[42] A. B. Varley, "The Generic Inequivalence of Drugs," *Journal of the American Medical Association*, 206:1745 (1968).

dissolution specification. It had not until then been *U.S.P.* practice to demand more than a "tablet disintegration time" test. Under standardized laboratory conditions, tablets had to be shown by the manufacturer to break up in artificial stomach juice into fragments small enough to pass through the holes in a piece of #10 wire screen. The assumption was that particles so small would be so much more fragmented by the time they reached the intestine that they could reasonably be expected to deliver up their active ingredient for solution in the intestinal juice. The Upjohn employee, therefore, made Orinase® tablets with one-half of the customary disintegrant, and the result was that they did barely manage to disintegrate within the limits of the *U.S.P.* bench standards. The Orinase® itself, however, being so insoluble, was not readily delivered up for solution even from the tablet fragments. This was proved by giving the tablets to "healthy, nondiabetic volunteer subjects at the Southern Michigan State Prison in Jackson, Michigan." Five prisoners were given the contrived tablets; the others, tablets taken from "a commercial production lot." [43]

The published data clearly show that the prisoners given the tablets that disintegrated poorly absorbed less Orinase® than the others. Because Orinase® is still patented, no generic counterpart is sold in the U.S. Thus, the title "The Generic Inequivalence of Drugs" in the AMA *Journal* article was, to be charitable, ill-written; the use of the general article "The" and pluralization of the word "Drugs" subtly conveyed the message that the author had uncovered a general truth which could attack the infrastructure of the *Pharmacopeia* of the United States of America. Had the Upjohn Company, the author of the article, and the Trustees of the American Medical Association made an effort to be constructive, they would have informed the *U.S.P.* and the *N.F.* of the need to tighten up the official specifications for tolbutamide and equally insoluble drugs and would have refrained from an attempt to downgrade the respect and esteem

[43] *Ibid.*

in which the *U.S.P.* is held throughout the entire world.

The affair has since taken an ironic twist which has trapped Upjohn in what could become a major financial problem. In August 1971, *Diabetes,* the official scientific journal of the American Diabetes Association, published the results of a ten-year, multi-university, cooperative, scientifically controlled trial testing the effectiveness of Orinase® treatment in persons with so-called "maturity-onset diabetes." By far the majority of the patients in the study are obese and over the age of forty. They have no symptoms of diabetes; they are discovered by chance, at physical examinations where blood is drawn for a sugar level or where urine is tested for sugar, to have either a higher than normal level or to be spilling some sugar in the urine. (My opinion is that these people are probably not true diabetics; that they do not suffer the obvious genetic abnormality which is the hallmark of the real diabetic, whose disease nearly always shows up in early life and makes itself apparent in weight loss, excessive thirst, and excessive hunger.) Whether or not it is necessary or even desirable to lower the blood-sugar levels of so-called "maturity-onset diabetes" patients is not known.

It was to discover if such a maneuver has any merit that the Multi-University Group Diabetes Program (UGDP) was conceived in 1960. Their findings surprised a lot of doctors and several pharmaceutical corporations, particularly the Upjohn Company. Although most physicians have the good training and good sense to treat real diabetics with insulin, a cult has grown in the past twenty years which believes that it is important to lower the blood sugar in "maturity-onset diabetes." Whether the cult has given any deep thought to what it does and to what extent the cult is motivated by a desire to "for goodness' sake, *do* something" are hard questions to answer. When the UGDP group published its results,[44] it was clear

[44] University Group Diabetes Program, "A Study of the Effects of Hypoglycemic Agents on Vascular Complications in

that (1) lowering the blood sugar in these patients causes no obvious benefit and that (2) if the popular oral blood-sugar-lowering drug Orinase® is used (providing an estimated $50 million in annual revenues for Upjohn) the patients' lives are probably shortened. The finding has stimulated a controversy within the medical profession that makes the argument over generic drugs appear like a tempest in a teapot.

Some physicians, many of whom refuse to believe the results of the UGDP study, are trying to discredit it by employing statisticians to poke holes in it. (But a detailed analysis of the UGDP study by the Biometric Society, a blue-ribbon international society of expert statisticians, upheld the results of the UGDP report. The biometricians' conclusions were published in the *Journal of the AMA* [February 10, 1975]. An authoritative estimate has been made that the use of Orinase® causes ten to fifteen thousand "unnecessary deaths" annually in the United States [*Present Status of Competition*, Part 25, p. 10775].) Note that even as they admitted they had no comparable statistics of the same quality and refinement as the UGDP group, many physicians based their opposition largely on "clinical experience." But the trouble with medical practice is that too much of therapeutics has been based for too long on "clinical experience" and "clinical impression." There is a very good chance now that the FDA will order a change in the extent to which Orinase® may be used by limiting its prescription to very special circumstances. Thus, according to the studies cited above, Orinase® performs no useful function for the patient and is likely a slow poison. Hence the benefit/risk ratio for Orinase® is zero, which is about as damning a statement as one can make about a medicinal agent.

Patients with Adult-Onset Diabetes, I. Design, Methods and Baseline Results," *Diabetes, 19*:(suppl. 2):747 (1970); "Mortality Results," *ibid.*, p. 789; "I.V. A Preliminary Report on Phenformin Results," *Journal of the American Medical Association, 217*:777 (1971).

VIII. The Modern FDA Is Indispensable to the United States [45]

There have been serious charges that the overly zealous implementation by the FDA of the 1962 Kefauver-Harris Amendment to the Pure Food and Drug Act has seriously stifled pharmaceutical innovation; the corollary of this charge is that Americans are being deprived of useful and new products that are available in foreign countries, a charge with little or no substance. The purpose of this chapter is to deal with the major charges one by one and to refute them.

In testimony before the Subcommittee on Monopoly, former Director of the Bureau of Drugs of the Food and Drug Administration, Henry E. Simmons, M.D., M.P.H., summarized certain specific charges made against the FDA by a number of sources, all inspired by the pharmaceutical industry. In summary, the charges were five in number and can be listed as follows:

1. That the requirement over the past fifteen years for proof of effectiveness of drugs (this is a requirement of the Kefauver-Harris Amendment of 1962) is counterproductive, too stringent, and should be repealed.

2. That the public and government are excessively concerned with drug safety.

3. That the approval procedures for new drugs in this country are causing the U.S. to fall behind the rest of the world in this important area of medical science and are responsible for a continuing decline in the number of new drugs introduced in this country each year.

4. That our safety and effectiveness requirements

---

[45] This chapter was abstracted from a thirty-eight-page statement authored by Henry E. Simmons, M.D., M.P.H., former Director of the Bureau of Drugs of the FDA, and given to the Nelson Subcommittee on Monopoly, February 5, 1973 (120 pages of reference material were appended to his report).

have kept from the citizens of this country access to important new drugs available to people in other countries.

5. That the regulatory system stifles creativity, needlessly escalates the cost of research, causes pharmaceutical firms to shift expenditure for research to more favorable climates abroad, and casts doubt on the future of drug development in this country.

Refuting Charge 1

In 1962, Congress required adequate, well-controlled clinical studies under which an objective, statistically valid determination might be made of drug effectiveness. Using this form of evaluation, the biases of clinicians, the differences that may randomly be found (*i.e.*, between patients, between diseases and between treatments), and the subjectivity inherent in "clinical impression" are reduced or eliminated. Properly designed trials safeguard the investigator from unwarranted conclusions and safeguard patients from unwarranted therapy. It is for want of adequately controlled trials that various forms of treatment have, in the past, become unjustifiably and sometimes painfully established in medical practice. The controlled clinical trial is virtually universally accepted today as the sole means by which scientifically valid conclusions can be reached about a drug's effectiveness. Leading scientists throughout the country testified in hearings leading up to the drug amendment in 1962 that any other standard is scientifically unreliable. Bear in mind that 1962 was the year of the thalidomide disaster. The public did not have to be strongly persuaded that prescription drugs needed to be tested for both safety and efficacy.

As a result of congressional adoption of effectiveness standards based on scientific data, 6300 drugs marketed in this country in twenty-four years between 1938 and 1962 were determined to be ineffective as of February 20, 1974.[46] By "ineffective," FDA meant it had been deter-

[46] *Competitive Problems in the Drug Industry*, Part 24, p. 9958.

mined, on the basis of National Academy of Sciences investigation, that insufficient scientific evidence existed to substantiate one or more of the claims made by the manufacturers. Many manufacturers have been granted grace periods in which to present additional evidence. Reasonable expectation is that eventually approximately one-third of all drugs in pharmacy inventories will have been removed by the FDA.

It is not surprising that a large number of marketed drugs whose claims were based solely upon "clinical impression" had to be eliminated from use. This is really nothing new in the history of medicine, which over the centuries has abounded in thousands of remedies used because of "clinical experience," remedies accorded an "indispensable place" but now known to be either useless or harmful.

The elimination of ineffective drugs represents perhaps as important an advance in medical therapy as the discovery of effective new drugs. If twenty drugs are available to treat a condition but only two are effective, it is critical to the medical profession, and to patients, that a scientific determination be required to make certain that only the two effective ones remain available.

Any requests for repeal of the law that a drug must be shown to be both efficacious and safe is entirely without merit, for if the request were successful we would reinstitute the errors of the past.

Refuting Charge 2

The United States Food and Drug Administration does require the most careful drug-safety testing of any regulatory agency in the world—and for good reasons.

First, a number of tragedies have occurred in other countries due to marketing of unsafe drugs in the recent past. Many tragedies also have occurred in this country from lack of consideration of safety: potentially lethal drugs have been used for minor, often self-limiting conditions. Second, there is an increasingly massive exposure of the public to drugs already numbering over two billion prescriptions and tens of billions of doses per year. Third, while everyone acknowledges the ability of certain drugs to affect favorably the course and outcome of previously serious, even fatal diseases, no one can dispute that drugs can themselves cause serious disease. Some authorities have suggested that as many as 18 to 30 percent of all hospitalized patients have a drug reaction of some sort and that the duration of their hospitalization is about doubled as a consequence. Also, studies of certain hospitals have shown that 3 to 5 percent of all admissions to hospitals (over 1,500,000 per year) are primarily for reactions caused by drugs.[47] The cost in both personal and financial terms staggers the imagination.

Obviously, no one can completely eliminate all drug reactions, but to the extent that this can be accomplished, every effort should be made to do so. No rational person can persuasively argue that the professional and the public should not be reasonably reassured (by the Amendment) that potential benefit must outweigh any risk inherent in the use of a pharmacologically active agent.

Doubtless, it might be possible to make some new drugs available sooner by relaxing requirements of proof of efficacy and safety, but recent experiences in other nations point out the hazards inherent in such a policy:[48] As examples, a drug developed to reduce appetite was found to cause so much constriction of blood vessels in the lung bed that the heart had to work extra hard to force the blood through the lungs; a sedative drug caused babies to be born without upper extremities; an "anti-inflammatory" drug caused jaundice; the introduction of a new kind of nebulizer for asthma which delivered highly concentrated drug by inhalation directly into the lungs caused a sudden sevenfold increase in deaths in asthma patients in England and Wales. This last was during the mid-

[47] K. L. Melmon, "Preventable Drug Reactions—Causes and Cures," *New England Journal of Medicine, 284*:1361–1368 (1971).

[48] *Ibid.*

1960s; 3500 deaths were caused to children ten to fourteen years old by the new form of nebulizer.[49]

The above incidents represent only a partial list. It is correct to say that the U.S. was spared every one of these disasters by the strict standards for safety testing demanded by the Food and Drug Administration as a result of the Kefauver-Harris Amendment of 1962. Any demand that the Amendment be repealed or its implementation be relaxed is nothing short of irresponsible.

Refuting Charge 3

The total number of "new" drugs being marketed in this country and throughout the world has been slowly decreasing for the past seventeen years. The phenomenon began six years before the passage of the 1962 effectiveness requirements. Since the U.S. has the most stringent requirements for proof of effectiveness of any nation, the falloff in new drugs has naturally been greater here. However, it must not escape attention that in countries where safety and effectiveness laws are less stringent and "miracle drug" development should, therefore, have been encouraged no miracle drugs have appeared. The major barrier to the development of important new drugs—such as a relatively non-toxic anticancer drug—is purely and simply a lack of basic knowledge of disease processes, secrets far less likely eventually to be uncovered in a pharmaceutical laboratory than in a large and sophisticated clinical or basic science research establishment, such as in a medical school or in, for example, the tax-supported National Institutes of Health in Bethesda, Maryland.

There is also valid reason to be grateful for any decrease in the plethora of new drugs being introduced, because most of this decrease is in trivial

[49] F. E. Speizer and R. Doll, "A Century of Asthma Deaths in Young People," *British Medical Journal*, 3:245–246 (July 27, 1968); editorial, *British Medical Journal* (November 25, 1972), pp. 443–444.

or duplicative items, or new mixtures, the use of which is considered by most experts to be incompatible with sound therapeutic practices. It can categorically be stated, on the basis of evidence supplied by the Food and Drug Administration (which is naturally sensitive to this particular charge number 3), that no marvelous or unique new miracle drugs have been discovered anywhere in the world which are not available as such, or as a counterpart equivalent, in this country.

Refuting Charge 4

National policy should be, and is rightfully, concerned only with the rate of introduction into this country of new drugs that promise significant medical advances. Between 1966 and 1970, several hundred new chemical entities were synthesized in England, France, and Germany. Only four of them, however, were introduced quickly for marketing in all three of those countries. None was introduced into the United States right away. But, in 1971, rifampicin, one of those four drugs, was introduced into the U.S. as a unique new antituberculosis drug to supplement others already marketed here. Canada accepted rifampicin in 1972; Sweden had already done so in 1970. The other three of the four presumably promising drugs had the following fates: one was voluntarily discontinued by its foreign sponsor because toxicity in animals began to show up; a second was never submitted for study or approval in this country by its manufacturer (an alternative drug is already available in this country); the third drug was subjected to some early preliminary testing here, but no application for marketing was submitted (with this third agent, too, there are at least four alternative drugs already being marketed in this country).

As one discusses this issue, it becomes clear that the health of the nation is not what is of primary concern to those who criticize FDA regulatory action. The cries are from manufacturers who can no longer introduce hundreds of supposedly "new" drugs advertised with hoopla and fanfare in order to make a lot of money from their sale—until doctors begin to discover that the "new drugs" are neither so remarkable nor miraculous after all. That is the point at which manufacturers cannot now, as they could prior to the new FDA policy, pull another molecule-manipulated "me too" drug out of their hats to be introduced with more bugles and fanfare in a never-ending march of drugs that are short-lived and inherently obsolescent but very lucrative for their manufacturers. The manufacturers feel cheated.

Refuting Charge 5

Clearly, Congress has determined that it is preferable to accept a delay in marketing, when necessary, in order to determine safety and effectiveness than to permit promiscuous and indiscriminate marketing of all new chemical entities for which corporations *hope* to prove safety and effectiveness. The goal of the 1962 Kefauver-Harris Amendment is to enable useful drugs to be introduced into this country as rapidly as possible, *consistent with public safety*. The policy has worked thus far.

If any individual can set forth substantial proof that any American has been deprived of a lifesaving drug because of the 1962 Kefauver-Harris Amendment or because of unconscionable delaying policies of the Food and Drug Administration, let him do so.

Finally, as proof that FDA *is* permitting the marketing of new and significant drugs in recent years, here is a table of them:

1969 mafenide acetate
1970 vasopressin nasal spray
  "   menotropins
  "   L-Dopa
  "   lithium salt
  "   carbenicillin injection
  "   ketamine

1971 spectinomycin
 " cephalexin
 " floxuridine
 " rifampicin
 " naloxone
1972 methyl methacrylate
1973 pancurium bromide
 " norethindrone mini-pill
 " diazoxide
1974 propranolol approved for use in angina pectoris

In other words, the FDA gave the green light to industry seventeen times in a period of five years.[50]

As for the related charge that pharmaceutical firms are being forced to invest elsewhere than in the U.S. for research, figures taken from Pharmaceutical Manufacturers Association annual surveys over the past years fail to give much substance to the claim. From 1960 to 1971, the percentage of their research and development expenditures in foreign countries has varied from 5.0 to 8.9 percent and the rise has not been continuous from year to year. It should not be unexpected, however, that pharmaceutical firms should begin to set up more and more plants in foreign nations where standards for efficacy and safety are still mediocre; since it is so easy to manufacture "me too" drugs by molecule manipulation, the firms could proceed to conduct themselves in many countries just as they did here prior to 1962, and could expect to turn in very large profits in those foreign nations.

[50] To market new drugs and to advertise a drug as useful for a new purpose. Obviously, it gave the green light *innumerable* times to companies wishing to market *their* versions of drugs whose patents had expired. In each of these cases, the company had to prove that they observe the Good Manufacturing Practices requirements of the Food and Drug Administration and that the product met the standards of the *U.S.P.* or *N.F.*, if the product was listed in either of those formularies. (If a product is not so listed, it is an unimportant product and probably has no business being prescribed, a rare exception being any vital discovery too new for inclusion.)

IX. The Bind the Pharmacist Finds Himself In

Probably very few citizens are aware of the plight of the average corner pharmacist in the complex relationship between the brand-name pharmaceutical industry and its undue influence over the medical profession, and the consumer whose pocketbook is too hard-hit by the need to buy necessary as well many unnecessary (but prescribed) medicines.

There are in the U.S. more than seventy-five schools of pharmacy, many with university affiliation. By and large their students come directly from high school and spend five or six years of hard work on a curriculum heavily loaded with scientific subjects. The well-trained graduate of a modern school of pharmacy probably knows as much chemistry—perhaps more—than the average medical school graduate. He has had courses in microbiology, bacteriology, inorganic and organic chemistry, and modern methods in quantitative chemical analysis and mathematics. These young men and women are a most important national resource. Upon graduation, they may enter hospital laboratories and undertake important responsibilities of a technical type. They may eventually run the complex photometers, photofluorimeters, gas chromatographs, or electrophoresis and other equipment that large hospitals use every day. What does happen to most of these young people, however? They end up in corner drugstores, taking things out of a big bottle and putting them into a little bottle.

Because of the oppressive "antisubstitution" laws in most states, the pharmacist is not even allowed the professional choice of which brand of a drug to dispense. The antisubstitution laws have forced him into carrying an unnecessary inventory—a very expensive one. The American Pharmaceutical Association has suggested a sensible solution to this problem for those who have already found themselves stuck with the task of trying to make a corner pharmacy run. The association suggests that pharmacists join consumer groups in enacting legislation to dismantle the "antisubstitution" statutes and regulations. If this were done, the pharmacist's inventory needs might drop by as much as two-thirds. He could buy inexpensive brands (there are some) or inexpensive generic counterparts and dispense them in lieu of the expensive brand written on the prescription. Instead of making a profit by taking a 40 percent markup, he could add a constant service fee to the actual cost of the medicine he dispenses. He could justify the service fee by pointing out to the public the long hours he remains open, his availability in emergencies, weekends, nights and holidays, the maintenance of delivery service, keeping of records, etc. (It is a fact that many pharmacists—but as yet a small minority—are conducting their business this way: they develop a reputation for providing good medications and good services at big savings to the consumer. The word gets around, and soon their businesses have grown by leaps and bounds.)

In my view, the repeal of antisubstitution laws and the institution by pharmacists of the service charge plus the cost-of-medication way of doing business will grow in popularity, although it will be a but transient phenomenon, one lasting a generation or two. I believe this because the pharmacist, though he may have lowered costs to the consumer, would still not be exercising all of the professional expertise of which he was once capable. He would still be taking things from a big bottle and putting them into a little bottle. The mortar and pestle that frequently ornament pharmacy windows are tools of a distant past whose use, except in very rare instances, is obsolete.

Schools of pharmacy ought gradually to begin to change their names to "schools of pharmacy and biological sciences" and eventually drop the "pharmacy" part. Their students ought to be using their scientific and technical know-how in the mainstream of medicine in ways suggested above or in research laboratories throughout the land. Many will ask, "How, then, will pharmaceuticals be distributed and doctors' prescriptions filled?" The answer would be to use existing health facilities, hospitals, and infirmaries throughout the country and to encourage doctors to carry in their offices a few items that are apt to be needed in an emergency and that are most commonly prescribed. The average doctor with a little knowledge of therapeutics would be very surprised to discover how few medications he needs to carry. (See the Basic Drug List.) I found, in my general medical practice, that fewer than thirty-four medications sufficed to provide for 95 percent of patients and that many of these thirty-four need be used only occasionally. Since most of them can be bought inexpensively by generic name, the doctor could give the items away at cost or figured as an extra 25 or 50 cents in his professional fee. Sometimes even this is excessive: it costs about 9 cents (!) to maintain a heart patient for three months on digitoxin taken at the usual rate of one tablet (0.1 milligram) daily.

It is disappointing that the United States of America, which has finally awakened to the misuse and squandering of its natural resources, continues to squander bright, eager, trained minds.

Finally, a word to the patient: Do bear in mind that the pharmacist, no matter what his age is now, was once an idealistic, hard-working student who was lured into pharmacy with the vision of being a professional person. The high cost of drugs is not primarily his fault; he is as much a victim of an oligopoly of big brand-name corporations as you are. If he is not as warm and friendly as you might like, reflect on the thousands of patients who have tormented him about "his" high prices. If he doesn't take to the idea of dispensing generic drugs, let it drop. He, as much as the physician, has been subjected over the years to propaganda and innuendo against them. Of this I can assure you, however: you are far more likely to discover a pharmacist who knows that there are accessible, inexpensive, and reliable generic drugs than you are a physician who knows as much.

As sympathetic as I am to the plight of professionalism in pharmacy, I find it regrettable that leaders of the American Pharmaceutical Association and the leadership of university-affiliated pharmacy students have suggested that pharmacists join the medical teams of major hospitals. Their argument is that they know more about the adverse side effects of the many drugs presently marketed and are more aware of the dangers inherent in giving more than one of certain drugs simultaneously than the doctors are. (Some drugs either potentiate or diminish the effects of other drugs; these phenomena are called "drug–drug interactions.") Drug–drug interactions are important to know about. However, it is the responsibility of *doctors* to know about them. Even though they are a recently popularized subject in medical circles, drug–drug interactions are likely less important than is currently believed may be the case. If doctors prescribed fewer drugs to patients, drug–drug interactions would certainly take on a less complicated appearance, and a comprehensive understanding of them would fall within the common knowledge of all practicing doctors.

I have myself heard the dean of a university-affiliated pharmacy school (who was discussing the reasons for the irrational prescribing practices of doctors) declare to the young doctors and their full-time mentors on the Harvard Medical Unit of the Boston City Hospital that the "pharmacist member of the team" making bed-to-bed rounds should guide the doctors in their decisions as to what drug or drugs would be best to administer to each patient. The statement was met with open hostility. One professor interrupted to ask if the pharmacists would also care to do the autopsies. Well motivated as the suggestion might have been, it was a ridiculous proposal, and continuing efforts to popularize such a role for pharmacists will never be treated seriously by good doctors. Good doctors understand all too well *how few effective drugs* even the average medical and surgical doctor need know about. The addition of a pharmacist to the hospital team would provide tacit acquiescence to the proliferation of unnecessary and duplicative "new" drugs whose existence ought correctly to be ignored; acquiescence to the existence of the artificially generated market for drugs; and acqui-

escence to the continuing handcuffing of the FDA
that allows a drug to be marketed if it can merely be
shown to be more effective than a sugar pill. The law
prevents the FDA from making its decisions on the
basis of whether new drug A is any *more* effective or
more safe than older drug B, which has been available for years and provides the same pharmacological
effect. An Omnibus Drug Law has been proposed by
Senator Gaylord Nelson. It, or a variant of it, will
become law; the handcuffs will be removed from the
FDA, which will then be free to make decisions on
the basis of *comparative* efficacy and *comparative*
safety. Nelson's proposed law is, of course, absolute
anathema to the Pharmaceutical Manufacturers Association, which will not be able so easily to exploit the
managers of their distribution depots—the pharmacists
—when the law is passed.

Pharmacists serve as pawns for PMA members,
whose relationship to pharmacy school deans .and
faculties is sorely in need of investigation by the
Congress. There has been considerable shuttling back
and forth of pharmacy teachers to and from industry.
There may be too much conflict of interest in the way
of "consultation fees" by pharmacy academicians with
the brand-name pharmaceutical industry.

PART TWO
Basic Drug List

Drugs that suffice to treat 95 percent of adult patients seen in office, outpatient clinic, or home by general practitioners or internists may be called "basic" drugs, and they are relatively few. They are listed here in twenty-three therapeutic categories; each drug is also discussed later in the Prescription Drug List pages. Medical students, doctors in training, and practicing physicians should use basic drugs wherever possible in writing prescriptions.

In this list only generic names are cited; if there is initial confusion over these names, reference to the Prescription Drug List will dispel it. For instance, the doctor who does not remember what diphenhydramine is need only look it up in the PDL to discover that he knows it well as Benadryl®. If the doctor learns the generic name for a drug and writes it on the prescription blank, this often makes it possible for the patient to save money when he has the prescription filled.

Readers with a medical education will recognize what the letters "U.S.P." and "N.F." stand for when they appear after drug names. U.S.P. stands for the *Pharmacopeia of the United States of America* (more commonly, *United States Pharmacopeia*) and N.F. for the *National Formulary*. Each is a highly respected, quasi-legal, authoritative volume. Each is published by the United States Pharmacopeial Convention. The purpose of the volumes is to supply continually updated drug standards, and to this end they are constantly revised and reissued (including frequent

publication of supplements) by outstanding leaders
in both medicine and pharmacy.

The histories of the *U.S.P.* and *N.F.* are worth
knowing. With the passage of the Pure Food and
Drug Act of 1906, both volumes were recognized by
the federal government as the official pharmacological
compendia for the nation: they provide legal standards of strength, quality, and purity *for the drugs
which they describe.* The *U.S.P.* contains a more
prestigious list of drugs than the *N.F.* because it has
been concerned from an earlier date (1820) with
listing only those drugs that reflect the best practice
and teaching of medicine. Therefore, the *U.S.P.* is
the single most valuable and reliable authority on the
quality, composition, and names of "blue ribbon"
drugs, which are listed in it only by generic name.
The *N.F.* has a format like that of the *U.S.P.,* and its
standards are as high; many good drugs in widespread
use which, for one reason or another, are not listed
in the *U.S.P.* are included in the *N.F.*

Until January 1, 1975, the *National Formulary*
had been published by the American Pharmaceutical
Association, an organization of pharmacy leaders
separate and distinct from the U.S. Pharmacopeial
Convention; the rights to own and continue to publish the *N.F.** were sold to the Pharmacopeial Convention on that date. The individual who will be in

* This is an appropriate point at which to pay respect to
the extraordinarily fine work done by Dr. Edward G. Feldmann, Director of Revision of the *National Formulary* for
many years. This careful scholar not only improved the quality
of the *National Formulary* to a point where its standards are
every bit as high as those of the *United States Pharmacopeia,*
but he has served a larger, national role that has gone little
recognized: using his numerous opportunities to testify as an
expert on pharmaceutics before Senator Nelson's Subcommittee
on Monopoly he quietly defended the truth whenever it was
treated casually by the Pharmaceutical Manufacturers Association. It was Dr. Feldmann's well-honed testimony that exploded
more PMA propaganda than any other single witness who has
appeared before Senator Nelson since his hearings began in
1967. The meticulous, effective Dr. Feldmann deserves the
plaudits of the nation.

charge of editing and updating both compendia will be Dr. Daniel Banes, a respected biopharmaceutical authority. The present plan is to continue publication of the *N.F.* for at least five more years. In 1980, a decision will be made as to whether to continue publishing. One possibility is that the *U.S.P.* and *N.F.* will be dovetailed into a single compendium.

One might think that the *U.S.P.* and the *N.F.* would be of great use to the doctor at the moment he writes his prescriptions. In fact, they are not. They are helpful, as they are meant to be, primarily to the *manufacturers* of drugs: they state in precise, technical terms the standards that a tablet or capsule or solution must meet in order to be marketed legally in interstate commerce in the U.S. Except for a brief notation as to the usual dose, and a mention of the therapeutic category to which a drug belongs, there is little in the two compendia that is of interest to the doctor *aside from the names of the drugs that are included.*

Many physicians might be surprised to discover how few of the drugs they are presently in the habit of prescribing are listed in the *U.S.P.* or *N.F.* They are reminded that under the Kefauver-Harris Amendment of 1962 a manufacturer need only prove *efficacy* (over a placebo) to market a drug. No test of *comparative efficacy* is required. *Most "new" drugs have not been shown to be more efficacious than U.S.P. and N.F. standbys.* It was pointed out earlier that "newness" is an inherent disadvantage in a drug because less can be known of its possible toxicity. That so many of the drugs doctors prescribe are not in the *U.S.P.* or *N.F.* attests to the ability of advertisers and drug salesmen to influence prescribing habits. Drug promoters understand their own power and would like to perpetuate and extend it; they are busily at work trying to undermine the authority of the official compendia through innuendo—usually by referring to *U.S.P.* and *N.F.* standards as "minimum standards." Wise doctors will pay little heed.

Neither the *U.S.P.* nor the *N.F.* considers cost in relation to the value of a drug, but the *Handbook* does. Therefore, if there is a category of drugs whose individual members have essentially the same therapeutic action, *Handbook* preference is usually given to the one most easily available at least cost. For example, among the host of thiazide and thiazide-like drugs (see category XI of the Basic Drug List) the 1975 *Handbook* prefers hydrochlorothiazide, a *U.S.P.* drug better known by the brand name Hydrodiuril®. The patent on hydrochlorothiazide has expired. Reference to the Price Lists (p. 362) will demonstrate how inexpensively this good drug is now available to both pharmacists and physicians if bought by its generic name. In rare cases a drug listed in neither the *N.F.* nor the *U.S.P.* is listed by the *Handbook* as basic—for example, flurazepam, a costly but unique new sedative which is preferred over others in category II in treating *certain* patients. In other cases, an *N.F.* drug is deemed preferable to its *U.S.P.* counterpart—for example, codeine sulfate over codeine phosphate, because the former tastes less bitter. The majority of the *Handbook's* basic drugs, however, are *U.S.P.* items.

It is important to note that most fixed-dose combination products are unacceptable to the two official compendia. (And prior to its dissolution by the governing group of the AMA that organization's important Council on Drugs also refused to give an imprimatur to such products.) The reason is simple: a tablet or capsule with two or more active drugs may be likened to a single shaker containing both salt and pepper—flexibility of dosage is lost. One cannot increase or decrease the dose of *one* drug without simultaneously increasing or decreasing the dosage of the *other* drug or drugs in the same tablet or capsule. The Drug Efficacy Study of the National Academy of Sciences advised the Food and Drug Administration to remove a large number of these fixed-dose combination products from the market, a decision that has contributed to a marked decline in their sale. At the time of publication of the 1970 *Handbook,* about 40 percent of all brand-name drug sales were of fixed-dose combination products. In 1975, these products are in much less wide use.

So-called "long-acting" dose forms are also unacceptable to the *U.S.P.* and the *N.F. because* no matter how well engineered the dose form is, gut-transit time is too unpredictable to warrant categorical claims that guarantee 8 or more hours of drug availability.

Most of the "basic" drugs listed below must be purchased with a doctor's prescription.

In reading comments on the value of certain drugs in the Prescription Drug List pages that follow the Basic Drug List, the patient should be aware that these apply to the *general* case, and that in special situations a doctor's decision to prescribe a drug of which the *Handbook* is critical may, indeed, be justified.

I. Drugs Used in Infectious Disease

THE PENICILLINS, NATURAL AND SYNTHETIC
POTASSIUM PENICILLIN G, U.S.P.
SODIUM DICLOXACILLIN
AMPICILLIN, U.S.P.

TETRACYCLINE AND CONGENERS
TETRACYCLINE HYDROCHLORIDE, U.S.P.

SULFONAMIDES AND DRUGS USED MAINLY FOR URINARY
TRACT INFECTION
SULFISOXAZOLE, U.S.P.
TRIPLE SULFAS TABLETS, U.S.P. AND N.F.

ANTITUBERCULOSIS DRUGS
ISONIAZID, U.S.P. (INH)
AMINOSALICYLIC ACID, U.S.P. (PAS)

ANTIFUNGUS DRUGS
GRISEOFULVIN, U.S.P.
TOLNAFTATE, U.S.P.
NYSTATIN, U.S.P.

ANTIPROTOZOAN DRUGS
CHLOROQUINE PHOSPHATE, U.S.P.
METRONIDAZOLE, U.S.P.

ANTIWORM DRUGS (ANTHELMINTICS)
PYRVINIUM PAMOATE, U.S.P.

II. Sedatives and Drugs for Sleep

SEDATIVES (SO-CALLED "TRANQUILIZERS")
PHENOBARBITAL, U.S.P.
CHLORAL HYDRATE, U.S.P. (capsules and syrup)

DRUGS FOR SLEEP (HYPNOTICS)
(SODIUM) PENTOBARBITAL, U.S.P.
(SODIUM) SECOBARBITAL, U.S.P.
CHLORAL HYDRATE, U.S.P.
FLURAZEPAM

III. Antipsychotic and Antidepressant Drugs

CHLORPROMAZINE, U.S.P.
AMITRIPTYLINE, U.S.P.

IV. Anti-Epilepsy Drugs

PHENOBARBITAL, U.S.P.
(SODIUM) DIPHENYLHYDANTOIN, U.S.P.

V. Antinausea Drugs

ANTIHISTAMINE WITH STRONG ANTINAUSEA AND ANTI-MOTION-SICKNESS EFFECT
DIPHENHYDRAMINE HYDROCHLORIDE, U.S.P.

PHENOTHIAZINE (ALSO AN ANTIHISTAMINE)
PROMETHAZINE HYDROCHLORIDE, U.S.P.

VI. Pain Relievers (Analgesics)

ASPIRIN, U.S.P.
CODEINE SULFATE, N.F.
ACETAMINOPHEN, N.F.
MORPHINE SULFATE, U.S.P.

VII. Antihistamines

CHLORPHENIRAMINE MALEATE, U.S.P.
DIPHENHYDRAMINE HYDROCHLORIDE, U.S.P.

VIII. Drugs That Suppress Cough (Antitussives)

CODEINE SULFATE, N.F.
DEXTROMETHORPHAN HYDROBROMIDE, N.F.

IX. Drugs for Asthma, or Bronchospasm (Bronchodilators)

AMINOPHYLLINE, U.S.P.
EPHEDRINE SULFATE, U.S.P.
ISOPROTERENOL INHALATION, U.S.P.
PREDNISONE, U.S.P.

X. Topical Nasal Decongestant

PHENYLEPHRINE HYDROCHLORIDE, U.S.P.

XI. Drugs for High Blood Pressure (Antihypertension Drugs)

INDIAN SNAKEROOT DERIVATIVE
RESERPINE, U.S.P.

THIAZIDES AND CONGENERS
HYDROCHLOROTHIAZIDE, U.S.P.

FIVE SOMETIMES USEFUL DRUGS
METHYLDOPA, U.S.P.
GUANETHIDINE SULFATE, U.S.P.
HYDRALAZINE HYDROCHLORIDE, N.F.
FUROSEMIDE, U.S.P.
PROPRANOLOL, U.S.P.

XII. Drugs for Heart Disease (Exclusive of Those Used to Treat High Blood Pressure)

DIGITALIS GLYCOSIDES
DIGITOXIN, U.S.P.
DIGOXIN, U.S.P.

BLOOD-VESSEL DILATORS
NITROGLYCERIN, U.S.P. (GLYCERYL TRINITRATE)

DRUGS FOR CERTAIN ABNORMAL HEART RHYTHMS
QUINIDINE SULFATE, U.S.P.
PROCAINAMIDE HYDROCHLORIDE, U.S.P.

THIAZIDES AND CONGENERS (See Section XI)

XIII. Drugs for Gastrointestinal Disorders, Including Peptic Ulcer

BELLADONNA TINCTURE, U.S.P.
ATROPINE SULFATE, U.S.P.
MAGNESIUM AND ALUMINUM HYDROXIDES SUSPENSION
PAREGORIC, U.S.P. (CAMPHORATED TINCTURE OF OPIUM)
DIOCTYL SODIUM SULFOSUCCINATE, N.F.

XIV. Adrenal Steroids

ORAL PREPARATION
PREDNISONE, U.S.P.

TOPICAL PREPARATION
HYDROCORTISONE CREAM, U.S.P. (or ointment) (1%)

XV. Thyroid Hormone

SODIUM LEVOTHYROXINE, U.S.P.
THYROID, U.S.P.

XVI. Drugs Used for Gout

COLCHICINE, U.S.P.
PROBENECID, U.S.P.
PHENYLBUTAZONE, U.S.P.

XVII. Drugs Used for Migraine

ERGONOVINE MALEATE, U.S.P.
ERGOTAMINE TARTRATE, N.F.

XVIII. Oral Contraceptives and Female Hormones

"THE PILL"

FEMALE HORMONES (NO CONTRACEPTIVE ACTION)
DIETHYLSTILBESTROL, U.S.P.
CONJUGATED ESTROGENS, U.S.P.

XIX. Vitamins

DECAVITAMIN TABLETS, U.S.P., and DECAVITAMIN CAPSULES, U.S.P. (See Addenda.)

HEXAVITAMIN TABLETS, N.F., and HEXAVITA-
MIN CAPSULES, N.F. (See Addenda.)
CYANOCOBALAMIN INJECTION, U.S.P. (VITA-
MIN B$_{12}$)

XX. Iron

FERROUS SULFATE, U.S.P.

XXI. Drug Used for Diabetes Mellitus

INSULIN INJECTION, U.S.P.

XXII. Anti-Parkinsonism

L-DOPA

XXIII. Anticoagulant

SODIUM WARFARIN, U.S.P.

PART THREE
Prescription Drug List

The commentary in the PDL applies primarily to prescribing for adults. (For a special section on prescribing for children, see Appendix A.) Not every doctor will necessarily agree with the statements made in the PDL commentary, but generally the opinions presented are the same as those in standard texts, in the most recent *AMA Drug Evaluations,* and in *Medical Letter,* a superb review on therapeutics published twice monthly for physicians. Unfortunately, therapeutic decisions must commonly be based on opinion, because little has been scientifically written for the profession about *comparative* efficacy and safety of drugs. This is the reason for honest differences of opinion. The PDL herein makes recommendations that lean always on the side of conservatism in therapy. This is because a very large percentage of patients' money is spent on unnecessary prescriptions and because many necessary prescriptions could cost the patient less if they were written differently.

In the PDL, drugs are discussed alphabetically, generally by brand name. For single-entity drugs, the generic name is indicated at the right of the brand-name heading, and the drug is also cross-listed under the generic name; however, commentary usually appears under the brand-name heading, as that is likely to be the name by which the drug is best known. Each discussion of a combination drug is accompanied, at the top right, by a breakdown of its active ingredients, indicating the amounts contained in each tablet, capsule, or other unit of dosage.

137

Patients should not expect a prescription from a doctor for every complaint, and ought to have the assurance that prescriptions will not be written: (1) to signal to the patient that his appointment is over; (2) where the patient's condition is self-limiting or trivial; (3) where a simple non-prescription item will suffice (*e.g.*, a cough syrup containing dextromethorphan instead of codeine or other expensive cough concoctions) or where a prescription is not required for the drug to be used (*e.g.*, acetaminophen, often prescribed as Tylenol®); (4) for products not acceptable to the *U.S.P.*, such as so-called long-acting dose forms and most fixed-dose combinations; (5) for a "new" drug when an older one has the same effect, unless there is substantial proof that the new drug is more reliably effective and as safe; (6) *unless it is known what the cost to the patient is likely to be.* Patients are often concerned about the cost of prescriptions, and they should discuss with their physician prescription drugs and their costs.

So much propaganda effort has been made over the past twenty to thirty years to prejudice doctors against using "generic" drugs and toward using "new" drugs instead of "old" that many excellent diagnosticians are reluctant to change their present prescribing habits. As a consumer, the patient has the right to ask about drug costs and to point out differential costs to the busy doctor who may be unaware of them. Most will welcome the information.

Until we have a mandatory national label law for pharmaceuticals, it is necessary for the doctor to *instruct* the pharmacist *to legibly display* the official name(s) of the active ingredient(s) in any drug along with the directions for its use. When the doctor hands a patient a prescription, the patient should check to see if it says "Label" after "Sig:".* If not, he might remind the doctor to instruct the pharmacist to put the official name of the drug on the con-

---

* This is the common way to write prescriptions. Actually it is redundant, for "Sig.," standing for the imperative *Signa*, literally means "Label!" But this is the traditional form.

tainer along with directions for use. The patient may be negligent of *his* own safety if he fails to do this.

ACETAMINOPHEN, N.F.
  See *Tylenol*®.

ACHROMYCIN®
  See Tetracycline Hydrochloride, U.S.P.

ACHROMYCIN® **V**   Tetracycline Hydrochloride,
                          U.S.P.
  See Tetracycline Hydrochloride, U.S.P.

ACTIFED®   triprolidine hydro-
                          chloride   2.5 mg
                         pseudoephedrine hydro-
                          chloride   60.0 mg
  See Antihistamines; Cough Remedies; Neo-Synephrine®.

This combination product is promoted for treatment of swollen nasal passage linings as in hay fever or the common cold. Recent review of this product by the National Academy of Sciences–National Research Council has classified the product as only "probably" effective for relief of nasal passage swelling and "lacking substantial evidence of effectiveness as a fixed combination."

Triprolidine is an antihistamine (see Antihistamines) with atropine-like side effects of drying up secretions. The same effect can be obtained by using other antihistamines at perhaps less expense (see Chlor-Trimeton®). As with all antihistamines, drowsiness may be a side effect of triprolidine.

One should not accept the casual systemic use of pseudoephedrine for treatment of a stuffy nose. The symptoms of the common cold are self-limiting and, if nasal stuffiness is troublesome enough to require treatment, phenylephrine (Neo-Synephrine®) nose drops, ¼ or ½ percent, may be used without side effects of systemic pseudoephedrine, including worsening of high blood pressure.

In 1967, Actifed® was one of the 100 most-prescribed drugs, and in 1973 it ranked 15th among all prescription items.

ACTIFED-C® EXPECTORANT	Codeine Phosphate,	
	U.S.P.	10 mg
	triprolidine hydro- chloride	2 mg
	pseudoephedrine hydro- chloride	30 mg
	glyceryl guaiacolate (per 5 ml, or 1 tsp)	100 mg

See Codeine Sulfate, N.F.; Codeine Phosphate, U.S.P.; Cough Remedies; Dextromethorphan Hydrobromide, N.F.

This product is recommended by the manufacturer for the relief of cough symptoms in the common cold and other similar conditions. Codeine alone is an excellent cough suppressant, and may be used alone just as effectively.

This combination of products combines triprolidine, which dries up secretions, with glyceryl guaiacolate, which is supposed to loosen them. It has already been mentioned above, under Actifed®, that the systemic use of pseudoephedrine is probably not necessary for simple colds and similar disorders.

In 1967, and again in 1973, this product ranked among the 150 most popular drugs prescribed to persons of all ages.

AFRIN® NASAL SPRAY AND SOLUTION	oxymetazoline hydro-	
	chloride	0.5 mg
	glycine	3.8 mg
	sorbitol	40.0 mg

phenylmercuric
  acetate   0.02 mg
Benzalkonium Chlo-
  ride, U.S.P.   0.2 mg
NaOH to raise pH to 5.5– 6.5
  (per ml of solution)

See Neo-Synephrine®.

Oxymetazoline, a constrictor of blood vessels, is
reputed to have a longer action than phenylephrine
(Neo-Synephrine®) when applied to the nasal passages. Like phenylephrine, oxymetazoline can cause
paradoxical, severe nasal congestion if taken regularly for a number of consecutive days. Most people
with a temporarily stuffy nose from a cold would do
well with hot liquids, steam mists, or with plain
phenylephrine nose drops, ¼ or ½ percent, which
can be bought without prescription at little cost (see
Neo-Synephrine®). See Phenylephrine in the Price
Lists.

In 1967, and again in 1973, Afrin® was among the
top 100 drugs prescribed.

ALDACTAZIDE®   Spironalactone,
                          U.S.P.   25 mg
                        Hydrochlorothiazide,
                          U.S.P.   25 mg

See Aldactone®; Hydrodiuril®.

Fixed-ratio dose combinations of drugs are best
avoided. The warning required by FDA regulation
in *Physicians' Desk Reference,* 1974 edition, for this
combination product, used to treat excess body fluid
or high blood pressure, reads (pages 1335–1336):

Fixed-dose combination drugs are not indicated
for initial therapy of edema or hypertension.
Edema or hypertension requires therapy titrated
to the individual patient. If the fixed combination represents the dosage so determined, its use
may be more convenient in patient management.

Both components of this product are excellent drugs. Spironolactone (see Aldactone®, below) is an ingenious medication which prevents loss of potassium salt that occurs with other "water pills" (diuretics) and is helpful in rare cases of liver cirrhosis, heart failure, nephrotic syndrome and hypertension. Unfortunately, this medication is expensive. Hydrochlorothiazide is a diuretic and among the most popular in use today. It is very effective (as is a closely related congener, trichlormethiazide), with substantial savings for patients (see Hydrodiuril® and Trichlormethiazide). The combination of the two does not add significantly to the already very high price of spironolactone alone.

While fixed-dose combinations should not be used to begin a program of treatment for a patient with high blood pressure or excess fluid, when it is later found that the best dose combination corresponds to that in a combination product, then such a product should be used *if* additional expenses are not engendered. Convenience and savings occasionally make the drug combination appropriate. More often than not, however, drug combinations encourage the use of unnecessary additional medications or more expensive ones than would otherwise be used.

While doctors are shy about writing for spironolactone (Aldactone®) alone, they were rather enthusiastic about the combination product, Aldactazide®. In 1973, the single product ranked 178th and the fixed-dose combination 60th among the most prescribed drugs in the U.S.

ALDACTONE®   Spironolactone, U.S.P.
See Aldactazide®.

The outer shell, or cortex, of the adrenal glands produces several hormones, including aldosterone. Aldosterone's effect is generally to encourage the retention of sodium and water and the excretion of potassium. Some diseases are occasionally associated with excessive aldosterone, either because of increased production or decreased destruction by the liver. Thus, most patients with accelerated (malignant) high blood pressure, some with the nephrotic syndrome (a kidney affliction), many with advanced liver disease (cirrhosis), and a very few with mild high blood pressure or chronic congestive heart failure owe something of their symptoms to the effects of too much aldosterone.

Spironolactone is an aldosterone antagonist with occasional usefulness in the diseases mentioned above. However, most patients with nephrotic syndrome, mild high blood pressure, cirrhosis, or heart failure do *not* need spironolactone. Rather, they can be treated with less expensive diuretics ("water pills") or with strict salt restriction. Aldactone® is more often than not given with another drug that causes increased urine production, usually a thiazide. The usual dose of Aldactone® alone is 4 tablets daily, which is very costly. If Aldactone® is to be used with a "thiazide" diuretic, generic hydrochlorothiazide is the preferable one because of its low cost, relative ease of availability (especially at larger drug chains), and proved efficacy.

Aldactazide®, a combination of Aldactone® with hydrochlorothiazide, is an expensive irrational prescription for most people to whom it is given.

ALDOMET®   Methyldopa, U.S.P.
    See Hydrochlorothiazide, U.S.P.

Methyldopa is included among basic drugs because, despite some toxicity, it has a unique and useful role in treating high blood pressure. Its price is high.

When high blood pressure of mild degree and unknown cause is first discovered, weight reduction, decreased salt intake, and mild diuretics may be indicated. If these measures do not improve the blood pressure readings, add reserpine to the diuretic to try the effect. When these measures have failed to lower blood pressure or the side effects of reserpine become troublesome, then methyldopa should be used. Diabetics and patients with gout may be made worse with thiazides, and in these patients methyldopa is an excellent drug.

When a thiazide is used in combination with reserpine or methyldopa, the least expensive is the most appropriate. This is usually hydrochlorothiazide.

Aldomet®, though useful, is surely overused. In 1973, it was the 21st most popular drug in the U.S.

ALDORIL®   Methyldopa, U.S.P.   250 mg
                          Hydrochlorothiazide,
                                U.S.P.   15 or 25 mg
    See Aldomet®; Hydrodiuril®; Trichlormethiazide.

Aldoril® is a fixed-dose combination of the high blood pressure medications methyldopa (Aldomet®) and the diuretic hydrochlorothiazide (Hydrodiuril®). Arguments against fixed-dose combinations in antihypertensive agents (at least at the beginning of therapy) have already been made (see Aldactazide®). Clearly, because of the popularity of methyldopa and its frequent use in conjunction with a thiazide diuretic, it has been marketed as a "convenience" product. Nonetheless, such combinations should *only* be used after the dosages are adjusted separately. The FDA warns against the use of this drug as follows: ". . . this fixed combination drug is not indicated for initial therapy of hypertension" (*Physicians' Desk Reference,* 1975 edn., page 1023).

Most people with mild elevation of blood pressure can be adequately treated with inexpensive generic hydrochlorothiazide either alone or in combination with inexpensive generic reserpine. The Aldomet® content of Aldoril® can cause impotence, by the way.

ALLOPURINOL
    See Zyloprim®.

ALUDROX®   magnesium and aluminum
                                oxides mixture

See Maalox®.

This antacid preparation is very similar to Maalox®.
Many less expensive, equally palatable antacids are
available in pharmacies.

AMBENYL®   Codeine Sulfate,
EXPECTORANT   N.F.   10 mg
                         bromodiphenhydramine
                           hydrochloride   3.75 mg
                         Diphenhydramine Hydro-
                           chloride, U.S.P.   8.75 mg
                         Ammonium Chloride,
                           U.S.P.   80 mg
                         Potassium Guaiacolsul-
                           fonate, N.F.   80 mg
                         menthol 0.5 mg, alcohol 5%
                           (per 5 ml, or 1 tsp)

*See Codeine Sulfate, N.F.; Codeine Phosphate,
U.S.P.; Cough Remedies; Dextromethorphan Hydrobromide, N.F.*

Why two antihistamines whose effect is to dry up
secretions are combined with two other drugs supposed to loosen secretions is hard to imagine. The
codeine in a tablespoonful of this concoction *alone*
ought to suppress most coughs; and codeine or dextromethorphan alone are the drugs of choice for suppression of troublesome coughing in viral illnesses.
Reputable medical literature does not support the
use of this irrational mixture and ones similar to it.

AMCILL®
See Ampicillin, U.S.P.

**AMINOPHYLLINE, U.S.P. (THEOPHYLLINE
ETHYLENEDIAMINE)**

Aminophylline is a "blue-ribbon" drug used mainly to treat mild recurrent asthma and asthma-like symptoms of bronchitis. In emergency situations it is given by slow intravenous injection, but most patients take it by mouth—100 or 200 milligrams four times a day. It is often said that many people are nauseated by aminophylline, but if it is taken with meals this side effect is less likely; and if it is given on an empty stomach together with an antacid, patients can often tolerate up to 300 milligrams at a time and will experience effects as profound as those produced by intravenous administration.

Aminophylline is a salt of theophylline. It is better absorbed and more effective than uncombined theophylline because the salt is much more soluble.

Aminophylline suppositories are available, but they have two drawbacks: absorption is unpredictable, and if used regularly they often cause rectal irritation. There are aminophylline solutions for administration by enema, but that is not practical in most cases.

Since there is little or no promotion of Aminophylline, U.S.P., for oral use, far too little of this fine, potentially inexpensive drug is prescribed in office practice.

See Aminophylline, U.S.P., in the Price Lists.

AMITRIPTYLINE HYDROCHLORIDE, U.S.P.
See Elavil®.

AMPICILLIN, U.S.P.

Ampicillin is a good, broad-spectrum antibiotic that is much prescribed when simple penicillins, sulfas, or tetracycline would do as well at a fraction of the cost.

Ampicillin is very commonly used in treating urinary tract (bladder and kidney) infections; triple sulfas or sulfisoxazole (Gantrisin® and others) would almost always suffice. Important but relatively uncommon exceptions include urinary tract infections due to unusual bacteria sensitive only to ampicillin.

Another common call for ampicillin is prevention of worsening respiratory symptoms of bronchitis in chronic lung disease patients. Tetracycline probably works as well in most instances and is cheaper.

Childrens' infections, especially ear infections; respiratory infections caused by *Hemophilus influenzae;* and some diarrheas are best treated with ampicillin. Also, ampicillin is now the therapeutic agent of choice for typhoid fever and *Hemophilus influenzae* meningitis, according to most experts, though some would still choose chloramphenicol (until recently, the only effective drug for these conditions). Ampicillin is as effective and less toxic.

Side effects from ampicillin are common; primarily these are rashes and diarrhea. Penicillin-allergic patients are also allergic to ampicillin.

Until recently, only five very expensive brands of ampicillin were available: Amcill®, Omnipen®, Penbritin®, Polycillin®, and Principen®. Generic ampicillin is now available at substantial savings from approximately twenty-five wholesale sources. Prices range from less than 10 cents to more than 35 cents per tablet.

ANTIHISTAMINES

Antihistamines block the effects of histamine. Histamine is a naturally occurring body substance that is released in certain allergic reactions. Unfortunately, antihistamines have no dramatic effects in people with asthma or other more severe diseases of an allergic nature. They may be effective in hay fever or mild recurrent "hives" of unknown causes.

Antihistamines abound in common-cold preparations. People who take antihistamines are likely to have less severe runny noses, but the other features of the common cold are not significantly affected. The reason is simple: antihistamines have atropine-like effects, one of which is to diminish the amount of secretions produced by the irritated lining of the nose or bronchial passages. The antihistamine di-

phenhydramine (Benadryl®) has been advertised as
a cough suppressant, but studies have shown that
antihistamines have no significant effect on the cough
reflex.* In fact, a carefully controlled study has
shown that antihistamines are no better than placebos
in relieving patients from the symptoms of the common cold†.

The side effects of antihistamines are noteworthy.
Drowsiness is the most common side effect. Therefore, antihistamines may be dangerous to patients
who are driving or operating machinery. They make
the mouth dry, and often impart an unpleasant,
metallic taste. In rare instances red blood cells can
burst (hemolytic anemia) or the bone marrow can
be depleted of blood-forming cells (agranulocytosis).
Many patients who are routinely given prescriptions
for antihistamines or who buy over-the-counter cold
remedies that include antihistamines might do better
without any treatment, or merely rely on some phenylephrine nose drops, aspirin, and bed rest.

The sedative side effects of antihistamines have led
to their inclusion in over-the-counter sleeping pills.
This group of drugs, including Compoz®, Nytol®,
Sominex®, and Excedrin®-PM, is among the most
abused in recent years. If sleep is a problem for patients, small doses of very inexpensive products available by prescription are much cheaper and more
effective. (See "Sedatives and Drugs for Sleep" in the
Basic Drug List, p. 131.)

Another important side effect of some members
of the antihistamine family of drugs is the prevention
of nausea and motion sickness, dizziness, and vertigo.
The various products sold primarily for this effect
include meclizine (Antivert®), diphenhydramine
(Benadryl®), and dimenhydrinate (Dramamine®).
Of these, dimenhydrinate is available without a prescription and non-brand-name products are available

* *Medical Letter, 13*:9 (1971).
† Feller, A. E., et al., *New England Journal of Medicine,*
242:737 (1950).

at a mere fraction of the cost of Dramamine® or Benadryl® (see Benadryl®).

Certain of the antihistamines are advertised as particularly effective against itching and are used most extensively by dermatologists (skin specialists). These include hydroxyzine (Atarax®, Vistaril®), cyproheptadine (Periactin®), and dexchlorpheniramine (Polaramine®). There is little or no evidence that any antihistamine relieves itching better than any other drug with equal sedative effects.*

Antihistamines, then, do have limited clinical usefulness *and* important side effects. Nearly every legitimate use to which their actions can be put will be served by one of these four: Tripelennamine Hydrochloride, U.S.P. (Pyribenzamine®), Diphenhydramine Hydrochloride, U.S.P. (Benadryl®), Chlorpheniramine Maleate, U.S.P. (Chlor-Trimeton®), and Dimenhydrinate, U.S.P. (Dramamine® and others). All of these medications are available at great savings if purchased by other than their brand names, and dimenhydrinate is available without prescription.

ANTIVERT®   Meclizine Hydrochloride,
                             U.S.P.   12.5 mg
See Antihistamines.

This product is the best-selling drug for dizziness in the country. The name of the product has undoubtedly helped its sales and made it more popular than cheaper and equally effective products.

Antivert® used to be a fixed combination of the antihistamine meclizine and nicotinic acid. However, a National Research Council panel of experts found the mixture "irrational." (Nicotinic acid is a vitamin whose deficiency causes the rare disease, pellagra. Also, 50 or 100 milligrams of nicotinic acid can cause a painless, perhaps pleasing, transient "warm-

* *Medical Letter, 13*:102–104 (1971).

all-over" effect, doubtless the reason why it used to be included.) The antihistamine meclizine is among the more expensive ones. Diphenhydramine (Benadryl®) can be expected to serve as well.

Antivert® is still allowed to be promoted nonspecifically for vertigo (dizziness), but may not be promoted for apprehension, mental confusion, etc. The drug *is* advertised for "dizziness" in older people. This kind of "dizziness" is most often due to inadequate circulation to the brain and almost invariably is not *true* dizziness but is better described as a "light-headedness." There is no specific treatment for this common symptom, but the doctor makes a gesture by prescribing something. Most of these patients would be satisfied by simple reassurance that "light-headedness" is common in people of advancing years and that there is not anything presently that can be done for it. Should a prescription be needed, doctors with an eye to economy should prescribe diphenhydramine. (See the Basic Drug List and p. 336 for Benadryl®.)

On the basis of National Research Council recommendations, the FDA has classified meclizine as "effective" only in "management of nausea and vomiting, and dizziness associated with motion sickness." (Any other antihistamine with as much sedative side effect would serve as well. An example: diphenhydramine.) The FDA has classified meclizine as only "possibly effective" in management of dizziness associated with diseases affecting the inner ear or any other part of the nervous system. (The "possibly effective" category was originally named the "probably ineffective" category.* A bit of lobbying from the pharmaceutical industry got the category's name changed to something more to their liking. Many people in government are aware of this farce, but most people—including most doctors—don't know.) (See Addenda.)

* *Competitive Problems in the Drug Industry,* Part 12, p. 5161.

ARISTOCORT® Triamcinolone, U.S.P.
See Hydrocortisone Cream, U.S.P.; Prednisone, U.S.P.; Kenalog®.

This is a "steroid" drug. Five milligrams of prednisone or prednisolone have the same effects as 4 milligrams of triamcinolone. Nearly without exception, patients requiring Aristocort® can be treated as well with prednisone or prednisolone and at much less expense.

Aristocort® is also sold as a cream or ointment for application to the skin; it is available as well under another brand name, Kenalog®. The *Handbook* recommends first a trial of hydrocortisone cream if a steroid cream is needed. (The patient should be instructed to rub the cream in very, very well.) Only when this is unsuccessful should the more expensive steroid creams like Aristocort® (which *do* diffuse into the skin a little more readily) be used.

ARTANE® Trihexyphenidyl Hydrochloride, U.S.P.

As predicted in earlier editions of this *Handbook,* the popularity of this drug and similar atropine-like drugs has waned. It was once used primarily for the treatment of Parkinsonism; now L-Dopa has replaced it. Currently the major use of this product and ones like it is in controlling the side effects of major sedatives given for emotional illnesses. In many cases where drugs such as trihexyphenidyl (sold as Artane®, Tremin®, Pipanol®), or its analogues, Kemadrin® (procyclidine), Pagitane® (cypcrimine), L-Dopa Akineton® (biperiden), and Cogentin® (benztropine), are used to control the side effects of major sedatives used to treat severe neurotics and psychotics, careful re-evalution of the need for such large doses of the sedatives should be undertaken. Indeed, most of the side effects controlled by these drugs—side effects that resemble the manifestations of Parkinsonism—are eliminated by discontinuing the sedatives.

Trihexyphenidyl is now available generically.

ASPIRIN, U.S.P.

A thousand 300 milligram aspirin tablets can have a wholesale cost from under $4 to over $30, depending on the manufacturer. Despite the plethora of marketed products containing aspirin, only a handful of manufacturers make the aspirin powder itself. *All aspirin powder and tablets sold in the U.S. must by law meet U.S.P. standards.* A recent listing of all commercially available products containing aspirin numbered over 200. The large retailers of aspirin argue too conspicuously on television to have a superior aspirin. This claim of superiority is unfounded; no conclusive proof based on controlled trials has demonstrated that the pain-relieving effect provided by any one brand of simple aspirin is better than another. Patients should buy the least expensive aspirin tablets available.

Recent increasing use of "fancier" aspirin products makes little sense. While aspirin dissolves better by the addition of a little baking soda ("acid buffer") to the tablet (as in Bufferin®), the amount of soda is not enough to cause a significant decrease in gastric acidity. Patients would do as well to eat food with their aspirin or take a full glass of water with each tablet if aspirin causes slight indigestion. Furthermore, ". . . it has never been established in patients with painful conditions . . . that there is a difference between buffered and non-buffered aspirin in time of onset of analgesia, duration or degree of relief of pain, or incidence of gastrointestinal distress."* The time-revered household remedy, Alka-Seltzer®, is an aspirin and "buffer" combination. While this product *does* contain a large amount of antacid and is rapidly absorbed, it is some 20 times more expensive than aspirin alone. In addition, Alka-Seltzer® is rich in sodium (the "buffer" is sodium bicarbonate), making it a poor drug for patients who must restrict their salt intake, including patients with high blood pressure and some heart disorders.

* *Medical Letter, 16:*58 (July 5, 1974).

Recent additions to the aspirin-antacid market include Ascriptin®, which combines the well-known antacid Maalox® with aspirin, and Excedrin®, a combination of aspirin with two other minor analgesics and caffeine; these are expensive and not significantly more useful than aspirin alone.

Timed-release and specially coated aspirin preparations allegedly delay and prolong the effects of aspirin, but with two important additional problems: first, the absorption of the aspirin into the bloodstream from the intestine is erratic and unpredictable; second, the cost is phenomenally high.

Aspirin, as with other drugs, has side effects: stomach irritation, bleeding from the stomach (making ulcers worse), and, less commonly, allergic reactions, liver damage, and interference with normal blood clotting. Cavalier use of the drug should be curtailed. When aspirin causes stomach upset—its most common adverse effect—the patient should buy acetaminophen (p. 330), which like aspirin requires no prescription. However, acetaminophen is not as effective in rheumatoid arthritis. The patient should be guided by his doctor.

ATARAX®   Hydroxyzine Hydrochloride, N.F.
See Antihistamines; Vistaril®.

This antihistamine drug was actively promoted as a "tranquilizer" in the early 1970s and most recently has been widely advertised as an anti-itching agent particularly useful in rashes. It has not been proved more effective than small doses of phenobarbital or other mild sedatives in treating itch. Its usefulness in preventing or controlling nausea and motion sickness is little different from that of less expensive preparations, primarily diphenhydramine hydrochloride (Benadryl®) and chlorpheniramine maleate (Chlor-Trimeton®). (See Diphenhydramine Hydrochloride, U.S.P., and Chlorpheniramine Maleate, U.S.P. in the Price Lists.)

ATROMID-S®   clofibrate

The purpose of this relatively new drug is to lower
the blood levels of lipids (fats), and cholesterol in
particular. Good evidence that either lowering the
cholesterol level or the use of Atromid-S® prolongs
life and decreases the incidence of heart attacks is
absent at this time. Studies made in reputable academic centers on the effects of the drug on deaths
from heart attacks show variable, unconvincing results.

The side effects of the drug are numerous and the
long-term safety of the product is uncertain, as is
always the case with newly marketed products. Nausea, rashes, and occasional serious blood disorders
have been reported.

Wise physicians will shy away from prescribing
Atromid® and will insist instead that the patient's
weight and diet be controlled. This drug will need to
be investigated much further before it will be known
if its therapeutic usefulness outweighs its potential
dangers.

ATROPINE SULFATE, U.S.P.

Doctors often overlook atropine sulfate or belladonna tincture in treating a variety of gastrointestinal
disorders ranging from peptic ulcer to "nervous stomach." Atropine is the active principle in belladonna
tincture.

Atropine is the prototype drug for blocking para-
sympathetic nerves to the stomach, which stimulate
acid secretion, and those to the gut, which stimulate
motility. However, doctors more commonly prescribe
drugs with atropine-*like* effects, which are newer and
more expensive but have not been convincingly
shown to be clinically superior to atropine or belladonna. Two of the best known are Pro-Banthine®
and Bentyl®, discussed elsewhere.

Considering how frequently patients with gastrointestinal symptoms present themselves, neither belladonna tincture nor atropine sulfate is much prescribed. The reason is that no one advertises and promotes these good, inexpensive drugs.

See Atropine Sulfate and Belladonna Tincture in the Price Lists.

AZO GANTRISIN®   Sulfisoxazole, U.S.P.   0.5 g
                            phenazopyridine hydro-
                                chloride   50.0 mg
  See Gantrisin®, Pyridium®.

The addition of phenazopyridine (Pyridium®), an orange dye that allegedly numbs the bladder, to the anti-infection drug sulfisoxazole, is of questionable value. In treating bladder infections and other urinary infections that are painful, phenazopyridine is only useful as a placebo. The patient takes a tablet and the next time he urinates his urine is orange-brown; he then "knows" that the drug is doing something! The dye is very expensive and increases the wholesale cost of sulfisoxazole by at least one-third. In the opinion of this *Handbook,* Azo Gantrisin® is an irrational product. When treating common acute urinary tract infections, the doctor merely has to inform the patient that it will take 12 to 24 hours before the anti-infection drug begins to diminish his discomfort. Such reassurance is worth ten times the cost of the placebo dye.

Yet, advertising, fixed prescribing habits, and too little awareness of cost kept Azo Gantrisin® the 123rd most-prescribed product in the United States, well within the top 200 in 1974.

AZULFIDINE®   salicylazosulfapyridine

Azulfidine® is a sulfonamide conventionally used to treat mild ulcerative colitis, a disease characterized by recurrent or chronic diarrhea. The drug does lessen the number of bacteria inhabiting the large bowel (although no drug known can "sterilize" the large bowel or even approach this feat). Poorly absorbed sulfonamide drugs other than Azulfidine® often used, in the past, for this purpose included the sulfathiazoles succinylsulfathiazole and phthalylsulfathiazole, which have been called "ineffective" by the National Academy of Sciences and subsequently by the FDA. Yet, Azulfidine® has inexplicably escaped proscription.

All of the poorly absorbed sulfonamides are converted in the bowel to more readily absorbed sulfonamides that cause the not uncommon side effects of headache, rashes, nausea, and blood disorders. The drug Azulfidine® also imparts a striking orange color to the urine—a placebo effect. This is caused by the same dye as in Azo Gantrisin®.

BELLADONNA TINCTURE, U.S.P.
See Tincture of Belladonna.

Belladonna Tincture, U.S.P., is the official name, but doctors usually refer to it as "Tincture of Belladonna" or "Belladonna."

BENADRYL®   Diphenhydramine Hydro-
                               chloride, U.S.P.
See Antihistamines.

This is the antihistamine most commonly used to combat nausea and seasickness. Major side effects are drowsiness and, as with other antihistamines, a dry mouth. It is readily available to all pharmacies by its official name at a lower cost than as Benadryl®, and should therefore be prescribed and purchased as diphenhydramine hydrochloride if more than a few doses are to be ordered at one time.

The pharmacologically active part of the diphenhydramine hydrochloride molecule is identical with the active part of the Dramamine® molecule, but it takes 50 milligrams of the latter to be as powerful as 25 milligrams of the former. Dramamine® is a brand

name for a different "salt" of diphenhydramine. For
reasons unknown to the *Handbook,* Dramamine® is
available as a non-prescription drug and is considerably more expensive than diphenhydramine unless
it is purchased in large lots under its official name,
dimenhydrinate.

Benadryl® is also used, as are the other antihistamines, for mild sedation and in minor allergies.

BENDECTIN®

Dicyclomine Hydro-	
chloride, N.F.	10 mg
doxylamine succinate	10 mg
Pyridoxine Hydro-	
chloride	10 mg
(with a special thick	
coating on the tablet)	

The manufacturer here has made changes in the
contents of the product in recent years but has not
changed the brand name for the mixture, which is
presently classified as only "possibly effective" (very
likely "probably ineffective"). Prudent doctors do not
give medications to pregnant women with morning
sickness!

Dicyclomine is better known as Bentyl®, just another atropine-like drug. Doxylamine is just another
antihistamine with all of the potential adverse effects
of others in its class. Pyridoxine is a vitamin that is
probably not harmful. However, when a pregnant
woman needs *a* vitamin, she must be assumed to need
all vitamins, and Decavitamins, N.F., is preferred.

It is simply incredible that physicians have not
heeded the warning of thalidomide. To provide doxylamine and dicyclomine to a newly pregnant woman
prompts these remarks:

1. Doctors are as busy as ever getting patients "off
their backs" by writing a prescription. (Many doctors
probably prescribe Bendectin® without knowing that
its contents has been changed only recently. They have

been so busy ordering Bendectin® that, in 1973, it was the 119th most-prescribed drug product sold in the U.S.A.)

2. Morning nausea is a tribulation suffered for millennia. It is self-limiting almost all of the time. Rarely is the vomiting prolonged and severe; and in these cases hospitalization is in order to provide intravenous fluids to prevent and/or treat dehydration. This is what to say to women with morning sickness in order to reassure them.

3. Doctors who prescribe more than some vitamins and iron for early-pregnant women must have nerves of steel. In this litigious era these men (and women) doctors still seem to be oblivious to the possibility of fetal deformities cropping up spontaneously. Why they should invite retrospective suspicion in their direction by the unfortunate mothers of deformed infants is beyond our comprehension.

4. Finally, look at the cost of Bendectin®. It is an outrage that a probably ineffective drug should command such a high price.

BENTYL®   Dicyclomine Hydrochloride, N.F.

See Atropine Sulfate, U.S.P.; Tincture of Belladonna (Belladonna Tincture, U.S.P.).

This drug fits in the category of antispasmodics and is prescribed primarily for ulcer patients and those with "irritable bowels." Related to atropine and belladonna in its effects, this synthetic product has side effects including dryness of the mouth, constipation, trouble with urination, and occasional trouble with sexual functioning in men.

As recommended previously, atropine or tincture of belladonna do as well with less cost to the patient. Bentyl® has recently reached the ranks of the 200 most-prescribed drugs in the U.S. primarily because of a large advertising campaign on the part of its manufacturer. It has no distinct advantages over the other synthetic antispasmodics or the fundamental substances atropine and belladonna. It has a disadvantage because it is newer and less is known about its possible long-term toxicity.

Bentyl® was the 176th most-prescribed drug in 1973.

BENTYL® WITH   Dicyclomine Hydrochloride,
PHENOBARBITAL   N.F., with Phenobar-
                             bital, U.S.P.   15 mg

This fixed-combination product combines the excellent sedative phenobarbital with dicyclomine. Mild sedatives such as phenobarbital are given patients with stomach difficulties since anxiety is so often related. However, fixed combinations do not allow for the adjustment of doses of the individual components independently. Use of fixed combinations such as this is, therefore, not recommended. The necessary dose of atropine or belladonna should be determined and, if sedation is necessary, a separate sedative dose of phenobarbital be given. The savings in using atropine and phenobarbital as opposed to Bentyl® with phenobarbital in a fixed-combination product are enormous.

Like its mother compound, Bentyl®, the new fixed combination, Bentyl® with phenobarbital, just recently entered the top 200 drugs (ranking 200th) prescribed in the U.S. in 1973 as a result of expensive and extensive advertising. When this *Handbook* decries the artificially induced market for superfluous and unnecessary drug products, it refers among many others to Bentyl® with phenobarbital.

This product is available generically; see the Price Lists.

BENYLIN®   Diphenhydramine Hydro-
EXPECTORANT   chloride, U.S.P.   80 mg

Ammonium Chloride,
   U.S.P.   720 mg
Sodium Citrate,
   U.S.P.   300 mg
Chloroform, N.F.   120 mg
   menthol   6 mg
   alcohol 5% (1.5 cc)
      (per 30 ml, or 2 tbsps)

See Antihistamines; Codeine Sulfate, N.F.; Codeine Phosphate, U.S.P.; Cough Remedies; Dextromethorphan Hydrobromide, N.F.

This is a cough mixture which is widely prescribed but whose purpose is an enigma. Diphenhydramine is an antihistamine whose side effect is to *dry up* secretions. Ammonium chloride's effect is to *loosen* secretions. The citrate is a flavored pharmaceutic aid. The small dose of chloroform, traditionally an ingredient of proprietary medications, might possibly act as a carminative—that is, help to expel gas—but proof is lacking. Menthol serves to make the preparation taste cool, a placebo effect. One and a half cubic centimeters (⅓ teaspoonful) of alcohol is unlikely to stimulate either euphoria or riotous behavior. A hot drink serves to loosen a cough pretty well, and an over-the-counter preparation of dextromethorphan will moderate ordinary degrees of cough. Patients who are racked with severe cough usually require codeine, but a prescription is needed for that.

BETAMETHASONE VALERATE, N.F.
   See Valisone®.

BROMPHENIRAMINE MALEATE, N.F.
   See Dimetane®.

BUTABARBITAL (SODIUM BUTABARBITAL, U.S.P.)
   See Butisol®.

BUTAZOLIDIN®   Phenylbutazone, U.S.P.

Phenylbutazone has anti-inflammatory and analgesic effects and is a very useful drug for certain
forms of arthritis and acute gouty attacks. The drug
is neither the preferred drug for these conditions
nor should it be used for sprains and other inflammations that normally are self-limiting.

The toxicity of Butazolidin® militates against its
being considered a first-choice drug. Doctors are well
aware that side effects include bleeding peptic ulcers
and serious (and sometimes fatal) abnormalities of
the white and red blood cells, but are less aware
that the drug also causes marked salt and water
retention, which can produce swollen legs or worsen
a high blood pressure problem. For these reasons, and
because the side effects are thought to be more severe
in older people, the drug should not be given to
elderly patients.

Phenylbutazone may work by "bumping" naturally
occurring hydrocortisone from its plasma-protein
carrier, making more natural hydrocortisone available
to act on tissues. This may also explain some of the
side effects, since bleeding peptic ulcer and salt retention are also side effects of prolonged and excessive
hydrocortisone treatment (but practically never when
the latter is merely used on isolated patches of skin).

BUTAZOLIDIN® ALKA   Phenylbutazone,
                        U.S.P.   100 mg
                        Dried Aluminum Hy-
                        droxide Gel,
                        U.S.P.   100 mg
                        Magnesium Trisili-
                        cate, U.S.P.   150 mg
See Butazolidin®.

This mixture was designed to appeal to those
physicians who want to prescribe phenylbutazone
(Butazolidin®) but fear a possible toxic side effect
of ulceration of the stomach or small intestine. While

the antacids provided in this combination product may mask the pain or discomfort of ulcers or gastric irritation, there is little evidence to suggest that these antacids in this even more expensive form of Butazolidin® prevent ulcers from occurring.

In recent years the popularity of this questionably more useful Butazolidin® has soared, ranking among the top 150 most-prescribed items for patients of all ages in 1967; it ranked 28th in both 1972 and 1973.

BUTISOL®   Sodium Butabarbital, U.S.P.
(BUTISOL SODIUM®)

Called by an easily remembered name, Butisol® is nothing more than the effective, old-fashioned barbiturate sedative butabarbital. Butabarbital offers little clinical advantage over phenobarbital, but if a doctor or patient feels that it does, it should be prescribed and bought by generic name. (See the generic equivalent, Butabarbital, in the Price Lists.)

CAMPHORATED TINCTURE OF OPIUM
See Paregoric, U.S.P. (Camphorated Tincture of Opium).

CEPHALEXIN MONOHYDRATE
See Keflex®.

CHLORAL HYDRATE, U.S.P.

One of the oldest and safest sedatives, excellent as a "tranquilizer" during the day (at a dose of 500 milligrams every 3 to 6 hours) and as a sleep-inducer in larger doses, chloral hydrate is available in capsule form from a large number of distributors at small cost to the patient. Many distributors sell the drug in liquid form (as syrup). One gallon of syrup contains approximately 800 teaspoonfuls (500 milligrams per teaspoonful), and cost to the druggist can be as little as a few pennies or less per dose. U.S.P. grade chloral hydrate crystals are very inexpensive, so large clinics that dispense the drug should consider making up their own syrup.

Chloral hydrate as well as many other prescription sleep preparations have been displaced in the past few years by a new sleeping pill, flurazepam, sold under the brand name Dalmane®. The advantage of Dalmane® that is advanced in the medical literature is that it preserves REM, or rapid-eye-movement, sleep; this stage of sleep is thought to be the most restful. Interestingly, of all the other common sleep preparations, chloral hydrate is the only one to preserve this stage of sleep, and it does so at a fraction of the cost.

Side effects from chronic use of chloral hydrate are few, but include occasional stomach irritation, smarting of the eyes, and a not unpleasant but acidic taste. Like all sleeping pills, it is presumably subject to abuse and overusage.* Chloral hydrate also interferes with the effect of warfarin (Coumadin®), a drug taken to prolong clotting time, and the two should not be used simultaneously. (See Dalmane®.)

CHLORDIAZEPOXIDE HYDROCHLORIDE, N.F.
See Librium®.

CHLOROTHIAZIDE, N.F.
See Diuril®.

CHLORPHENIRAMINE MALEATE, U.S.P.
See Chlor-Trimeton®; Teldrin®.

CHLORPROMAZINE HYDROCHLORIDE, U.S.P.
See Thorazine®.

---

* Suicide with chloral hydrate must be difficult. A dose large enough to kill an adult would probably cause vomiting.

CHLORPROPAMIDE, U.S.P.
  See Diabinese®.

CHLORTHALIDONE, U.S.P.
  See Hygroton®.

CHLOR-TRIMETON®   Chlorpheniramine Maleate, U.S.P.
  See Antihistamines.

Chlorpheniramine is an excellent antihistamine that many patients with seasonal hay fever and nasal congestion like because it may make the patient less sleepy than Benadryl® (diphenhydramine) or other antihistamines. But it is not economical to buy it as Chlor-Trimeton® or Chlor-Trimeton® Repetabs®. It should be purchased instead by its generic name, chlorpheniramine maleate, which is less expensive. (See the Price Lists.) Repetabs® are reputedly long-acting, but generally are not recommended because their longer action is uneven and their additional cost is unnecessary.

Among the various antihistamines, effects are similar. It matters very little which among the several single-product preparations you purchase of the numerous ones available. Polaramine® (dexchlorpheniramine), Dimetane® (brompheniramine), and others are clinically equivalent to chlorpheniramine, but more expensive.

Chlor-Trimeton® was the 42nd most popular name written on prescription pads by doctors in 1973.

CLEOCIN®   clindamycin hydrochloride
  See Dynapen®.

Clindamycin, sold as Cleocin® by its only manufacturer, Upjohn, is an antibiotic that has very specific and very limited uses. Unfortunately, the drug has been vastly overused and overprescribed in its initial years on the market. (See Addenda.)

The manufacturers have recommended clindamycin for minor upper respiratory infections, lower respiratory tract infections (chronic bronchitis and pneumonias), skin and soft-tissue infections, and dental infections. Most of these infections are caused by bacteria that can be eradicated as well by one or another form of penicillin or by tetracycline with less cost and less possible toxicity. If a patient is allergic to penicillin, clindamycin is *still* not the preferred drug; rather, erythromycin would be the drug of choice since it causes fewer side effects and is considerably less expensive. In severe infections caused by unusual organisms, including some that grow only in oxygen-free environments, clindamycin is probably the drug to use; but such infections are often severe enough to require hospitalization.

Infections caused by staphylococci, often involving bone, skin, or soft tissue, can be treated with clindamycin in patients allergic to penicillin G, or when the staphylococcus is penicillin-resistant. Otherwise, dicloxacillin is the treatment of choice.

In general, clindamycin should only be used in *rare* instances, and definitely not in simple respiratory infections and dental infections. Cost and effective action are the major considerations, but serious side effects have also been reported. The most serious of these include severe diarrhea and colitis with bleeding from the bowel, and rashes. Deaths have been reported. *In a recent study* approximately 21 percent of people developed diarrhea while taking the drug, and 10 percent had inflammation of the bowel wall.*

Cleocin® is obviously a drug with limited usefulness, yet it has soared from relative anonymity to the 84th and 49th most frequently prescribed drug in 1972 and 1973, respectively. Advertising and promotion to doctors are responsible for this irresponsible overuse.

Cleocin® costs a small fortune compared to penicillin G (or V) or tetracycline, especially if these drugs are prescribed and dispensed as generic drugs.

* *Medical Letter, 16*:73–74 (August 30, 1974).

CLINDAMYCIN HYDROCHLORIDE
See Cleocin®.

CLOFIBRATE
See Atromid-S®.

CLORAZEPATE DIPOTASSIUM
See Tranxene®.

CODEINE SULFATE, N.F.
CODEINE PHOSPHATE, U.S.P.

The manufacture and sale of this narcotic substance and its price are controlled by the United States government. Despite the ominous categorization of this drug as a class II narcotic, it is one of the most useful drugs available for both pain control and cough suppression.

While Darvon® compounds of various descriptions, Demerol®, and Percodan®, as well as codeine in combination with acetaminophen (Tylenol®) and APC-like preparations (Empirin®), all ranked within the 200 most-prescribed drugs, codeine in its cheapest form did not. Yet, codeine in adequate dosage taken with 2 aspirin tablets rivals any of the above preparations in its ability to kill pain.

An adequate dose of codeine is often 60 or 120 milligrams every few hours. The cost of such an aspirin and codeine combination is far less than that of Darvon® preparation, oral Demerol®, or Percodan®.

Similarly, codeine is an excellent cough suppressant taken in smaller doses. While dextromethorphan is preferred, codeine works well and is available usually for far less than the extravagant concoctions prescribed so often by physicians. Of course, coughs have their place, especially in bacterial pneumonias, where they help clear the accumulated materials from the lungs. But, in viral illnesses and in the usual cold, cough suppression is helpful for restful sleep and comfort. Cough suppression doses are 15 or 30 milligrams every 3 or 4 hours.

Side effects of codeine are not uncommon, and include constipation and occasional dependence. Thus, codeine is likely to cause habituation if used to excess for prolonged periods; but rarely is addiction a problem within 2 or 3 weeks. The addictive potential of narcotic-containing drugs like Demerol® and Percodan® is worse.

There is no known advantage of APC preparations with codeine over aspirin and codeine alone. Tylenol® lacks the anti-inflammatory effects of aspirin and is more expensive, unless shopped for and bought as acetaminophen. Therefore, aspirin and codeine is a better preparation for all except those who cannot abide the side effects of aspirin.

COLCHICINE, U.S.P.

Colchicine is the drug of choice for the treatment of acute gout. A very old drug with a complicated molecular structure, it comes from the bulb of the autumn crocus—whose leaves appear in spring and flowers in late summer. It is not patented and need not be costly. See Colchicine, U.S.P., in the Price Lists.

Persons with sudden, painful attacks of gout nearly always experience relief if they take 0.5 milligrams of colchicine every hour. A limit of 8 doses is set for any single attack to avoid possible toxicity, but 8 doses are rarely required; usually the attack abates by the third or fourth dose. Colchicine causes watery diarrhea with cramps; a good way to stave off this effect is to take a teaspoonful of paregoric with each dose.

The possible serious toxic effects of colchicine are kidney and bone-marrow damage, but these are highly unlikely to result from only 8 doses. In the rare case where a gout attack persists after 8 doses, Butazolidin® or Indocin® might be useful. People with gout sometimes have a premonition of an impending attack and, by taking 1 or 2 doses of colchicine, can prevent a moderate attack. Some take colchicine regularly, 0.5 milligrams twice daily, a routine said to be "preventive." It is emphasized that colchicine affords only symptomatic relief and fails to affect the underlying abnormality in gout.

It is fascinating to reflect on how earlier generations discovered the effectiveness of certain plants in treating disease. Such specifics as opium, digitalis, reserpine, and ergot were discovered in this way, to name a few, and so was colchicine. Preparations of the autumn crocus were used in Europe and Asia Minor in the sixth century for treating joint pains, and its specificity for gout was recognized in 1763. Benjamin Franklin had gout, and he is reputed to be the one who introduced the use of the drug into America. But the active chemical in the autumn crocus that gives it its unique pharmacologic property was not isolated in pure form until 1820.

How colchicine works its benefit in gout has been partially elucidated only recently by Seegmiller and colleagues at the National Institutes of Health in Bethesda, Maryland. When uric acid crystals precipitate out of solution (often in the base joint of the big toe), white blood cells swarm into the area to "eat them up" (phagocytosis). In the process, these cells get much of their energy by using a kind of metabolism which temporarily requires little oxygen; they make less carbon dioxide and water than do oxygen-breathing cells. Instead, they make a lot of lactic acid, which diffuses out of them into the local joint tissues, and the resulting acidity causes inflammation: redness, swelling, heat, and pain. Colchicine prevents phagocytosis and thus aborts the attack. Certain obvious questions have not yet been answered: What happens then to the uric acid crystals deposited in the joint? And is it ill-advised to give colchicine to a person with infection elsewhere in the body? Will colchicine interfere with its resolution, which is normally due in part to white-blood-cell phagocytosing action on bacteria? These would be good research projects.

Aside from treatment of acute attacks with colchicine, gout is well worth treating prophylactically over the long term to avoid insidious, life-endangering deposits of uric acid crystals in the kidneys. To accomplish this, probenecid (Benemid®) is the drug of choice. See Probenecid, U.S.P.

COMBID® SPANSULES® *	Prochlorperazine	
	Maleate, U.S.P.	10 mg
	isopropamide iodide	5 mg

Combid® is a preparation for ulcer, irritable bowel, and functional diarrhea therapy. Combining an antinausea sedative (prochlorperazine) with an atropine-like drug (isopropamide) is a traditional way to treat these disorders, but the choice of 15 milligrams of phenobarbital three or four times daily with a 0.4 milligram atropine sulfate tablet would work as well in most cases and at significant savings to the patient.

Spansules® are not acceptable to the *United States Pharmacopeia* or the *National Formulary* because gut transit time is too unpredictable to reproducibly provide 10 or 12 hours of drug availability. And the multiple little granules that make up a Spansule®, because of increased production costs and other reasons, add considerably to the retail cost of the product. Also, prochlorperazine, because it belongs to the so-called phenothiazine class of drugs (such as Thorazine® and its imitations), is inherently more toxic than small doses of phenobarbital.

COMPAZINE®   Prochlorperazine Maleate, U.S.P.
See Antihistamines; Benadryl®; Phenergan®.

Compazine®, a member of the phenothiazine family, is most commonly used as an antinausea drug. Many prescriptions for antinauseants are unnecessary since most bouts of nausea and vomiting are short-lived

---

* The word "Spansule®" is a clever trademarked neologism for a capsule that is supposed to release its active ingredient over a span of time.

and self-limiting. Persistent nausea and/or vomiting is reason for careful evaluation of the cause. Infections, drugs, X-ray or cobalt therapy, early pregnancy, alcoholic gastritis, painful stimuli, emotional disorders, or motion, as well as other conditions, may all cause nausea. When possible and if necessary, the cause of the nausea should be treated. If no obvious cause is known, persistent nausea or vomiting is reason for hospitalization.

For chronic nausea, phenothiazines usually bring relief. However, the possible toxicity of phenothiazines (jaundice, decreased production of white blood cells, Parkinsonian symptoms, rashes) ought to serve as a damper on the enthusiasm of doctors for using them in minor illnesses. The non-phenothiazine antinauseants are the drugs of first choice, even though they may have a less pronounced effect and shorter action: antihistamines, such as diphenhydramine (Benadryl®), are preferred as first-line drugs. Promethazine (Phenergan®), a phenothiazine with many antihistamine properties, is an excellent second-line drug; one or two 25 milligram suppositories of promethazine is a highly effective, safer alternative to Compazine® for helping vomiting patients for a few hours.

Drug cost is not really a factor in acute cases, where only a few doses are requested. It becomes important when patients, for whatever reasons, must take Compazine® in large amounts over long periods of time.

CONJUGATED ESTROGENS, U.S.P.
See Premarin®.

CORDRAN®   Flurandrenolide, N.F.
See Hydrocortisone Cream, U.S.P.

This very effective topical steroid, like most others, is expensive, especially for use in treating chronic skin diseases that require daily application of a drug for long periods. For such chronic conditions, it may be useful and economical to find a pharmacist who is willing to prepare either a ½ or 1 percent hydrocortisone cream. See Hydrocortisone Cream for a way to purchase this inexpensively. While it is true that flurandrenolide is sometimes effective when hydrocortisone is not, the latter is usually adequate if rubbed in well.

**CORTISPORIN®
OINTMENT**

polymixin B 5,000 units
zinc bacitracin 400 units
neomycin sulfate 5 mg
Hydrocortisone, 10 mg (1%)
  U.S.P.
white petrolatum
(per gram ointment)

See Mycolog®.

This ointment is a mixture of three antibiotics and a steroid. These topical antibiotic mixtures are intended by the manufacturers and physicians who use them to improve wound healing and resolution of skin infections. There is very little evidence, however, to suggest that this preparation or others like it (*e.g.,* Mycolog®) are effective in shortening wound-healing time or in preventing skin infection. Minor cuts, bruises, abrasions, and small infections involving the skin usually heal without antibiotic or steroid treatment. If serious skin infections exist, antibiotics should be given by mouth or by injections (but preferably by mouth). In burns, orally administered antibiotics can be very useful in preventing infection.

The side effects of each of the four components of Cortisporin® Ointment are numerous. Consider only one component, neomycin, which has been shown to cause skin reactions in 6 to 8 percent of users, deafness if repeatedly applied to deep wounds, and kidney disease, and may make the use of certain related life-saving antibiotics impossible because of similar toxicities.

The addition of hydrocortisone to antibiotics applied to the skin is not useful. An excellent study comparing a steroid skin ointment with a steroid-plus-antibiotic skin preparation showed no difference between the two in 27 patients with inflammations and infections involving the skin.*

COUGH REMEDIES

See Antihistamines; Codeine Sulfate, N.F.; Codeine Phosphate, U.S.P.; Dextromethorphan Hydrobromide, N.F.

There are more prescription products available for treatment of coughing than for any other symptom. Furthermore, over-the-counter (non-prescription) items abound. These products usually contain mixtures of drugs in a sweet syrup.

Most coughs are associated with viral infections of the upper respiratory tract and these infections are usually self-limited, brief in duration, and do *not* require medications. In fact, the cough reflex is a protective mechanism that helps rid the respiratory tract of secretions.

When coughing is very severe and troublesome, when little secretion is being produced, or when coughing leads to pain, codeine is the most useful drug. Codeine acts not only to reduce the cough reflex but has mild pain-relieving and sedative effects as well. Codeine is available either as a tablet or as terpin hydrate and codeine elixir. While codeine does come under the narcotic drug category, its potential for abuse is low and physical dependence is uncommon. Codeine is among the cheapest drugs available.

The common throat tickle or throat irritation can be treated with candy drops.

Medical Letter (*13*:9-11; 1971), perhaps the physician's best practical reference on drug prescribing, comments on the multitude of cough remedies as follows:

* C. M. Davis, et al., *Journal of the American Medical Association, 203*:298 (1968).

. . . there is no justification for using four or more drugs simultaneously, some having opposing effects on the cough reflex. Multiple fixed-ratio drugs also multiply adverse effects and prevent flexibility in dosages of the individual drugs. Another objection to multiple drug mixtures is the increased risk of interactions between drugs in the mixtures with other drugs simultaneously prescribed. . . .

There are no reports of well-controlled trials showing that these multiple-drug preparations, which frequently contain suboptimal and ineffective concentrations of useful drugs, are superior to placebos, candy demulcents, or selected single drugs in controlling a troublesome cough or in improving expectoration.

If thick, tenacious secretions are a problem, hot drinks should be encouraged and inhalation of steam or cool mists is sometimes helpful. Drugs like glyceryl guaiacolate (Robitussin®) present in many cough preparations have NOT been proved effective as expectorants. In fact, guaiacolates are derivatives of the obsolete compound creosote, used in the primitive days of modern medicine for treatment of tuberculosis.

In sum, only the most severe coughs should be treated, and codeine is the cheapest and most effective drug. Candies are best for dealing with throat irritation of colds. And hot drinks are the most effective expectorant for the garden variety of viral illnesses that comprise the great majority of colds.

It is an unfortunate fact that cigarette smokers, most of whom have chronic bronchitis from the habit, are prone to develop "chest colds" whenever they have a common upper respiratory infection. (So do children.) Adults who are known to have chronic bronchitis should have a supply of a good, broad-spectrum antibiotic on hand (tetracycline is the agent of choice) to start taking immediately when a common cold begins in order to prevent secondary bacterial infections in the lungs. These are marked by an increase in the amount of sputum raised and a change in its color from clear to yellow or green. Every time a smoker with bronchitis goes through this ordeal of a "chest cold" he is, aside from being likely to lose time from work, probably suffering from small patches of bronchopneumonia scattered throughout the lungs. Usually these infections resolve themselves spontaneously, but as this happens multiple small scars are left. The scars derange the fine architecture of the lung, leaving the patient with a little less respiratory reserve than he had after recovery from his previous "chest cold." Unchecked and unprevented, each episode brings him closer to the day when, as a respiratory cripple, he is said to have "emphysema." "Emphysema" and "chronic bronchitis" are two different words used to describe the same class of patients. Death for them is slow, expensive, and miserable.

COUMADIN®   Sodium Warfarin, U.S.P.

Coumadin® is a "blood-thinner" or, more correctly, an anticoagulant. At present, the usefulness of this drug is proved in conditions such as severe thrombophlebitis, and in certain heart diseases.

While several different anticoagulant drugs are available, only Coumadin® is very widely used and remains the largest-selling drug of its kind. Coumadin®, not warfarin, is the everyday word for physicians, and this means that price competition is limited and that Coumadin® can remain high-priced. Other companies could produce warfarin, but it would cost too much to alert physicians and doctors to its availability. Dicumarol®, another and older drug with the same effects, is sold by many companies and therefore can be purchased for much less. (Although Dicumarol® is a trademarked name, it is a curious fact that many companies sell it by this name. The *Handbook* does not know why.)

The side effects of warfarin are minimal, with one important exception. Warfarin and any other anticoagulant can cause spontaneous bleeding. By depleting certain clotting substances in the blood, the drug prolongs the clotting process. Careful regulation of dosage must be made at frequent intervals by monitoring "prothrombin time" with blood tests in order to make certain that the blood's clotting factors have not been so much depleted as to predispose the patient to serious bleeding.

Coumadin® and Dicumarol® metabolism can be severely affected by the simultaneous administration of other drugs in such a way that their anticoagulation effect goes out of control. Some of these medications may include chloral hydrate, clofibrate (Atromid-S®), phenylbutazone and oxyphenbutazone (Butazolidin® and Tandearil®), and diphenylhydantoin (Dilantin®).

The importance of careful dosage control is demonstrated by widespread use of the drug as rat poison; lack of odor and taste makes it easy to put large amounts of warfarin in bait attractive to rodents. Its lethality, of course, resides in its ability to cause widespread spontaneous hemorrhages. Rats with excessive internal hemorrhage develop a craving thirst for water. They relinquish their hidden indoor nests to venture outside in search of water, and usually die outside of buildings. This is advantageous to those who wish to exterminate rodents—they then do not have to deal with the bodies.

CYANOCOBALAMIN
See Vitamin B₁₂.

CYCLANDELATE
See Cyclospasmol®.

CYCLOSPASMOL®   cyclandelate

Cyclospasmol® is recommended by the manufacturer, according to the package insert, as "adjunctive therapy" for vascular disorders causing decreased blood flow to the legs, arms, and brain; thrombophlebitis; leg cramps at night; and Raynaud's phenomenon. Raynaud's phenomenon may be described as blanching of the fingers or hands in response to cold and may be associated with one of several arthritis-like diseases but most commonly has no serious significance; it is more common in women than men.

While cyclandelate has the effect of relaxing the smooth muscles lining medium-sized and small blood vessels, the evidence that the drug works to improve *any* of the conditions for which it is sold and advertised is poor at best. The AMA Council on Drugs finds the evidence for its usefulness provided in studies and articles "unacceptable." * The FDA has evaluated it as only "possibly effective," which means that it is probably ineffective. In 1973, Cyclospasmol® was the 191st most-prescribed drug in this country.

CYPROHEPTADINE
See Periactin®.

DALMANE®   flurazepam hydrochloride
See Chloral Hydrate U.S.P.; Nembutal®; Seconal®.

Dalmane® is a sleeping pill that is chemically related to diazepam (Valium®) and chlordiazepoxide (Librium®) and manufactured by the same firm, Roche Laboratories. It shares with these products rather substantial price tags and massive advertising efforts.

Flurazepam is an effective sleeping pill, works rapidly, and has a prolonged action—making a good night's sleep likely. Advertisements claim that it causes less "hangover" than other such agents. But other drugs that are much cheaper often do as well. Barbiturates, such as secobarbital (Seconal®) or pentobarbital (Nembutal®), and chloral hydrate usually are perfectly adequate as sleeping pills and cost a small fraction of the price that flurazepam does. In patients likely to abuse sleeping pills, there is little evidence to suggest that flurazepam will not be abused

* *AMA Drug Evaluations*, 2nd edn., page 28.

like the rest. There is, however, the suggestion that flurazepam is less likely to be a successful suicidal agent if taken in large doses; furthermore, flurazepam does not interact with warfarin, as do the barbiturates and chloral hydrate.

DARVOCET-N®	propoxyphene	
	napsylate	50 mg
	acetaminophen	325 mg
DARVON®	Propoxyphene Hydrochloride, U.S.P.	
DARVON® COMPOUND-65	Propoxyphene Hydrochloride, U.S.P	65.0 mg
	Aspirin, U.S.P.	227.0 mg
	Phenacetin, U.S.P.	162.0 mg
	caffeine	32.4 mg
DARVON-N®	propoxyphene napsylate	
DARVON-N® WITH A.S.A.®	propoxyphene	
	napsylate	100 mg
	aspirin	325 mg

Darvon® and its variants include at least 9 or 10 different products that together comprise the largest-selling prescription pain reliever. Darvon® Compound-65 ranked 3rd among the most prescribed prescription drugs in 1973. Eli Lilly, who makes Darvon® in all its various formulations, has only Hoffmann-LaRoche (Roche Laboratories) as rival for sales of single-drug products. Roche makes Valium® and Librium®.

Propoxyphene is a mild pain killer. The napsylate (Darvon-N®) salt was more recently introduced, and is more stable than the hydrochloride (Darvon®). A 100 milligram dose of the napsylate provides precisely the same amount of propoxyphene as a 65 milligram dose of the hydrochloride. The effects of both preparations, therapeutic and adverse, are similar, so separate discussions are not necessary.

Most careful studies of propoxyphene using the most reliable techniques of drug study show it to be no more effective than a placebo in its usual dose and in no way as effective as either aspirin or acetaminophen alone. Most drug experts agree that 32 milligrams of Darvon® or 50 milligrams of Darvon-N® does no more than a placebo pill,* and an excellent study of cancer patients with pain showed that even 65 milligrams of Darvon® was no better than a placebo.†

Side effects from Darvon® alone are usually mild, but an ever-increasing number of overdoses are being reported, and the effects of an overdose resemble those of narcotics. Dependence, usually milder than that with narcotics but similar in nature, is seen. The drug is well known among adolescents and is widely abused. Several deaths have been reported.**

Perhaps the most important "side effect" of all is its cost. The cost of simple aspirin to the pharmacist is usually less than one-tenth that of Darvon® Compound-65.

Darvon® in its various forms is unquestionably among the most popular drugs taken by patients. Patients are often eloquent about its excellent pain-relieving effects. Certainly, the gray-and-pink Pulvule®, which is a trademark for Lilly's capsules, has come to have wide placebo effect; and many physicians simply cannot convince a long-time user that it is not better than aspirin or acetaminophen (Tylenol®).

The combination products of Darvon® make sense only insofar as they contain effective drugs in addition to the Darvon® or Darvon-N® products. Darvocet-N® contains acetaminophen, which is an effective agent in relieving pain and lowering fevers. Darvon®

---

* R. R. Miller, et al., *Journal of the American Medical Association,* 213:996 (1970).

† C. G. Moertel, et al., *New England Journal of Medicine,* 286:813 (1972).

** W. Q. Sturner and J. C. Garriott, *JAMA,* 223:1125 (1973).

Compound-65 contains APC, or aspirin in combination with phenacetin and caffeine (a long-standing pain reliever*). Finally, Darvon-N® with A.S.A.® contains nothing more than Lilly's brand of aspirin.

For effective pain relief, as with severe toothaches or other pains that keep one awake, codeine sulfate, 30 to 60 milligrams, plus a couple of aspirin tablets is recommended. Despite their devotees, both among physicians who prescribe them and patients who ingest them, Darvon® products are of dubious efficacy and should be avoided because of their expense.

DBI-TD®   phenformin hydrochloride

As an oral blood-sugar-lowering drug most commonly used in elderly diabetics, DBI® or DBI-TD® (a timed-release preparation) probably should never be used. All of the oral medications for treating diabetics have come into disrepute primarily because they increase the probability of heart attacks and other cardiovascular problems. Like Orinase®, Diabinese®, and Tolinase®, DBI-TD® should never be used to treat severe cases of diabetes, juvenile diabetes, or any complications of diabetes, or prophylactically to treat diabetes patients undergoing stressful experiences such as a severe infection or an operation.

Before any therapeutic agent is used in mild "diabetes," † serious attempts at weight control, dietary discretion, and regular daily exercise are of the first order. If they fail to lower the blood sugar, insulin therapy may be initiated.**

* In the view of many authorities on therapeutics, APC is an irrational combination.

† Everyone should know that merely lowering a mildly elevated blood-sugar level is probably a useless exercise. Lowering the blood-sugar level to normal is like a religion for many people, including many doctors. (See Addenda.)

** It cannot be said with any certainty that so-called "maturity-onset diabetes" is properly classified as true diabetes. If any figures exist to show that people with "maturity-onset diabetes" (who are usually overweight) live less long than a

It is the opinion of the *Handbook* that oral blood-sugar-lowering agents are poisonous and should not be used. Should these agents be used with the full knowledge (as of February 1975) that the risk of death from a heart attack is probably increased thereby, the doctor may be putting himself in a position where he could be sued for malpractice.

It has been said that DBI® and DBI-TD® (phenformin), because they commonly cause a metallic taste in the mouth and take away appetite, can help a patient lose weight. One should be very wary about long-term administration of a foreign substance whose side effect is to take away appetite.

A recent ten-year study by the University Group Diabetes Program involving approximately a dozen medical schools and clinics has demonstrated that DBI-TD® is likely poisonous in that it decreases the length of life in those who take it regularly. (See Addenda.)

DECADRON®

See Prednisone, U.S.P.

Dexamethasone Sodium
Phosphate, N.F.

---

matched population of people who are also overweight but do not tend to run somewhat higher than "normal" blood sugars, they are not known to the *Handbook*. Nor are there any autopsy studies conclusively demonstrating the characteristic tissue changes nearly always seen in the blood vessels in real diabetes, where insulin is necessary to prolong life.

The 1970 *Handbook* clearly warned that these oral agents were experimental drugs and refused to list them as Basic Drugs. This skepticism, it seems, has been borne out by the UGDP Study. Now the *Handbook* suggests that the next logical step is for the FDA to remove the oral blood-sugar-lowering agents from the market. The authors of the *Handbook* are aware that this would cause a major decrease in sales for a certain few large brand-name drug corporations with immense lobbying powers. Therefore, the likelihood that agents Orinase®, Dymelor®, Tolinase®, and DBI® will be removed from the market is very small—even though the experts have estimated that upward of 10,000 Americans die yearly from the prototype of three. Such a scandal is more obnoxious than the one involving Chloromycetin®.

Decadron® is a more potent but not more powerful steroid drug than prednisone. The distinction is important. "Potency" refers to the *amount* of drug required to cause a certain effect, and "power" to how much *effect* a drug can cause if given in a large-enough dose. Decadron® is high in potency but is not the steroid drug of choice for treating the usual office patient who needs one. Prednisone (prednisolone is harder to obtain as a generic), in a 5 milligram dose, is equal in effect to Decadron® of 0.25 milligrams, and is much less costly. It used to be bruited about —and still is—that, where retention of fluid is a problem, Decadron® is superior to prednisone. There is no convincing evidence that this is true. Prednisone, in large doses, is often successfully used by internists to treat nephrotic syndrome, the archetype of abnormal fluid retention. Of course, the patent is now off dexamethasone, and it is relatively cheaply purchased from distributors of generic drugs. Even so, it is more costly than prednisone.

DECAVITAMIN CAPSULES, U.S.P. (OR TABLETS)

Decavitamin is the only *official* multiple-vitamin preparation listed in the *United States Pharmacopeia,* and hexavitamin the only one in the *National Formulary*. Most doctors are unaware of this because commercial sources of information about drugs have not bothered to let them know. No "therapeutic" concentrate inordinately rich in multiple vitamins is listed in either the *U.S.P.* or the *N.F.,* as the value of such concentrates is dubious. Nearly every patient who buys them is making an uneconomical decision.

Each component of a decavitamin tablet or capsule is present in an amount which approximates the Recommended Daily Allowance of the National Academy of Sciences–National Research Council. Each tablet or capsule contains:

Vitamin A	4000.00 U.S.P. units
Vitamin D	400.00 U.S.P. units

Vitamin C (ascorbic acid)	75.00 mg
Vitamin B complex	
thiamine (B₁) hydrochloride	1.00 mg
riboflavin (B₂)	1.20 mg
nicotinamide (niacinamide)	10.00 mg
folic acid	0.25 mg (250 mcg)
calcium pantothenate	5.00 mg
cyanocobalamin (B₁₂)	2.00 mcg

The *U.S.P.* has chosen to design a multiple-vitamin preparation because persons who for any reason are truly vitamin-deficient rarely lack only one. Pernicious anemia cases, which are due to vitamin B_{12} deficiency, may be cited as an exception, but here the diet may contain adequate B_{12}; the patient is simply unable to absorb it from the intestine. (The amount of B_{12} in decavitamin is not enough to have a favorable effect on a patient with pernicious anemia, and the amount of folic acid is not sufficient to produce an unfavorable effect.)

No prescription is needed to purchase decavitamin, and it is inexpensive in comparison with most other multiple-vitamin formulas. Hexavitamin Capsules, N.F., also a non-prescription item, are sold by a larger number of manufacturers than Decavitamin, U.S.P. and therefore may be easier for the patient to buy. See Hexavitamin Capsules, N.F., for details. (See also Addenda.)

DECLOMYCIN®   Demethylchlortetracycline Hydrochloride, N.F.
(Also, Demeclocycline Hydrochloride, N.F.)

See Tetracycline Hydrochloride, U.S.P.

This is a broad-spectrum antibiotic related to tetracycline. Its chemical composition causes it to be excreted more slowly from the body than other members of the tetracycline family. Therefore, 150 milligrams usually suffices to provide as high a blood level of antibiotic as 250 milligrams of tetracycline. This is of no major clinical importance.

Aside from its high price, Declomycin® is disadvantageous because it too often sensitizes patients to sunlight and severe blistering is not uncommon. When need for a tetracycline is indicated, doctors should prescribe tetracycline instead of Declomycin®. Undoubtedly, doctors have come to use this drug less as years pass, since it fell from the 95th most-prescribed drug in 1972 to the 139th in 1973.

DEMECLOCYCLINE HYDROCHLORIDE, N.F.
 See Declomycin®.

DEMEROL®   Meperidine Hydrochloride, U.S.P.

Demerol® is a very popular narcotic-like pain reliever used widely by physicians for shots to relieve pain. As a drug given by mouth, it is far less effective than either its "shot" form or other oral agents used to control severe pain.

Meperidine-like drugs used orally should be limited to patients suffering severe and excruciating pain. As examples, patients with cancer involving bone or internal organs, patients with severe injuries or recent surgery, and occasional patients with intractable headaches *should* receive drugs of narcotic potency. In the case of patients with pain from cancer, the addiction potential of the drugs is not important; rather, control of pain is what is important. In the case of patients having had surgery or having been in serious accidents, the pain usually lets up within a few days and the likelihood of addiction is small.

Most severe pain is as well controlled by large doses of codeine as it is with oral meperidine. If codeine is unable to suppress pain, methadone is the drug of choice for oral use. While other oral narcotic-strength pain relievers are available, including dihydromorphinone (Dilaudid®), anileridine (Leritine®), and Percodan®, methadone is usually cheaper and more effective. Methadone is best known for its use in getting heroin and other narcotic drug abusers off their habits. In smaller doses it is the most effective and cheapest oral pain reliever available to us.

DEMETHYLCHLORTETRACYCLINE HYDROCHLORIDE, N.F.
See Declomycin®.

DEMULEN-28®
See Oral Contraceptives.

DEXAMETHASONE SODIUM PHOSPHATE, N.F.
See Decadron®.

DEXCHLORPHENIRAMINE MALEATE, N.F.
See Polaramine®.

DEXTROAMPHETAMINE SULFATE, U.S.P.

Amphetamine, a synthetic, has a relatively simple molecular structure, resembling that of epinephrine. Epinephrine, better known as adrenaline (its best-known brand name is Adrenalin®), is the hormone which comes in a spurt from the inner part of the adrenal gland when one is suddenly frightened. It causes pallor, a pounding heart, and sweating and makes one suddenly forget that one is feeling tired. Amphetamine reproduces the effects of adrenaline, but its actions are more sustained and there is relatively more of the "alerting" and "antifatigue" effects. When a person is suddenly frightened, he loses interest in food. That is the effect of adrenaline. Amphetamine does the same.

When Smith Kline & French synthesized amphetamine many years ago, they thought (or so the story goes) that it would have little medical usefulness; they were experimenting with variants of the adrena-

line molecule in the hope of finding a drug that might
be useful in cardiovascular diseases. Someone in the
organization had the idea of marketing the drug as
an appetite suppressant. It was later noticed that the
pharmacologic attributes of amphetamine reside entirely in the "right-handed" (dextro-) molecules; that
the "left-handed" (levo-) mirror-image molecules are
inactive. (Molecular mirror-images were first discovered by Pasteur, who separated right-handed and
left-handed tartaric acid crystals from each other
with a tweezers, then demonstrated that a solution of
one caused a beam of light to rotate one way, whereas
a solution of the other made it rotate the opposite
way.) So, Smith Kline & French removed the "molecular dross,"* namely 50 percent of every batch of
newly crystallized amphetamine, and marketed the
pure dextro- form as Dexedrine®. The official name
is dextroamphetamine sulfate.

The patent on dextroamphetamine expired years
ago. Large and small drug corporations market dextroamphetamine at low cost, but most doctors seem
not to know this. They continue to refer to the drug
as Dexedrine®, they write "Dexedrine®" on prescription blanks, and their patients are locked into a
transaction requiring them to buy a drug that costs
the pharmacist about fifteeen to twenty times more
than is necessary.

Dextroamphetamine is a powerful agent that many
people have become dependent on for its ability to
make them feel ebullient. There is a danger that they
may keep increasing the dose in order to keep on
getting the same antifatigue and euphoria effect, and
then they are likely to get into trouble. The dependent person on high dosage often experiences toxic
effects on the brain, including hallucinations, commonly visual. There is a famous story of a truck
driver on the night shift who took dextroamphetamine
regularly to stay awake. One night he was barreling

* A term coined by the Schering Corporation to describe the
levo- form of chlorpheniramine. By eliminating "molecular
dross," they were able to market chlorpheniramine (Chlor-
Trimeton®) as dexchlorpheniramine (Polaramine®).

down the highway when he spied a trailer truck carrying a cabin cruiser jackknifed across the road. He slammed on his brakes to avoid disaster, only to realize that the vision was all in his mind. He decided not to pay attention to the increasingly occurring occasions when his mind played tricks with his eyes. So, another time when he was barreling down the highway, he ignored an "illusion" and at 65 miles an hour slammed into a trailer truck jackknifed across the road . . .

Other effects that can occur in those regularly taking large doses include auditory hallucinations, paranoid ideas, and flagrant toxic psychosis, which is like schizophrenia. When the drug is stopped, the mind straightens out in about a week.

In years past, the most widely advertised use for dextroamphetamine was as an appetite suppressant. One of the most common reasons for going to see the doctor was for a prescription "to help me lose weight." In the days of Rubens, women with ample breasts and thighs and buttocks were "beautiful." Standards of beauty have changed.

For patients who are really obese and simply cannot screw up the willpower to push themselves away from the table while still a little hungry, medications are unlikely to be helpful. Some physicians would argue that brief courses of treatment with dextroamphetamine might be helpful. One-half of one 5 milligram tablet a couple of hours before the one or two largest meals may diminish appetite. But, it is well documented that most patients who lose weight on a crash diet with the help of an appetite suppressant subsequently regain it. To lose weight and remain thin, one must adopt a way of life that includes eating less food, avoiding certain kinds of foods, and taking regular exercise.

DEXTROMETHORPHAN HYDROBROMIDE, N.F.

Too many over-the-counter medications containing this good cough reliever contain additional, unnecessary drugs that add to cost and may cause unpleasant side effects. There is a plethora of such non-prescription remedies available at every pharmacy. Two popular ones are Romilar® CF and Robitussin®-DM.

A single adult dose of dextromethorphan could cost only pennies if a pharmacist made up the syrup himself, although this is practical only for large clinics or municipal medical facilities. Here is how a pharmacist may make it:

Dextromethorphan Hydrobromide, N.F.   1/000
Syrup of Wild Cherry q.s. ad.   500 cc (or 1 pint)

A teaspoonful (5 cc), taken every 4 to 6 hours, will contain 10 milligrams of drug. This is the usual adult dose. The dextromethorphan powder is sold by Robinson Lab., Inc., 355 Brannan St., San Francisco, Cal. 94107.

DIABINESE®   Chlorpropamide, U.S.P.
See Orinase®.

When Upjohn was licensed by a German manufacturer to be the sole source of tolbutamide (Orinase®) in the U.S., Pfizer decided that there was room for others in the oral blood-sugar-lowering drug market. Their chemists synthesized a related member of the sulfonylurea family, chlorpropamide. While it works, it is generally associated with more toxic side effects (such as stomach and bowel upsets, rashes, dizziness, muscular weakness, headache, unpleasant taste, jaundice, rare blood disorders, and alcohol intolerance) than tolbutamide. It is not significantly cheaper than other sulfonylureas, and though Diabinese® was not in the UGDP study that found Orinase® life-shortening, it seems prudent to avoid Diabinese®.

Adult-onset diabetics who may seem to require

blood sugar-lowering medications would do better by losing weight, watching diet, and exercising regularly to avoid these medications. If medications are necessary, small doses of insulin are de rigueur. Some say that, should a diabetic have an insulin allergy or be so severely blinded by his diabetes as to be unable to administer his own insulin correctly, there is then a place for these oral medications. The *Handbook* refuses to underwrite this compromise, which is only an excuse for keeping drugs like Diabinese®, Orinase®, Dymelor®, and Tolinase® on the market. The oral blood-sugar-lowering agents are going to have to disappear from general use. This will not be hard to accomplish if courses in clinical pharmacology stress the need to unlearn superficialities and return to the basics.

DIAZEPAM
See *Valium®*.

DICLOXACILLIN (SODIUM DICLOXACILLIN)
See *Dynapen®*.

DIETHYLPROPION HYDROCHLORIDE
See *Tenuate®*.

DIETHYLSTILBESTROL, U.S.P. (STILBESTROL)

The discovery that this synthetic chemical, easy and cheap to make, mimics all of the effects of natural female hormones, can be taken by mouth, and does not have to be injected to be effective is one of pharmacology's fascinating chapters. Physicians and others interested in this story are referred to Sir Charles Dodd's review in *The Scientific Basis of Medicine* (London, Athlone Press, 1965). The efforts of a group of dedicated scientists interested in structure-activity relationships among female hormones attracted little attention until 1938, when they demonstrated the properties of diethylstilbestrol, which until then had never been synthesized.

Diethylstilbestrol has a well-defined place in medi-

cine even though its use is associated with the development of cancers in the female organs of daughters
of mothers using it.* Its newest use at this time is as
the "day after" pill to prevent pregnancy after intercourse. When given in daily 25 milligram doses for 3
days following intercourse, it usually prevents pregnancy. It also causes serious nausea and, not infrequently, troublesome vomiting.

DIGOXIN, U.S.P., AND DIGITOXIN, U.S.P.

Digoxin and digitoxin are essential for treating heart
diseases. Both are purified derivatives of the *Digitalis
lanata* plant, and each has the same effects on the heart.
The only significant difference lies in the time it takes
for the body to excrete them. One-half of a body store
of digoxin is excreted in three days; excretion of the
same amount of digitoxin takes seven or eight days.

The major effects of each are to cause the heart to
beat more efficiently and to slow transmission of elec-
trical impulses from the upper chambers (atria) to the
lower (ventricles). Side effects from overdosage are
not uncommon. Usually loss of appetite is the first
symptom, but extra-beats are common, too. Less often
encountered·are the complaint of pink or yellow vision
and the illusion of halos around lights.

Digoxin must never be confused with digitoxin. If
a patient has been taking digoxin daily for years and
suddenly switches to digitoxin, he might become *under*-
digitalized because of their different excretory rates.

Five years ago it was discovered that the one important brand name by which digoxin tablets are known,
Lanoxin®, was providing better dose uniformity and

* While it is true that diethylstilbestrol given to pregnant
women to prevent miscarriage has caused vaginal carcinoma
14 years later in the female issue of these pregnancies, stilbestrol remains an important therapeutic agent. Its usefulness
in the treatment of menopausal symptoms is well known. Used
for this purpose, it is fully as effective as conjugated estrogens
(usually sold as Premarin®, see page 389) and is very much
less expensive than either Premarin® or its generic equivalents.

better absorption of the active drug than some unbranded digoxin tablets. (The latter represented about 2.5 percent of the digoxin market.) The cause for the discrepancy was soon found and corrective measures were taken by the *U.S.P.* and FDA. At present, there is no reason to buy expensive Lanoxin® in place of an unbranded digoxin, because it is a drug which is usually taken for years. Cumulative savings with the generic will be considerable. Digitoxin can also masquerade under expensive brand names. Patients taking either should see their entries in the Price Lists.

DILANTIN® SODIUM   Sodium Diphenylhydantoin, U.S.P.

After phenobarbital had been shown to diminish the frequency of epileptic seizures in many patients, diphenylhydantoin, which is related structurally to barbiturates, was developed. It probably has less anticonvulsive relative to sedative effect than phenobarbital, and it likely is not as powerful an anticonvulsant. The two are often used together. Occasionally the drug is used for certain heartbeat irregularities.

The side effects of diphenylhydantoin include loss of balance, dizziness, slurred speech, visual difficulties; rashes; and enlargement of the gums. Since the drug must be used daily for many years—perhaps a lifetime—long-term cost is an important consideration. Should a doctor write for large quantities of the drug (*e.g.,* 1000 tablets) and use the generic name, Sodium Diphenylhydantoin, U.S.P., and should the patient know something about prices and be willing to price the drug with different pharmacists, there is little doubt that he will be able to save large amounts of money.

DIMENHYDRINATE, U.S.P.
  See Dramamine®.

DIMETANE®   Brompheniramine Maleate, N.F.

This is an example of what the HEW Task Force on Prescription Drugs has referred to as "me too" drugs—"substances which are not significantly different from other drugs, nor significantly better," but which can be marketed at a high price with a special brand name in order to siphon off a portion of the market for a certain class of drugs. The only difference between Dimetane®, an A. H. Robins product, and Chlor-Trimeton®, a Schering product, is in the substitution of bromine atoms for chlorine atoms. (High-school chemistry students know how similar bromine is to chlorine.) It is the "pheniramine" part of the molecule in each one that is pharmacologically active as an antihistamine. It matters little whether bromines or chlorines are attached, but the slight molecular change allows A. H. Robins to put out a "differentiated" product that sells for as much as or a little more than Chlor-Trimeton®. Chlor-Trimeton's® active principle is available at low cost by its official name, Chlorpheniramine Maleate, U.S.P. (see this name in the Price Lists.)

As for Extentabs®, neither the *United States Pharmacopeia* nor the *National Formulary* recognizes them as an official dosage form.

DIMETAPP®

Brompheniramine Maleate, N.F.	12 mg
Phenylephrine Hydro-chloride, U.S.P.	15 mg
phenylpropanolamine hydrochloride	15 mg

See Antihistamines; Neo-Synephrine®.

See comments on Dimetane®. It is extravagant to purchase a combination of brompheniramine, phenylephrine, and phenylpropanolamine, three of the most common chemicals available to drug manufacturers, from a retailer who must in turn spend $75 per 1000 doses. Vasoconstrictor drugs (phenylephrine and phenylpropanolamine) should not be taken systemically for something as trivial as a stuffy nose.

Phenylephrine nose drops are available without a prescription for a dollar or less and are usually preferable treatment. Extentabs® are not officially recognized by the *U.S.P.* or the *N.F.*

Dimetapp® is one of the nation's most popular preparations. It ranks 14th among the most frequently prescribed drugs in the U.S., a scandalous matter that necessarily must indicate either abject ignorance or an I-don't-give-a-damn attitude on the part of the medical leadership. The leadership is where the corrupt medical politicians are to be found; the vast majority of practicing doctors are only honest dupes.

DIPHENHYDRAMINE HYDROCHLORIDE, U.S.P.
See Benadryl®.

DIPHENOXYLATE HYDROCHLORIDE
See Lomotil®.

DIPHENYLHYDANTOIN (SODIUM DIPHENYLHYDANTOIN, U.S.P.)
See Dilantin®.

DIUPRES®

Chlorothiazide,
N.F.   25 mg and 50 mg
Reserpine, U.S.P.   0.125 mg

See Diuril®; Reserpine, U.S.P.; Enduron®.

Diupres® is widely prescribed for high blood pressure. It is a fixed combination in two different dosage forms of a diuretic, or water-eliminating pill, and the drug reserpine that is commonly used to control blood pressure.

Products that combine two different drugs have been in disrepute for many years. The manufacturer of these products is compelled by federal controls to print the following warning both on the package insert accompanying all physician's samples of the drug

and on the drug description in the *Physicians' Desk
Reference,* the most frequently used guide to drugs:

This fixed combination drug is not indicated for
initial therapy of hypertension. Hypertension requires therapy titrated to the individual patient.
If the fixed combination represents the dosage
so determined, its use may be more convenient
in patient management. The treatment of hypertension is not static, but must be re-evaluated as
conditions in each patient warrant.

For the convenience of taking 1 pill rather than 2,
the patient with high blood pressure usually pays a
high premium. See comments on Hydrodiuril®, where
it is explained how to achieve the same antihypertension
and diuresis effects at lower cost.

DIURIL®   Chlorothiazide, N.F.
See Potassium Chloride, U.S.P.; Hydrodiuril®.

This drug, when taken orally, causes increased urination and, especially when taken along with reserpine or other drugs, may lower elevated blood
pressure.
Diuril® and its related compound Hydrodiuril® are
very expensive. Patients can receive the same diuresis
and antihypertension effects with less costly generic
hydrochlorothiazide. The latter is now widely available.
An alternative to hydrochlorothiazide is Metahydrin®,
but it is considerably more costly unless it, too, is
bought in its generic form (trichlormethiazide). The
latter is far less well distributed than generic hydrochlorothiazide.
Side effects from the "thiazide" diuretics, including
all of those discussed above, are numerous. Often*
potassium and chloride salts are lost in the urine and
must be replaced with foods rich in potassium or
with potassium chloride pills. Diabetes patients taking
the widely used oral blood-sugar-lowering agents are

* But less often than is currently believed to be the case.

often influenced in their requirements for such drugs by the addition of "thiazide" diuretics. This need cause no commotion; simply discontinue the blood-sugar-lowering drug because it is in any event dangerous. Mild stomach upsets and dizziness occasionally occur with chlorothiazide. As with any thiazide, abdominal pain with or without jaundice may occur. This can be a very serious matter, a sign that toxic pancreatitis has developed. Inflammation of the pancreas is one of the least suspected but most serious of the toxic hazards of thiazide drugs.

DONNATAL®

Hyoscyamine Sulfate, N.F.	0.1037 mg
Atropine Sulfate, U.S.P.	0.0194 mg
hyoscine hydrobromide	0.0065 mg
Phenobarbital, U.S.P.	16.2 mg*

See Atropine Sulfate, U.S.P.; Phenobarbital, U.S.P.; Tincture of Belladonna (Belladonna Tincture, U.S.P.).

This is one of the most commonly prescribed tablets for patients with gastrointestinal symptoms ranging from possible peptic ulcer to "nervous stomach." For most adults the hyoscyamine and hyoscine components can be little more than placebos in these small amounts ("homeopathic" doses), and the dosage of atropine sulfate is also very small (the usual dose is 0.2 to 0.4 milligram). The advertising claim of A. H. Robins (*Physicians' Desk Reference,* 1968) is that hyoscyamine, hyoscine, and atropine are "synergistic" in their action, but it is likely that they mean "additive." The potential effects of the three are essentially the same as far as stomach and intestines are concerned. The phenobarbital part of the mixture is probably useful, and might well account for

---

* It is absurd to measure the amounts of these drugs to the fourth decimal place since the number of tablets prescribed per day is usually the same, regardless of the patient's weight.

the slight dryness of mouth that many Donnatal® recipients report. Donnatal® is not a *U.S.P.* or *N.F.* drug.

Many doctors who prescribe Donnatal® may be unaware of how little atropine and atropine-like drug it contains and of the cost. The doctor can make Donnatal® even more costly to the patient if he writes down "Donnatal Extentabs®". (Neither the *United States Pharmacopeia* nor the *National Formulary* lists Extentabs® nor approves of sustained-action forms of pills.)

There is little doubt that 15 milligrams of pheno-barbital (sometimes 30) with belladonna tincture or atropine sulfate is useful. By ordering these drugs separately, one can avoid high cost and provide greater flexibility of dosage.

If there is any instance of widespread, thoughtless prescription practice, it is with Donnatal®. This agent was the 13th most-prescribed drug in the United States in 1973!

DOPA (L-DOPA [LEVODOPA]; DIHYDROXYPHENYLALANINE) *

Dopa is an essential body substance but is present in the blood and tissues in such small concentrations as to be difficult to detect. This is because a new molecule of dopa is converted to another substance almost as soon as it is made. Dopa's immediate chem-ical antecedent is the common amino acid tyrosine, a lot of which is normally present in blood and tis-sues. Dopa is converted to dopamine. Another chem-ical step makes dopamine into noradrenaline, the nerve transmitter chemical, and another step makes some of the noradrenaline into adrenaline, which is stored in the adrenal gland to be released at times of fright. There is a lot of dopamine in the brain. Re-

* Dopa has been commonly known to chemists for genera-tions as dihydroxyphenylalanine. German chemists have called it dioxyphenylalanine, and took to referring to it as "dopa."

cently it has been discovered that certain brain centers normally rich in dopamine are dopamine-poor in patients who have suffered from Parkinsonism during life.

Dopa is widely used and is often effective in the treatment of Parkinsonism, relieving some or most of the distressing symptoms. The drug has had widespread use for several years and is relatively safe. When begun for the first time, the drug must be given in slowly increasing doses until the symptoms of shakiness, difficulty walking, and so forth are gone and/or until the side effects prohibit increasing the dose. Side effects common with the drug include nausea (very common), low blood pressure with occasional faintness, involuntary movements and muscle jerks, and agitation or restlessness.

Cost of the drug, despite at least three major producers in the United States, is relatively high. A day's dose often costs between $1 and $2; annual costs to the patients are several hundreds of dollars. One might argue that the improvements in mobility and mentation afforded by the use of this drug outweigh its costs, but it is an undeniable fact that L-Dopa was for many years a very inexpensive common laboratory reagent and is an unpatentable product. How a very few companies have succeeded in charging so much for such a universally available laboratory reagent is a scandal that should have been investigated some time ago.

DORIDEN®   Glutethimide, N.F.
    See Chloral Hydrate, U.S.P.; Dalmane®; Nembutal®; Seconal®.

This is a sedative commonly used as a "sleeping pill."

In the past, advertisements for this drug have emphasized its nonbarbiturate chemical structure. This is no advantage except to the rare person who gets a rash from barbiturates, or is excited by them, and who also finds chloral hydrate unsatisfactory. Doriden® lends itself in excessive usage or dosage to the very same abuses as barbiturates: habituation, addiction, and suicide. Doriden® overdosage can be a particularly nasty kind of poisoning to treat. "Tolerance" to Doriden® can develop just as it does to barbiturates.

It is hard to justify a doctor's "routine" selection of Doriden® for a sleeping pill when pentobarbital, secobarbital, and chloral hydrate are available so inexpensively.

DORMETHAN®
See Dextromethorphan Hydrobromide, N.F.

DOXEPIN HYDROCHLORIDE
See Sinequan®.

DOXYCYCLINE HYCLATE
See Vibramycin®.

DRAMAMINE®   Dimenhydrinate, U.S.P.
See Antihistamines; Benadryl®.

Dramamine® and Benadryl® have the same active component, diphenhydramine. Diphenhydramine is available by that name at little cost. So is dimenhydrinate. As is often the case with small numbers of drugs purchased at a single time, there will be little or no saving of money by ordering diphenhydramine if less than 16 or so tablets are prescribed. When a larger number is needed, the patient will obtain the same effect at lower cost from 25 milligrams of diphenhydramine.

Dramamine® ranks among the 200 most-*prescribed* drugs, even though it is available over the counter without prescription, albeit at a high price!

DRIXORAL®   Dexbrompheniramine
                                       Maleate, N.F.   6 mg
                                 d-isoephedrine sulfate   120 mg

See Antihistamines; Neo-Synephrine®.

Drixoral® is a fixed combination of an antihistamine and phenylephrine-like (Neo-Synephrine®) drugs prepared in a timed-release long-acting tablet. Fixed combinations and timed-release tablets are generally to be frowned upon because they prevent the adjustment of individual doses of each of the components and they make it difficult to sort out the side effects that may result from either of the components. They are also usually quite expensive.

This drug includes a special form of the brompheniramine maleate molecule (Dimetane®); dexbrompheniramine comprises only those crystals that polarized light rotates in one direction. These crystals are the more active, but purification to obtain these crystals is expensive and adds to the cost of the drugs without providing known benefit to the patient. As recommended previously, the least expensive antihistamine is most appropriate, and this is usually diphenhydramine hydrochloride (Benadryl®) or chlorpheniramine maleate (Chlor-Trimeton®).

The addition of a oral phenylephrine-like drug is common in cold preparations such as this. However, simple phenylephrine (Neo-Synephrine®) nose drops would do better to relieve nasal congestion.

DYAZIDE®   Hydrochlorothiazide,
                                        U.S.P.   25 mg
                                    triamterene   50 mg

See Trichlormethiazide.

Triamterene (Dyrenium®), a drug developed by Smith Kline & French, can increase the production of urine (diuresis) but, unlike thiazide drugs, does so without causing an associated outpouring of potassium. It can, on the contrary, cause *retention* of potassium. Because continued use of thiazides can lead to potassium depletion, which can be harmful and even fatal if the patient is not taking a diet rich enough in potassium, the company marketed a product combining a small dose of hydrochlorothiazide (Hydrodiuril®) with triamterene (Dyrenium®) in order to obtain a good diuresis with a minimum of potassium retention. Foods rich in potassium include oranges, bananas, figs; and the medication potassium chloride elixir in combination with generic hydrochlorothiazide is a far cheaper way of treating patients in need of diuretics.

Triamterene is not without toxicity of its own. Its most frequent side effects, in addition to retention of potassium, include nausea, diarrhea, headache, rash, and mouth dryness.

For the moment it is well to use it only for patients who cannot tolerate thiazides alone. It is hard to believe that there is frequent-enough reason for giving this drug to warrant Dyazide's® inclusion among the top 30 drugs prescribed in the United States in 1973. It is easier to believe that successful promotion and advertising are the causes of this travesty.

DYNAPEN®   sodium dicloxacillin

Dicloxacillin is one of the newer semisynthetic penicillins, drugs whose principal use must, for the sake of the public health, be restricted to the treatment of infection by staphylococcus strains of bacteria that are known or suspected to be penicillin-resistant.

When antibiotics were introduced, few anticipated that certain bacteria would become resistant to their effects, but that is what has happened. In the early 1950s, staphylococcus was found to have become in some cases resistant to penicillin, to all of the tetracycline antibiotics, to erythromycin, chloramphenicol, and others. The problem became acute primarily in large municipal hospitals. Suburban and rural hospitals were not affected.

The mechanism of resistance to penicillin is now fairly well understood. Some staphylococcus strains are "born" resistant to penicillin, because they can manufacture and secrete penicillinase, a substance which splits the penicillin molecule and inactivates it. In hospitals where a lot of penicillin is in constant use, naturally resistant strains appear in increasing numbers and displace their weaker cousins who are unable to make penicillinase. Infections with these organisms were often fatal—scores of them were observed at Boston City Hospital—until British investigators found a way to manipulate the penicillin molecule so that it was no longer as susceptible to destruction by penicillinase, while retaining some of its antibacterial activity. These newer penicillins are called "semisynthetic, penicillinase-resistant" penicillins. Methicillin was the first and oxacillin the second. There are now several others that are less expensive than oxacillin, and these include dicloxacillin and cloxacillin.

The possibility for emergence of staphylococcus strains resistant to these drugs remains. It is, therefore, important for drugs of this type to be used only in situations where they are known to be needed or where there is strong reason to suppose they might be. Such instances include severe infections caused by staphylococcus germs that are resistant to simple and older forms of penicillin, such as penicillin G and V.

Semisynthetic penicillins are, like all penicillins, able to kill the pneumococcus and hemolytic streptococcus, but doctors are advised not to use them for this purpose because:

1. Milligram for milligram they are less effective than penicillin G or penicillin V.

2. Cost relative to penicillin G or V is astronomical.

3. Most important, the public health might be endangered if we should spend our antistaphylococcus ammunition indiscriminately.

Dynapen® is one of three commonly prescribed brands of dicloxacillin, including Wyeth's Pathocil® and Ayerst's Veracillin®. Cloxacillin, sold by Bristol as Tegopen®, is usually prescribed in a dose double that of dicloxacillin but similar in cost for a day's treatment. Other semisynthetic antistaphylococcus oral penicillins are uniformly more expensive and they should be avoided. These more expensive forms include nafcillin (Unipen®) and oxacillin (Bactocill® and Prostaphlin®), all of which are approximately twice the cost of cloxacillin or dicloxacillin. These more expensive forms have no advantages.

None of these semisynthetic antistaphylococcus antibiotics is any longer among the most frequently prescribed 200 drugs in America. This is precisely as it should be, and undoubtedly reflects the results of a controversy in the late 1960s that required one of the major manufacturers of these drugs to revise its recommendations for use. When one is given a prescription for treatment over several days for one of these products, he should be prepared to spend as much as $10.

ELAVIL®   Amitriptyline Hydrochloride, U.S.P.

It is common practice to prescribe this as a "mood elevator" for depressed patients. While perhaps helpful to some, it is not universally effective. The name undoubtedly confers a degree of placebo effect on both patient and doctor. (If "amitriptyline" doesn't make you feel better, perhaps "Elavil®" will.) Some psychiatrists prescribe Elavil®, not because they are convinced that it is effective, but because many patients and referring physicians expect them to. One psychiatrist friend frankly admits to being afraid of possible lawsuits or "trouble" should any of his depressed patients harm themselves and it be demonstrated that he had "withheld" this or related drugs. This subtle pressure to conform is not healthy.

For whatever reasons, psychiatrists and others are prescribing mammoth amounts of Elavil®, which in 1973 was the 34th most-prescribed drug in the nation. The elderly buy much of it. One can seriously question whether there is enough depression to warrant such widespread use of relatively difficult-to-prove-useful drugs. If depression stems from severe psychiatric disorders and mental derangements, this and related drugs may be of use. If depression stems from external circumstances, such as death in the family, disillusionment, disappointment, or anxiety over having too little income, the drug will not be effective.

ELIXOPHYLLIN®	Theophylline, N.F.	80 mg
	alcohol 20%	3 cc
	(per tbsp)	

See Aminophylline, U.S.P. (Theophylline Ethylene-diamine).

Elixophyllin®, which is theophylline in alcohol, is promoted for asthma and asthma-like symptoms. It would be far cheaper and as effective to buy a large quantity of aminophylline tablets and take 100 or 200 milligrams 4 times a day with meals. There may be some value to the alcohol in Elixophyllin®, but there are less expensive ways to take alcohol (a *U.S.P.* drug, incidentally).

EMPIRIN® COMPOUND	Aspirin, U.S.P.	3½ gr
WITH CODEINE	Phenacetin, U.S.P.	2½ gr
PHOSPHATE	Caffeine, U.S.P.	½ gr
	Codeine Phosphate,	
	U.S.P. ⅛, ¼, ½, or 1 gr	

See Aspirin, U.S.P.; Codeine Sulfate, N.F., Codeine Phosphate, U.S.P.; Tylenol®.

Empirin® Compound is an expensive APC tablet. Ask the druggist for something less expensive. Pharmacists can buy APC tablets from any one of a number of manufacturers for less. No prescription for APC alone is required. It is unwise to use APCs habitually over a period of years because the phenacetin has known toxic effects on the kidney. Aspirin alone is preferred to APC.

While acetaminophen (Tylenol®) has rather good analgesic effects, it is less likely to control inflammation as well as aspirin alone and is not only more expensive but also may do the kidneys harm, much like phenacetin. (Only chronic use for years is suspect.)

The addition of codeine makes an APC tablet a "big-league" pain reliever. For the common case of a patient who needs a very few doses to tide him over a toothache or a throbbing finger, a dozen tablets of Empirin® Compound with 15 or 30 milligrams of codeine should cost no more than the pharmacist's minimum prescription price and should provide good pain relief when taken as the doctor orders. The product is basically cheap, but when its use is to continue for many weeks, codeine and aspirin purchased separately and in their cheapest forms may afford some savings.

E-MYCIN®   Erythromycin
                           Stearate, U.S.P.   250 mg
See Erythrocin® Stearate; Ilosone®; Pediamycin®.

This Upjohn product is not a salt of erythromycin, as are so many erythromycin products; E-Mycin® is erythromycin base, enteric-coated in order to minimize destruction of the drug by stomach acids. The hope is that the tablet will reach the alkaline juice of the small intestine and that absorption will take place from that safer vantage point. Such enteric-coated tablets are generally unnecessary, and add to the expense and often to the uneven absorption of the product. In patients with rapid movement of food and pills through the stomach and bowel, enteric-coated E-Mycin® is more likely than others to pass from mouth to anus without being absorbed. Obviously, E-Mycin® should be avoided, and generic erythromycin should be prescribed and dispensed instead.

ENDURON®   methyclothiazide
See Trichlormethiazide.

This "thiazide" diuretic acts to increase urine formation and enhances medications that lower blood pressure in patients with high blood pressure. It is very similar to all the other "thiazide" diuretics, both in action and side effects.

Enduron® is expensive. The cheapest forms of "thiazide" diuretics should always be used. Although trichlormethiazide (brand name: Metahydrin®) was until recently the least expensive *brand* generally available for substitution, the patent on the very effective diuretic hydrochlorothiazide (Hydrodiuril®) has expired and generic hydrochlorothiazide is widely available at enormous savings.

EPHEDRINE SULFATE, U.S.P.

An interesting basic drug, ephedrine is the active component of mahuang, a Chinese herb medicine resurrected for the Occident in the 1920s. It has the effect of adrenaline but is longer-acting and not as powerful. Its uses are many, but the major one is in treating asthma. It dilates the air passages. A less common use is for persons whose heart disease manifests itself in a heart rate so slow as to disable; ephedrine, if taken regularly, may speed up heart action. One drawback is that it may cause jitteriness, like adrenaline and amphetamines. This is why it is commonly given with some phenobarbital.

In recent years, part of the mechanism by which ephedrine exerts its pharmacological effect has been elucidated. It acts in two ways:

1. It "releases" a nerve-transmitter substance, noradrenaline, from the terminals of certain nerve fibers where they have contact with the muscle elements of the heart, air passages, and small blood vessels, thereby stimulating these structures to do what a real nerve impulse would make them do. It acts on muscle elements directly.

2. Continuous exposure to ephedrine leads to its becoming less and less effective—a not unexpected consequence of its first mode of action, through which it may deplete the chemical transmitter stores in nerves.

Big brand-name manufacturers probably do not really wish to market ephedrine—it is too cheap and plentiful. There are many, many firms who are purveyors of the product; and there is, accordingly, some healthy price competition. But a clever firm can use a device to exact a higher price; thus, Lilly markets ephedrine in specially shaped capsules that are trade-marked and cost the patient significant sums. A more lucrative device is to market the ephedrine in combination with other drugs, to give the combination an easily remembered brand-name, and to advertise it very widely. This is what Warner/Chilcott has done: it has taken three common, inexpensive, and useful drugs—theophylline, ephedrine, and phenobarbital—put them into the same tablet, and named it Tedral®; it is now being sold to pharmacies for a preposterous price. The *Handbook* believes this combination contains too little theophylline and too little phenobarbital, but doctors and patients wishing to have the item should know that it can be purchased at a fraction of the cost of Tedral®. There is little doubt that ephedrine is the most important component.

EQUAGESIC®

Aspirin, U.S.P.	250 mg
Meprobamate, N.F.	150 mg
Ethoheptazine Citrate, N.F.	75 mg

Wyeth Laboratories has combined a small dose of the sedative meprobamate with aspirin and a very mild analgesic, ethoheptazine. Two or 3 aspirin tablets and 15 milligrams of phenobarbital will usually work as well as Equagesic® at a fraction of the cost. Seventy-five milligrams of ethoheptazine is a very mild analgesic; if it were otherwise, it would stand on its own as an important, single-entity drug.

If a patient has muscle pain, for which this drug combination is often prescribed, a hot bath, 15 to 30 milligrams of codeine sulfate, and 2 aspirin tablets will be at least as effective an analgesic as Equagesic®.

EQUANIL®   Meprobamate, N.F.
See Meprobamate, N.F.

Meprobamate, the first non-barbiturate sedative to be discovered, was very widely overused shortly after its discovery. In its usual dosage of 200 to 400 milligrams every 4 to 6 hours, meprobamate is probably no more effective than small doses of barbiturate. If you must have it, do not buy it as Equanil® or Miltown® if you wish to save money; buy it as meprobamate and insist on the savings this makes possible.

ERGONOVINE MALEATE, U.S.P.
ERGOTAMINE TARTRATE, N.F.

The severe epidemics that swept medieval Europe were mostly caused by infection, but some were probably cases of mass poisoning by ergot, a fungus that infects rye as it grows. Ergot has a number of pharmacologically powerful constituents. One is ergotamine, a poison (or a drug, depending on your point of view) that causes prolonged constriction (even complete closure) of small arteries throughout the body and severe uterine contractions capable of causing abortion. Epidemic abortion, excruciating pain, and gangrene in hands and feet (due to cutoff of the arterial blood supply) were known to medieval people as "Saint Anthony's Fire." Outbreaks were due to a bad rye crop and the ingestion of ergot-poisoned rye bread. Chemical and pharmacologic studies of ergot and its constituents, of which ergonovine is one, and ergotamine another, constitute fascinating research.

No one knows the cause of migraine headache, an agonizing, one-sided affair whose onset is often heralded by hard-to-describe visual disturbances or subtle feelings known as "aura." When the aura of an impending attack is sensed, it is often possible to lessen the severity of the headache by taking one of these drugs at once. Part of the pounding pain of migraine is due to the throbbing of distended, dilated arteries; these drugs help relieve symptoms by causing the main arteries in the scalp and cranium to become narrower.

Either drug must be taken as the doctor orders, never freely and indiscriminately. Now and then a case of poisoning results from ergonovine overdose; there is no effective treatment. Gangrene with loss of fingers and toes is a danger.

Institutions buying ergonovine or ergotamine in large amounts would do well to purchase them by generic name. However, for the average person who has an occasional migraine headache, it is probably not worthwhile to shop for the less expensive generic. Eli Lilly sells ergonovine as Ergotrate® and Sandoz sells a combination of caffeine and ergotamine tartrate as Cafergot®. Recently a form sold as Ergomar® for use under the tongue became available; in this form the active drug is rapidly absorbed and claims are made that it relieves migraine more rapidly. However, Ergotrate® and Cafergot® are usually effective within 15 to 30 minutes; suppositories of both have been available for a long time and are more rapidly active than the oral forms.

Considering the usual minimum cost of a prescription, it is not going to save much to buy the drugs generically. However, if bought in lots of 100 tablets, some savings may be accomplished. As long as the pills are kept dry, they do not lose their potency.

ERYTHROCIN®   Erythromycin Stearate, U.S.P.
STEARATE
   See *E-Mycin®; Ilosone®; Pediamycin®.*

This antibiotic has a spectrum similar to penicillin G or V, but the cost is much higher. It is the drug of choice for patients who have a penicillin allergy. Erythromycin is relatively non-toxic. As is the case with tetracycline, erythromycin too has been useful in the treatment of pneumonias caused by mycoplasma, a bacteria-like organism. (This pneumonia mimics virus pneumonia.)

For clinical purposes, Erythrocin® should *not* be

confused with Ilosone®. Ilosone® is a different erythromycin salt with a particularly severe side effect;
viz., jaundice. (For this reason Ilosone® should be
avoided; it was, however, the 20th most-prescribed
drug in the United States in 1973.)

ERYTHROMYCIN STEARATE, U.S.P.

*See E-Mycin®; Erythrocin® Stearate; Ilosone®;
Pediamycin®.*

ESIDRIX®   Hydrochlorothiazide, U.S.P.
See Hydrodiuril®.

This is only another expensive brand name of
hydrochlorothiazide (Hydrodiuril®). Esidrix® ranked
104th among the drugs prescribed in the nation in
1973, while Hydrodiuril® ranked 13th. The cheaper
"thiazide" diuretics, such as generic hydrochlorothiazide
and trichlormethiazide, are not found among the most
prescribed 200 drugs in 1973 despite their equivalent
efficacy and significantly lower price.

ESTROGENS
See Oral Contraceptives; Premarin®.

ETHAMBUTOL
See Myambutol®.

ETHCHLORVYNOL
See Placidyl®.

ETRAFON®	Perphenazine Hydrochloride, N.F.	2 or 4 mg
	Amitriptyline Hydrochloride, U.S.P.	10 or 25 mg

This fixed-combination drug combines varying doses of an allegedly antipsychosis phenothiazine drug, perphenazine (Trilafon®) with the antidepressant amitriptyline (Elavil®). The former drug is said to be useful in treating more severe nervous disorders; simply stated, perphenazine is used to treat psychotic people.* Statistics show that amitriptyline is probably effective in many people suffering from a non-situational depression, and has not been proved useful for depression due to the trials and tribulations of life.

As with all fixed-dose combination products, the adjustment of each component's dose is impossible —a distinct disadvantage. Another disadvantage is Etrafon's® cost.

It would be of enormous importance to know if there really are enough "crazy" people in this country to warrant Etrafon's® popularity. It ranked 177th in the hit parade in 1973.

FEOSOL®   Ferrous Sulfate, U.S.P.
See Ferrous Sulfate, U.S.P.

Feosol® is ferrous sulfate from which the water has been evaporated. Since one-third of the weight of a Ferrous Sulfate, U.S.P., tablet is water, an equivalent tablet of Feosol® weighs one-third less.†

If iron is prescribed as generic Ferrous Sulfate, U.S.P., the patient can save significant sums. Furthermore, iron pills may be purchased without prescription. (N.B.: probably not in all states.)

FERROUS SULFATE, U.S.P. (IRON SULFATE)
See Feosol®.

* A universally precise definition of psychosis does not exist.
† Evaporating the water is a senseless exercise. When a patient swallows a Feosol® tablet, he generally takes some water to wash it down; what ends up in his stomach is, therefore, Ferrous Sulfate, U.S.P.

One of the most important drugs in medical practice, ferrous sulfate is used in the treatment of iron-deficiency anemia.

Red blood cells can carry oxygen only to the extent that they contain hemoglobin. An essential part of a hemoglobin molecule is an atom of iron. A healthy person keeps using the same iron over and over as red blood cells and their hemoglobin are continually broken down and remanufactured. For healthy males, therefore, iron deficiency is nearly impossible unless there has been chronic blood loss over a period of time and the iron intake in the diet has been insufficient to replace the loss. For females in the child-bearing years, things are different; if menstrual loss of blood is regularly very heavy, iron loss can exceed usual dietary intake and iron deficiency can readily occur.

Iron-deficiency anemia is common. It is easy to diagnose, but in every case it is necessary to discover why there is a deficiency. The doctor is likely to subject the patient to extensive questioning and some tests before he gives him a prescription for ferrous sulfate. It would do no good to replace the iron and ignore a bleeding but curable cancer somewhere.

An official *U.S.P.* ferrous sulfate tablet weighs 300 milligrams, of which 60 milligrams are elemental iron, 133 water, and 107 sulfate. It is effective and very inexpensive. Preparations containing a mixture of iron, vitamin B_{12}, and other vitamins and minerals, stomach concentrates, etc., are often extremely expensive and by discouraging careful diagnosis may actually be harmful.

To avoid the gastrointestinal symptoms that may sometimes accompany the taking of iron, the daily dose of ferrous sulfate should be increased gradually from 1 tablet a day taken at the end of a meal to 2 tablets a day after a week or ten days. It is rare for 3 tablets a day to be necessary, because in the presence of iron deficiency the intestine takes up iron with more than usual avidity.

FIORINAL®

Butalbital, N.F.		50 mg
Aspirin, U.S.P.		200 mg
Phenacetin, U.S.P.		130 mg
Caffeine, U.S.P.		50 mg

This is merely an APC tablet with a little barbiturate sedative. It is named for the Monte*fiore* Hospital in New York City, where the drug was at one time widely used.

A review of the indications for this product carried out by the prestigious National Academy of Sciences —National Research Council has listed this drug as only "possibly" effective for its numerous advertised uses, including "conditions in which combined sedative and analgesic action is desired, such as, nervous tension and sleeplessness associated with pain, headache, or general malaise." The 1975 *Physicians' Desk Reference* also lists as indications such entities as ". . . rheumatic and arthritic conditions, neuralgia, aches and pains [sic], dysmenorrhea, respiratory infections and febrile conditions (common colds and grippe), dental extractions and minor surgical procedures and headaches."

Given its cost, patients would do as well with a couple of inexpensive aspirin tablets and a small dose of phenobarbital for headaches associated with anxiety or "tension." In no case can a reasonable rationalization account for this drug's rank as 30th among the most prescribed drugs in the United States.

FLAGYL® Metronidazole, U.S.P.

Flagyl® is used for treatment of infection with trichomonads, one-celled creatures that are a common cause of intense vaginal itch and discharge. Males frequently harbor the organism in the urethra, so sexual partners ought to be treated at the same time. Flagyl® is a good drug with a low incidence of serious adverse side effects.

Recently there has been speculation that one serious side effect may be cancer of the cervix of the uterus. Although this has not yet been confirmed, some doctors are reverting to an older remedy for trichomonad infection: vinegar douches, which are safer but less likely to bring about a cure.

FLUOCINOLONE ACETONIDE
  See Synalar®.

FLURANDRENOLIDE, N.F.
  See Cordran®.

FLURAZEPAM
  See Dalmane®.

FUROSEMIDE
  See Lasix®.

GANTANOL®   sulfamethoxazole
  See Gantrisin®; Triple Sulfas.

Gantanol® is a sulfonamide promoted for and ordinarily used for treatment of garden-variety urinary tract infections. However, there is little reason for it to be prescribed. Its major breakdown product in the body is insoluble enough to make kidney blockage a more serious possibility than with some other sulfonamides. Also, its cost is high.

The doctor who wishes to prescribe a sulfonamide for urinary tract infection ought to think first either of triple sulfas (Trisulfapyrimidines, U.S.P., or the N.F. counterpart) or of Gantrisin® (Sulfisoxazole, U.S.P.). If he prefers Gantrisin®, he should know that it is sold by its official name at lower cost. See Sulfisoxazole, U.S.P., and Triple Sulfas in the Price Lists.

Let us examine why Gantanol® is being marketed so aggressively and why it has the brand name it does. Roche, a giant drug corporation, had a patent monopoly on Gantrisin® for seventeen years. During that time nearly every prescribing doctor was trained to think "urinary infection—Gantrisin®." Most of them never learned Gantrisin's® official name. Several years ago the patent monopoly on Gantrisin® expired, but few doctors became aware of its availability at lower cost if bought by generic name. Moreover, the company had its chemists slightly change the molecule into sulfamethoxazole (which is less soluble and therefore not as good a drug as sulfisoxazole) and gave it the brand name Gantanol®. It has been easy to train many doctors' tongues to make the switch from Gantrisin®. No one who takes the view that selling drugs is just another business can blame Roche, but medical journals should not lend their pages for advertisements which do not deal with the issues of comparative efficacy and comparative cost.

A great deal of Gantanol® is being prescribed. It ranks within the top 150 drugs prescribed in the U.S.

GANTRISIN®   Sulfisoxazole, U.S.P.

Sulfisoxazole is a good sulfonamide for treating the majority of urinary tract infections. Nearly all of these are due to *E. coli,* and most (though not all) of these organisms are so sensitive to sulfisoxazole that there is a wide permissible dose range. Reflex tendency on the part of doctors to think "urinary tract infection—Gantrisin®" is due to effective promotion and advertising. Trisulfapyrimidines Tablets, U.S.P., or the *N.F.* counterpart (doctors need only write "Triple Sulfas Tablets") will serve as well. Both triple sulfas *and* generic sulfisoxazole are available at significant savings to the patient. The dose of sulfisoxazole to treat a patient is the same as the dose of triple sulfas.

Gantrisin® is widely advertised and enormously popular. It is one of the 50 most commonly prescribed drugs for all age groups. Hardly anyone advertises triple sulfas and, therefore, very little is prescribed.

The recent trend to use ampicillin-related drugs to treat urinary tract infections makes no sense, and adds phenomenal expense to the patient's drug bill. Thus, ampicillin, cephalexin (Keflex®), and carbenicillin (Geocillin®) have to be used only when complicated kidney problems or repeated infections with unusual bacteria occur. If you receive a prescription for one of these, you ought to ask your doctor why he did not use generic sulfisoxazole or triple sulfas.

GLUTETHIMIDE, N.F.

See Doriden®.

GRISEOFULVIN, U.S.P.

Also sold as Fulvicin®, Grifulvin V®, and Grisactin®, this drug is effective in combating certain fungus infections of hair and skin. Used mostly for the treatment of ringworm infections and tinea, the drug has use only in special instances with certain fungus organisms and is relatively expensive. Side effects on blood-cell production can be extremely serious, although they are rare. Also, griseofulvin has a greater than usual propensity to interreact and interfere with the actions of other drugs given concomitantly. *Handbook* advice is to approach the use of griseofulvin gingerly.

GUANETHIDINE SULFATE, U.S.P.

See Ismelin®.

HEXAVITAMIN CAPSULES, N.F. (OR TABLETS)

Hexavitamin is the only multiple-vitamin compound listed by the *National Formulary*. It is highly recommended for use where indicated. For related comments, see Decavitamin Capsules, U.S.P. (or Tablets), and Addenda.

Each hexavitamin capsule or tablet contains:

Vitamin A	5000 U.S.P. units
Vitamin D	400 U.S.P. units
Vitamin C (ascorbic acid)	70 mg

Vitamin B Complex
thiamine hydrochloride 2 mg
riboflavin 3 mg
nicotinamide (niacinamide) 20 mg

Three components of Decavitamin, U.S.P., are not included in Hexavitamin, N.F.: folic acid, calcium pantothenate, and vitamin B_{12}. For the overwhelming majority of adults who need a multiple-vitamin preparation (the number is small in the United States), Hexavitamin will be fully as satisfactory as Decavitamin. It is easier to purchase (wider distribution) and can be as inexpensive. No prescription is necessary.

HYDERGINE®

dihydroergocornine
methane sulfonate 0.167 mg
dihydroergocristine
methane sulfonate 0.167 mg
dihydroergokryptine
methane sulfonate 0.167 mg

This curious drug, given 4 to 6 times daily under the tongue and allowed to dissolve over several minutes, is of very questionable usefulness.

Panels of medical experts under contract to the National Academy of Sciences—National Research Council recently studied many drugs and ranked their indications as "effective," "probably effective," "possibly effective," and "ineffective." In reviewing Hydergine®, the group could find it neither "effective" nor even "probably effective" used as its manufacturer advertises to ease senile mental changes.

Simply stated, the *Handbook* finds no reason to use this drug at any time. Nonetheless, it ranked within the most frequently prescribed 200 drugs in America in 1974. It is not inexpensive.

HYDROCHLOROTHIAZIDE, U.S.P.
See Esidrix®; Hydrodiuril®.

HYDROCORTISONE CREAM, U.S.P.

In office practice, one of the most useful preparations for treating many skin disorders is washable cream containing a steroid. A number are marketed by brand name in collapsible tubes, and they are all high-priced. The least costly way to obtain a substantial amount is to have a pharmacist make it up. He disperses hydrocortisone powder·in a water-soluble base (cream). Even with a relatively substantial compounding fee from the pharmacist, the cost of the hydrocortisone or cream ointment can be a small fraction of that of similar products sold by brand name. (However, see Hydrocortisone in the Price Lists.)

It has been claimed by consulting dermatologists that hydrocortisone is not as effective when applied topically as are newer steroids such as flurandrenolide (Cordran®), triamcinolone (Kenalog®), fluocinolone acetonide (Synalar®), or betamethasone valerate (Valisone®). Perhaps so, but for the majority of persons treated by the general practitioner and internist, hydrocortisone is an excellent first-line drug and is highly effective. (The skin specialists' view· is skewed; they see so many of the hard-to-manage cases.) Side effects of topical steroids, including darkening of skin and increased blood vessel growth (telangiectasis) and absorption into the bloodstream, are less likely with hydrocortisone than with the newer steroids. For economy's sake, it is sensible to think of hydrocortisone as the first-line topical steroid. *The doctor must carefully instruct the patient to rub the cream in so well that it "disappears."*

HYDRODIURIL®   Hydrochlorothiazide, U.S.P.
See Esidrix®; Trichlormethiazide.

Hydrodiuril® and Esidrix® are different brands of hydrochlorothiazide, a diuretic. Diuretics cause increased urine formation and help in the control of high blood pressure and certain heart disorders. Side effects of all the thiazides are similar. The patent on hydrochlorothiazide recently expired, and a glance at comparative price lists will show for how little money this useful drug is available.

As is the case, when an individual takes any diuretic of the thiazide family, it is important not to deplete the body of potassium. The easiest way to do this is to eat an orange each day.

See also Kaon®.

HYDROPRES®   Hydrochlorothiazide,
                                         U.S.P.   25 and 50 mg
                                  Reserpine, U.S.P.   0.125 mg
See Diupres®; Hydrodiuril®; Reserpine, U.S.P.

Hydropres® is analogous to Diupres®. Hydropres® is a fixed combination in two different dosage forms of a diuretic and the blood pressure medication reserpine.

Fixed combinations have come into disrepute; the warning published in the *Physicians' Desk Reference* and printed on the package insert accompanying the drug hints that Hydropres® is not a good drug for initiating treatment for high blood pressure.

The patient pays a very large premium for the convenience of taking 1 pill rather than 2; a similar antihypertensive and diuretic effect may be accomplished with significant savings by using reserpine and generic hydrochlorothiazide separately.

HYDROXYZINE HYDROCHLORIDE, N.F.
See Atarax®; Vistaril®.

HYGROTON®   Chlorthalidone, U.S.P.
See Potassium Chloride, U.S.P.; Hydrodiuril®.

This is a diuretic and high blood pressure medication related to the thiazides but slightly different in structure. It has side effects similar to thiazides, however, and like thiazide drugs is useful as an adjunct to reserpine and other antihypertensive medications. The only significant advantage that chlorthalidone is claimed to hold over to other "thiazide" diuretics is a longer effect; often it is necessary to take the medication only once daily or every other day. However, because of the longer-lasting effect it may cause patients the inconvenience of having to awaken at night to urinate.

As with the other diuretics, cost should be the major determinant of what is prescribed and purchased.

ILOSONE®   Erythromycin Estolate, N.F.
   See E-Mycin®; Erythrocin® Stearate; Pediamycin®.

Erythromycin rarely causes side effects. However, this form of the drug has a major disadvantage when compared with other erythromycin products: it causes jaundice due to changes in the liver. It seems that many doctors are unaware of this danger, for the product Ilosone® ranked 20th among the drugs prescribed in 1973. Erythrocin®, a safer, equally effective form of the same drug ranked among the top 25 drugs. Unspecified (generic) erythromycin ranked 68th despite its being potentially cheaper than either Erythrocin® or Ilosone®, and distinctly safer than Ilosone®.

IMIPRAMINE HYDROCHLORIDE, U.S.P.
   See Tofranil®.

INDERAL®   Propranolol Hydrochloride, U.S.P.

Propranolol has recently come into very widespread use for patients with high blood pressure, angina pectoris, abnormal heart rhythms, and unusual heart abnormalities. Some explanation is necessary to understand how it can have so many different uses.

The human body produces adrenalin and adrenalin-like chemicals. These chemicals are secreted by certain nerve fibers in the heart, and serve as transmitters to stimulate and influence the heart muscle cells. Heart muscle cells have on their surface two types of sites (receptors) where the nerve chemical molecules can attach themselves, thereby altering the function of the cells. Similar receptor sites are located in blood vessels, lungs, stomach, and intestines. When the nerve transmitter stimulates one type of receptor, the various organs react differently than when the other type is stimulated.

In actual fact, receptors have never been seen; but their presence is theorized because of extensive experimental observations made in the pharmacology laboratory on isolated organs, on whole laboratory animals, and on man. Drug receptor theory supposes that there are on the surface of cells—muscle cells, gland cells, and others—special chemical sites that are ultramicroscopic in dimension. How many such receptor sites there are on any one cell, how evenly such sites are distributed, how specific (*i.e.*, how discriminating), what the actual chemical composition is, and what the ultramicroscopic shape is have all been subjects of intense speculation and study since shortly after the mid-nineteenth century.

The observable fact that a relatively few thousand molecules of many chemicals (drugs) can trigger highly specific physiological changes is remarkable. It is remarkable that organic chemists can synthesize molecules structurally similar to though not exactly identical with drug molecules known to be active drug molecules. It is presumed that the chemist's new molecule has a configuration enough like that of the real drug to fit into the receptor site, but that because of its minor alteration it lacks the ability of the real drug to trigger a physiologic action. Theory holds that this is how antihistamines block histamine's effects, how atropine blocks acetylcholine's effects, and how propranolol blocks chemical nerve transmitter effects.

In the case of atropine, a large enough number of molecules of this chemical can always overcome any

concentration of molecules of acetylcholine. Conversely,
there is no concentration of atropine which cannot be
overcome by a high enough concentration of acetylcholine. The same relation holds true for antihistamines
and histamine, and for propranolol and the nerve transmitter it "blocks." Such a relation between drugs is
called "competitive antagonism."

Propranolol acts by usurping those receptor sites
whose stimulation by the nerve-secreted drugs will increase force of heart contraction, rate of heartbeat, and
constriction of small arteries. Therefore, propranolol
can make the heart beat less vigorously and more
slowly and dilate the small arteries.

The most serious unwanted side effect is to weaken
the heartbeat enough to cause "heart failure." However, a properly controlled dose is unlikely to make
this happen, and is likely to diminish the frequency and
severity of "heart pain" (angina pectoris). The drug
may often lower blood pressure, too, by its dilating
effect on small arteries. Severe diabetics and asthmatics
require particularly careful regulation of dose; the
reasons are beyond the scope of this book. Like most
new drugs, propranolol is going through a popular
phase—it is being widely used and perhaps overused.
When data have been accumulated, more will be known
of the specific indications for its use and of its true value.

INDOCIN®   Indomethacin, N.F.
See Aspirin, U.S.P.; Butazolidin®; Tandearil®.

Indocin® is an anti-inflammation drug that lowers
fevers and relieves pain, especially in the joints.
However, it should not be used for inflammatory
arthritis until other drugs have been tried and have
failed. Side effects of Indocin® are frequent and serious;
they include headache, dizziness, nausea, vomiting,
peptic ulcers and bleeding peptic ulcers, and, more
rarely, serious blood disorders.

Indocin® and aspirin are about equally effective
in the treatment of rheumatoid (the more severe

form of) arthritis. Aspirin should be tried first, since it is usually better tolerated, has less far fewer serious potential side effects, and is very much less expensive than Indocin®. When aspirin fails to control joint problems, an alternation of aspirin and Indocin® is reasonable, although the drugs should not be taken simultaneously, since aspirin may interfere with indomethacin absorption from the stomach and intestine. Indocin® is probably safer than Butazolidin® and Tandearil® *for long-term use* and may be more useful in the unusual arthritis affecting the neck and spine, ankylosing spondylitis.

In the far more common arthritis of older people, osteoarthritis, Indocin® is of questionable value. When aspirin is not tolerated, it is alleged that Indocin® *may* help with osteoarthritis of the hip; evidence for this claim is poor. The severe potential side effects of Indocin®, and the possible very serious side effects of Butazolidin® * and Tandearil®,* should make any prudent doctor think twice or more times before prescribing them. If a patient cannot tolerate aspirin, he should try other modes of treatment: hot baths, hot packs, and acetaminophen (p. 139).

In acute gout attacks, Indocin® is not the drug oı choice. Since the attacks are usually brief, most physicians should use colchicine (p. 167), but Butazolidin® may be used as a backup drug. The best long-term preventive treatment for gout is probenecid (Benemid®) (p. 288).

It cannot be emphasized strongly enough that Indocin® should never be used simply to relieve nonspecific pains or fever; its serious side effects are far too serious for that. Yet, Indocin® ranked 11th among the drugs prescribed in the United States in 1973!

INDOMETHACIN, N.F.
  See Indocin®.

  * Bone marrow poisoning.

INSULIN INJECTION, U.S.P.

The backbone of diabetes therapy is insulin. The history of this drug's discovery goes back to 1889, when two German investigators, Von Mering and Minkowski, studying the digestive function in dogs, surgically removed the pancreas of several. Flies were more attracted to the cages of these animals than to those of unoperated ones, and this was discovered to be because the operated animals had large amounts of sugar in their urine. It was the first recorded intimation that the pancreas might have something to do with "sugar diabetes," at that time a fatal disease in young persons. After unsuccessful attempts on the part of many others, Drs. Banting and Best at the University of Toronto succeeded in isolating from fresh pancreas tissue a principle called "insulin," which on injection into an adolescent dying from diabetes caused dramatic improvement. Subsequently isolated in crystalline form, insulin's complicated protein structure has been unraveled (1960) and has actually been synthesized (1964). Its three-dimensional complexities were further elucidated recently. For commercial purposes insulin must still be extracted from slaughterhouse-animal tissue, which makes it expensive, though no more so than the newer oral blood-sugar-lowering drugs, whose price has been artificially set high. Insulin is the agent of choice in every respect except convenience, since it must be injected by the patient himself or by someone else.

The oral blood-sugar-lowering agents are not insulin and are not to be used in its place for treating juvenile or severe diabetes, or for any patient with complications of diabetes. The diabetes patient must not try to pressure his doctor to switch him from insulin to an oral drug.

A recent change in the purification and packaging of insulin has come about. Insulin is currently available in 100 units per milliliter. This form is preferred for one major reason: there is less likelihood of mistakes with dose. Cost should be approximately the same as with U-80 and U-40 forms. During the changeover from older preparations to U-100, patients should be careful to use the appropriately calibrated syringes (which have recently been in short supply).

For prices, see Insulin Injection, U.S.P., in the Price Lists.

IONAMIN® phentermine resin
See Dextroamphetamine Sulfate, U.S.P.

This product is promoted for weight loss. It is only "possibly effective," according to the National Academy of Sciences—National Research Council. Appetite suppressants have fallen into disrepute among the medical community and probably should not be used. If they are used, they must be used briefly and with full knowledge of their numerous side effects, including dryness of the mouth, nervousness, sleeplessness, headache, and drug dependence. Drug abuse, stemming from the availability of appetite suppressants, has become a significant social problem.

ISMELIN® Guanethidine Sulfate, U.S.P.

This is a very interesting drug, useful for some persons with severe high blood pressure.

Guanethidine (known commonly as Ismelin®) acts like reserpine in causing the stores of chemical transmitter in sympathetic nerves to be depleted. It is unlikely that this is its only action, however, because it is more powerful at lowering blood pressure than reserpine. Probably it has a "bretylium-like" effect at the terminals of these same nerve fibers. (Bretylium is a drug which prevents the release of nerve transmitter chemical from sympathetic nerves, thus rendering them inactive.) When guanethidine is combined with a thiazide drug, the blood-pressure-lowering effect is enhanced.

In treating severe high blood pressure, guanethidine has largely replaced ganglion-blocking drugs like Inversine® (mecamylamine), Ecolid® (chlorisondamine), and Ansolysen® (pentolinium) because it has fewer adverse side effects. Still, it has *some* side effects, including dizziness on suddenly standing up (especially in the morning), faintness, urinary incontinence, blurred vision, and stuffy nose.

The dose must be carefully adjusted for each patient. It is customary to do this by starting treatment with 10 milligrams a day for a week, then increasing the daily dose by 10 milligrams. After another week, the dose might have to be increased again. Some persons require and can tolerate as much as 50 milligrams a day. Less usually suffices if a thiazide drug is taken at the same time. Generic hydrochlorothiazide is the drug of choice.

Ismelin®, though losing in popularity, is still widely used and can be very costly. At present Ismelin® is the only available brand of guanethidine.

ISONIAZID, U.S.P. (INH, ISONICOTINIC ACID HYDRAZIDE)

The discovery that this organic chemical is a powerful but relatively non-toxic antituberculosis drug that can be taken by mouth was one of the most important medical observations of our time. As with most other discoveries, the usefulness of isoniazid was determined by chance, educated guessing, and trial and error. In 1945 it had been noted that nicotinamide (niacinamide, one of the B vitamins) interfered moderately with the growth of the tuberculosis germ in test-tube cultures. The molecular configuration of nicotinamide is strongly reminiscent of isoniazid.

Isoniazid (also called INH) can be bought very inexpensively. This is important to know and to take advantage of, because isoniazid is the keystone of antituberculosis treatment and must ordinarily be taken for a long time—even years.

Isoniazid is widely used to treat children who are found to have a positive tuberculin skin test even though they are healthy and have a normal chest X-ray. It has been shown that such prophylactic treatment diminishes the likelihood of active tuberculosis appearing later in adulthood. Recent studies have shown that liver damage is very rarely related to INH, and for this reason the practice of treating all children and adults whose TB skin test turns positive has been under some discussion. The *Handbook* votes for continuing the use of "prophylactic" INH. The minor risk is well worth the benefit.

For comparative prices, see Isoniazid, U.S.P., in the Price Lists.

ISOPTO CARPINE®　　　　Pilocarpine Hydrochloride, U.S.P., 0.25, 0.50, 1, 2, 3, 4, 5, 6, 8 and 10%

Pilocarpine is the best drug for beginning and continuing therapy in glaucoma, a disease of the eye in which the pressure within a portion of the eyeball builds up. The drops rarely cause irritation of the eye, and allergic reactions are uncommon.

Eye preparations are not inexpensive, but if purchased in large quantities generic forms of pilocarpine eye drops may lead to some savings. Your ophthalmologist can probably direct you to a place where you can buy this important medication inexpensively. If you are in the age group eligible for membership in the American Association for Retired Persons, ask your doctor to write the prescription in his usual fashion. Append *"please dispense the least expensive equivalent,"* and you ought to save considerable money.

ISORDIL®　　　　　　　　　isosorbide dinitrate
See Nitroglycerin, U.S.P.; Peritrate®.

Isordil® was introduced enthusiastically as a long-acting prophylactic treatment for heart pain (angina pectoris). As with other drugs developed for this purpose (Peritrate® and Peritrate® SA) the achievement of prophylaxis has been elusive. Many of these items are now sold in mixtures with sedatives or "tranquilizers," but always the patient is instructed to carry some plain, old-fashioned nitroglycerin too, "just in case."

Most patients with angina pectoris find that sublingual (under the tongue) nitroglycerin relieves pain within minutes; other nitroglycerin-like compounds, such as Isordil®, have similar effects when used sublingually, but cost considerably more than plain "nitro."

Oral Isordil® and other long-acting nitrite preparations, although widely used—and suggested for use a few minutes before physical, emotional, or other stressful situations, to prevent the onset of angina—have *not* been shown to prevent attacks of angina, and should be avoided because of their expense and questionable efficacy. Indeed, there is some evidence that persons taking long-acting nitrites might get *less* benefit from nitroglycerin when they need it.*

ISOSORBIDE DINITRATE
See *Isordil*®.

ISOXSUPRINE HYDROCHLORIDE
See *Vasodilan*®.

KAON®
potassium gluconate
See *Potassium Chloride, U.S.P.*

Kaon is a liquid or tablet preparation of the gluconate salt of potassium. Potassium supplementation is often necessary in patients receiving "thiazide" or related diuretics, including Hydrodiuril®, Hydropres®, Diuril®, Diupres®, Esidrix®, Hygroton®, Metahydrin®, and others. There are also some other situations where potassium supplements may be required. When potassium supplementation is required, diet can

* J. L. Schelling, et al., *Clinical Pharmacology and Therapeutics, 8*:256 (1967).

usually supply adequate amounts without the added cost of commercial potassium preparations. When foods are unable to provide adequate potassium supplementation, generic potassium chloride (10% elixir) is preferred and cheap.

Foods rich in potassium are plentiful and, if taken in adequate quantities, can obviate the need for potassium supplements in the form of medicinals. Examples of potassium-rich foods include dried apricots, dates, raisins, dried peaches, cantaloupe, dried figs, bananas, and prunes and oranges and their juices. Fig leaves are a specially rich source.

If these foods do not provide adequate potassium, patients should have potassium chloride 10% elixir because, although unpalatable, it is cheaper and better absorbed than potassium chloride tablets.

KEFLEX®   cephalexin monohydrate

Keflex® is an antibiotic that only rarely is appropriate for use outside a hospital setting. It is a broad-spectrum antibiotic that is *not* the first-line drug for most bacterial infections. It happens also to be extraordinarily costly.

Three kinds of infections most commonly *inappropriately* treated with Keflex® are those involving the respiratory tract and throat, skin and soft tissue, and the urinary tract. In respiratory and throat infections, penicillin (see Penicillin G Tablets) is cheaper and preferred; in patients with penicillin allergy, there is also a high chance of allergic reaction to Keflex®, and, therefore, erythromycin should be used. In skin and soft tissue infections, where staphylococcus has been found to be involved, semisynthetic penicillins like dicloxacillin (Dynapen®) should be used; Keflex® is less effective against this organism and has a broader spectrum, making the likelihood of "superinfection" or overgrowth with new kinds of bacteria more likely. In urinary tract infections, a sulfonamide such as sulfisoxazole is preferred; when resistant organisms are found, ampicillin should be used if it kills these organisms. Only after culture and special sensitivity studies where bacteria are found resistant to sulfa and ampicillin but sensitive to Keflex®, should Keflex® be used. Another uncommon reason for using Keflex® in capsule form is to complete a course of intravenously administered Keflex® begun in the hospital, when the patient leaves the hospital.

Keflex® has been widely and aggressively advertised and publicized, accounting for its rank as the 64th most frequently prescribed drug in the United States in 1973. A 10-day course of treatment using 4 tablets daily costs approximately four or five times the same course of penicillin or sulfa.

KENALOG®   Triamcinolone Acetonide, U.S.P.
See Hydrocortisone Cream, U.S.P.

Topical steroids are very useful in certain skin problems. Somewhat less potent, non-fluorinated steroids are usually quite effective and cheap. Stronger compounds, like triamcinolone, and the strongest compounds, like Synalar,® are useful when the less expensive and less powerful formulations do not work. Bear in mind that stronger forms should be avoided because skin changes and suppression of the adrenal gland are possible complications.

Despite the suitability of hydrocortisone cream for most cases where Kenalog® is effective, the brands are much more widely prescribed.

LANOXIN®
See Digoxin, U.S.P.

LASIX®   furosemide
See Potassium Chloride, U.S.P.; Trichlormethiazide.

Furosemide is a potent diuretic, faster and more powerful than thiazide and related diuretics (Diuril®,

Hydrodiuril®, Esidrix®, Enduron®, Hygroton®). For patients with heart failure, high blood pressure, and other diseases that call for "water pills," furosemide is a *second-line* drug that should be prescribed only after the less expensive and less toxic thiazides, such as generic hydrochlorothiazide or trichlormethiazide, have been tried for adequate periods of time.

Side effects from Lasix® resemble those of the thiazides, to which it is a close chemical cousin. Of primary concern is potassium loss in the urine, which is more severe than in the thiazides. Excessive loss of water and body salts may be so rapid and severe when the drug is given as to cause collapse, but this usually occurs when the drug is given as a "shot." The usual need to supplement one's diet with potassium-rich foods or potassium chloride holds for Lasix® as well as for the less potent "thiazide" diuretics.

In the late 1960s, Lasix® skyrocketed into use with a series of sensational ads appearing first in 1966; complaints lodged by the FDA ensued, and the ads were revised. But physicians have undoubtedly been persuaded by the promotional material to use furosemide as a routine, first-choice oral diuretic in office practice. This can be the only explanation for the drug's current rank of 8th among the most prescribed drugs in the United States in 1973. In most instances where it is used, hydrochlorothiazide or trichlormethiazide would do as well.

L-DOPA
   See Dopa   (Levodopa; Dihydroxyphenylalanine)

LEVODOPA
   See Dopa   (L-Dopa; Dihydroxyphenylalanine).

LEVOTHYROXINE (SODIUM LEVOTHYROXINE, U.S.P.)
   See Synthroid®.

LIBRAX®   Chlordiazepoxide Hydro-
                                    chloride, N.F.   5.0 mg
                                    clidinium bromide   2.5 mg
     See Atropine Sulfate, U.S.P.; Librium®; Phenobar-
bital, U.S.P.; Tincture of Belladonna (Belladonna
Tincture, U.S.P.)

Librax® is a combination product comprised of
Librium® and an atropine-like drug, clidinium bromide. Roche has succeeded in marketing what for
clinical purposes is a duplicative product that adds
little of importance except confusion and cost. It is
recommended for relief of "hypersecretion, hyper-
motility and anxiety and tension states associated
with organic and functional gastrointestinal disorders
and . . . in the management of peptic ulcer, gastritis,
duodenitis, irritable bowel syndrome, spastic colitis
and mild ulcerative colitis" (*Physicians' Desk Reference*, 1974 edn., p. 1224).
Evidence that the product has any influence or
significance on irritable colon or peptic ulcer disorders is slim. If a patient has an ulcer, and gastric
motility should be slowed, atropine or related drugs
alone should be used. If a patient needs sedation,
sedatives alone should be used. Librax® has no advantage over inexpensive belladonna tincture or
atropine sulfate plus 15 milligrams of phenobarbital.
Yet it was the 32nd most frequently prescribed drug
in the United States in 1974.

LIBRIUM®   Chlordiazepoxide Hydrochlo-
                                    ride, N.F.
     See Phenobarbital, U.S.P.; Valium®.

Librium® was the first of a series of benzodiazepines that are now the most frequently prescribed
sedatives in the nation. Librium® ranked 2nd among
the prescribed drugs in the United States in 1973,
and its close relative, Valium®, ranked 1st. Serax®
and Tranxene®, drugs of the same family with similar
effects, are increasingly popular.

Chlordiazepoxide initially caught the attention of investigators when it was alleged to have the power to "tame" vicious animals. Hundreds of articles and, now, at least one complete book have been published on Librium® and related drugs.

Careful experiments studying the efficacy of Librium® compared to alternative drugs for sedation and their effects are few. While most physicians in the United States prefer Librium® or Valium® to other mild sedatives, the *Handbook* feels that phenobarbital works as well or better in most situations. For the usual patient with mild anxiety, it is reasonable to begin treatment with phenobarbital if any medication is needed at all. Before deciding that phenobarbital is ineffective, the doctor should increase the dose to as much as 30 milligrams 4 times daily. In some cases it might then be helpful to switch to Librium® or another similar sedative. In disabling neuroses or frank psychoses, however, no *drug* is a substitute for adequate and wise attention from physicians and friends.

One advantage of Librium® over the barbiturates and many other sedatives is important: it is probably more difficult to commit suicide with an overdose of Librium®. However, where a patient is thought to be so depressed as to be contemplating suicide, he ought to be hospitalized. Dependence on Librium® is well known and its sudden withdrawal can cause serious symptoms.

While Librium® and its closely related drugs may sometimes be useful when phenobarbital is not, it is also true that far too much Librium® is unnecessarily prescribed. Some evidence exists suggesting that the use of tranquilizers and other drugs in parents predisposes children to abuse stronger drugs in their adolescence. Good statistical evidence exists that a new market for tranquilizers has emerged over the past decade that accounts for a very large percentage of our drug costs. At the risk of being old-fashioned, the *Handbook* recommends to physicians and their patients that so-called "tranquilizers" (sedatives) be avoided for psychological, economic, and social reasons. It is indeed frightening that over half of adult Americans "pop" these sedatives regularly.

LINCOCIN®

See Addenda.

LOMOTIL®   diphenoxylate hydro-
                                  chloride   2.5 mg
                                Atropine Sulfate,
                                  U.S.P.   0.025 mg
                                  (per tablet or tsp liquid)

See Paregoric, U.S.P. (Camphorated Tincture of Opium).

A drug for loose bowels with a name designed to be catchy, Lomotil® is comprised of an opium-like synthetic narcotic and atropine. The atropine is added presumably to prevent abuse of the product by narcotics users who are inclined to self-inject the material. (The atropine, by the way, is probably present in too small a quantity to prevent such abuse).

Careful studies of the effectiveness of this product have shown 2 tablets approximately equal to 15 milligrams of codeine and 8 milliliters of paregoric. Comparable to codeine and paregoric in effect, Lomotil® also has similar side effects when used for prolonged periods of time: addiction, overdosage, sedation, nausea, and vomiting.

Because of cost, Lomotil® is not recommended by the *Handbook* for either acute or chronic diarrhea; paregoric should be used. Despite its cost—some four or five times that of an equivalent dose of codeine and some two or three times that of paregoric—Lomotil® ranked 25th among the most prescribed drugs in 1973.

MAALOX®   magnesium and aluminum
                                hydroxides mixture

See Mylanta®.

Antacids, such as Maalox®, are very widely used preparations that can be purchased without prescription. They are used for treatment of ulcers, reflux of acid into the esophagus ("heartburn"), and irritable or "nervous" stomach. Whether antacids help with healing of ulcers is unclear, but they certainly improve the discomfort.

Some antacids cause constipation, while others can cause diarrhea. Some antacids are very rich in sodium, which must be avoided in patients with high blood pressure, heart failure, cirrhosis, and kidney diseases. Others can damage kidneys because of excessive absorption of calcium and formation of kidney stones.

Most preparations, including Maalox®, combine aluminum and magnesium hydroxides. Other preparations commonly used include calcium carbonate (better known as Tums®) and sodium bicarbonate ("sodamint" tablets).

Many patients take Maalox® regularly and in large amounts. They would save considerably if they bought the same or similar mixtures by another name. Many drugstores carry their own brand, which is usually less expensive than Maalox®.

Liquid antacid preparations are probably more effective if less convenient to carry around. If one has a great deal of discomfort despite antacids, probably too little is being used. A reasonable routine is to take antacids one hour after meals, when gastric acid is highest. If that alone does not work, the antacids should be used at very regular intervals, such as every 2 hours or even every hour. Since pain is often most severe at night, the *Handbook* suggests that a liquid antacid be kept right at the bedside; when awakened by discomfort, the patient should simply take a swig. Calcium carbonate (Tums®) may be effective during the day but should not be used at night, since it causes a "rebound" of gastric acid secretion in several hours.

Since antacids are taken in such large quantity and for such prolonged periods of time, the patient is advised to shop around for the one that is most efficacious for him, palatable, cheapest, and causes the least diarrhea or constipation or other side effects, and to buy in bulk after perhaps some bargaining with the local pharmacist. Those preparations with aluminum tend to cause constipation, while those with magnesium tend to cause diarrhea. A patient might like to have both kinds on hand to alternate swigs and keep his bowels normal.

MACRODANTIN®   Nitrofurantoin, U.S.P.
See Ampicillin, U.S.P.; Gantrisin®; Triple Sulfas.

Macrodantin® is a trademark for nitrofurantoin, sold widely for years as Furadantin®. One of Furadantin's® major drawbacks is the ease with which it causes nausea and vomiting, so the manufacturer, Eaton Laboratories, marketed Furadantin® with larger (macro-) crystals. This change was alleged to decrease associated nausea and vomiting, but the evidence for this is poor.

Nitrofurantoin (as either Furadantin® or Macrodantin®) has been on the market for over twenty years and the exclusive patents have expired. Many far cheaper generic forms are available, such as McKesson's Trantoin®.

Nitrofurantoin is used in urinary tract infections as a second- or third-line drug. Since most urinary tract infections are caused by *E. coli,* sulfa should be the first-line drug, and when sulfa is ineffective, ampicillin is probably more effective, with fewer side effects than nitrofurantoin. In unusual infections with enterococcus, nitrofurantoin is quite effective.

In chronic urinary tract infections, nitrofurantoin has some role in suppressing the growth of bacteria. Again, in these cases, other drugs are preferred. Either methenamine mandelate, with 4 to 8 grams of ascorbic acid daily, or methenamine hippurate is a better drug. Methenamine mandelate should be purchased generically and not as Mandelamine®, which is very much more expensive. (See Addenda.)

Extensive use of nitrofurantoin in children with

chronic urinary tract infections has led to countless cases of chronic crippling inflammation of the nerves that innervate muscles, a serious effect of the drug that has been given too little attention. Despite the adverse side effects and the availability of generic forms usually about half as expensive as Macrodantin®, it was among the 100 most-prescribed drugs in the United States in 1973. The medical profession has got to find an effective means to educate its members about rational prescribing. Public tolerance has its limits.

MAGNESIUM HYDROXIDE
See *Aludrox®; Maalox®; Mylanta®*.

MANDELAMINE®
See *Addenda*.

MARAX®		
	Theophylline, N.F.	130 mg
	Ephedrine Sulfate, U.S.P.	25 mg
	Hydroxyzine Hydro-chloride, N.F.	10 mg

See *Ephedrine Sulfate, U.S.P.*

Marax® is a variant of the theophylline-ephedrine-phenobarbital combination for asthma of which Tedral® is the brand name most well known. In Marax® the phenobarbital component is replaced by hydroxyzine (Atarax®), a minor antihistaminic sedative. The amounts of theophylline and ephedrine are similar to those in Tedral®. The *Handbook* recommends generic combinations of theophylline-ephedrine-phenobarbital or use of the separate components as aminophylline and ephedrine. Savings can be substantial; see the Price Lists for what these combinations need cost.

As with so many of the very popular drugs in this *Handbook* that are of questionable usefulness, the National Research Council found Marax® only "possibly effective" (as opposed to "effective" or "probably effective") for controlling asthmatic conditions.

MECLIZINE HYDROCHLORIDE, U.S.P.
   See Antivert®.

MEDROL®   Methylprednisolone, N.F.
   See Decadron®; Prednisone, U.S.P.; Predisolone, U.S.P.

Medrol® is a cortisone-like drug; 4 milligrams of Medrol® is equivalent to 5 of prednisone or prednisolone. Prednisolone can always be used in place of Medrol®. See Prednisone in the Price Lists.

MEDROXYPROGESTERONE ACETATE, U.S.P.
   See Provera®.

MELLARIL®   thioridazine
   See Thorazine®.

Mellaril® is a phenothiazine drug that is often used for treating psychoses. Psychosis might be defined here as an illness in which there is altered emotion, confusion about sexual identity, altered thought processes interfering with normal logic and thinking, and inappropriate mood. A classic example of psychosis is schizophrenia. The drug should not be used for minor or self-limiting illnesses, neuroses, or nervousness not associated with severe mental derangement because it is a drug with an extraordinarily large list of possible toxic side effects, including sudden death.
   Mellaril® was among the 50 most-prescribed drugs of 1973. Are there really so many psychotic people in this country?

MEPERIDINE HYDROCHLORIDE, U.S.P.
   See Demerol®.

MEPROBAMATE, U.S.P.

When meprobamate was introduced in the early 1950s, the public and the doctors were sold on "tranquilizers" by every conceivable promotional device, including reference to them by TV comics. Even the United States Pharmacopeial Convention was caught up in the enthusiasm, and listed meprobamate in its roster of blue-ribbon drugs, though at a later date it was forced to demote the drug from its position because it was found to have a relatively high addiction potential. Wallace Laboratories, the company with the patent on meprobamate, named it Miltown®, after a small town in New Jersey. Wallace was not large enough to exploit the potential market for the drug as well as it wished, and it therefore licensed Wyeth to sell its product under the brand name Equanil®.

Some pharmacologists, not excluding those with a financial interest in its sale, say that meprobamate is a "tranquilizer," not a "sedative," because there is evidence that it affects a part of the animal brain which sedatives like phenobarbital, chloral hydrate, and alcohol do not affect. Perhaps this is correct. But for most human beings who need a little calming down, phenobarbital, butabarbital, amobarbital, or a small dose of chloral hydrate usually works well.

Meprobamate certainly exerts sedative effects; 400 to 800 milligrams at night puts one to sleep with as much ease as a barbiturate. Those who maintain that it is not a "sedative" explain this by saying that meprobamate "fosters" sleep. So do barbiturates. Meprobamate is not non-toxic, and it can be addicting.

If patient and doctor are for any reason convinced that meprobamate is the drug they want, the doctor should prescribe it and the patient buy it at the lowest possible price as meprobamate. For what it need cost by this name, see Meprobamate, N.F., in the Price Lists.

METHAQUALONE
  See *Quaalude®*.

METHYCLOTHIAZIDE
  See *Enduron®*.

METHYLDOPA, U.S.P. (ALPHA-METHYLDOPA)
  See *Aldomet®*.

METHYLPHENIDATE HYDROCHLORIDE, N.F.
  See *Ritalin®*.

METHYLPREDNISOLONE, N.F.
  See *Medrol®*.

METHYPRYLON, N.F.
  See *Noludar®*.

METRONIDAZOLE, U.S.P.
  See *Flagyl®*.

MILTOWN®
  See *Meprobamate, N.F.*

MINOCIN®   minocycline hydrochloride
  See *Tetracycline Hydrochloride, U.S.P.*

  Minocin® is a form of tetracycline that is longer-
acting than plain tetracycline, so that one need theoretically take only 1 or 2 doses daily instead of 3 or 4.
This longer action takes place also with demeclocycline (Declomycin®) and doxycycline (Vibramycin®).
These longer-acting tetracyclines are among the more
expensive of all the tetracyclines, and Minocin® is
the *most* expensive of them all.

Minocin® is the tetracycline most poorly concentrated in the kidney and urine and, of all the tetracyclines, is least likely to be of use where there is infection in these places. Despite clever advance promotion, Minocin® is not a drug to be used against staphylococcus resistant to tetracycline itself. The manufacturer was "requested" by FDA to make this clear in a "Dear Doctor" letter of February 10, 1975.

Side effects include nausea and stomach upset, not unusual for a tetracycline. However, unlike with other tetracyclines the manufacturer was asked by the FDA to warn of an unusual toxic effect: light-headedness and true dizziness (vertigo). Hence, the drug is not to be given to those who must drive cars or work with hazardous machinery.

In summary, the manufacturer itself (Lederle), which admits that its product is no better and probably less desirable than other tetracyclines, has the audacity to keep it on the market and charge an exorbitant price for it. They have already got doctors prescribing enough of it so that it ranks among the 200 most-prescribed pharmaceuticals in the country!

MINOCYCLINE HYDROCHLORIDE
See Minocin®.

MULTIPLE VITAMINS
See Decavitamin Capsules, U.S.P.; Hexavitamin Capsules, N.F.

For economy's sake, it is well worth knowing that there is only a single multiple-vitamin preparation in the *United States Pharmacopeia:* Decavitamin; and only a single one in the *National Formulary:* Hexavitamin. Decavitamin, U.S.P., is not as widely available as Hexavitamin, N.F.

MYAMBUTOL®   ethambutol
    See Isoniazid, U.S.P. (INH, Isonicotinic Acid Hydrazide).

Ethambutol is an addition to the group of drugs for treating tuberculosis. Ordinarily, the ambulatory patient is cared for very well with isoniazid plus aminosalicylic acid (PAS). Despite its astronomically higher cost, ethambutol has somehow come to replace PAS as the drug usually paired with isoniazid. This is because PAS is not infrequently associated with nausea, vomiting, and other gastrointestinal upsets. However, by starting with small doses of PAS and increasing them weekly, the nausea is eventually overcome. Side effects of ethambutol, on the other hand, may include serious visual changes including loss of acuity, color vision, and field of vision. PAS has no such serious side effects.

Almost any patient who has to take daily ethambutol is soon in "financial straits" and should be switched to PAS as an adjunct to isoniazid (INH) whether for treating tuberculosis prophylactically or for treating active tuberculosis. Where tax-supported institutions maintain tuberculosis treatment centers, the use of the costly and potentially toxic ethambutal should be discontinued forthwith.

MYCOLOG®   Nystatin, U.S.P. 100,000 units
                               Neomycin Sulfate,
                                   U.S.P.   2.5 mg
                               gramicidin   0.25 mg
                               triamcinolone aceto-
                                   nide (per g)   1.0 mg
    See Cortisporin®; Mycostatin®; NeoDecadron®.

This ointment is analogous to Cortisporin®, discussed earlier in the *Handbook*. It combines two antibiotics, neomycin and gramicidin, with an antifungus drug, nystatin (see Mycostatin®), and a steroid cream. While used for wound healing and resolution of skin infections, there is little evidence to support the contention that it works. If serious infections exist, antibiotics specific for the implicated bacteria should be given orally or intravenously. Only in burns and unusual skin infections have topically applied antibiotics been shown useful, and even in the instance of burns there is doubt that the topical medication is the equal of one given either by injection or by mouth.

Nystatin is useful for fungal infections; the most common among these is a yeast, *Candida albicans*. There are some occasions when the physician will want to treat a yeast infection with nystatin, but *not* in combination with two antibiotics and a steroid cream. Neomycin and gramicidin are antibiotics with serious side effects that "cover the waterfront" of bacterial infections on the skin. Neomycin is proved as one of the most common causes of skin rashes, occurring in 6 to 8 percent of normal people and in 49 percent of patients with previous reactions to other topical drugs.*†** More significantly, if rarely, it may cause serious hearing losses and deafness if adequately absorbed from wounds or from application to the skin with occlusive dressings, such as diapers on infants with diaper rash treated with neomycin-containing ointments or creams. Furthermore, neomycin allergy may make impossible the treatment of lifesaving antibiotics like gentamicin. In two careful studies, comparisons between neomycin and the cream base used to make neomycin creams and between neomycin with steroids and the steroid alone show that omitting the neomycin changes nothing.‡***

The National Academy of Sciences–National Re-

* North American Contact Dermatitis Group, *Archives of Dermatology, 108*:537 (1973).

† J. Patrick and J. D. Panzer, *Arch. Dermatol., 102*:532 (1970).

** E. Epstein, *Journal of the American Medical Association, 198*:517 (1966).

‡ National Academy of Sciences–National Research Council, Drug Efficacy Study Group, *Federal Register, 37*:12857 (June 29, 1972).

*** C.M. Davis et al., *JAMA, 203*:298 (1968).

search Council has found this preparation only "possibly effective" for the various claimed indications. The *Handbook* does not recommend its use. When yeast or fungus infections involve the skin, nystatin creams should be used. When yeast or fungus infections involve the skin with associated inflammation and scaling of skin, combinations of nystatin with steroids (like hydrocortisone) may be of use for brief periods.

MYCOSTATIN®   Nystatin, U.S.P.

Nystatin is one of three very effective drugs used to treat "thrush," an infection due to a species of yeast called *Candida albicans*. Thrush is usually localized to the mucous membranes of the mouth or vagina.

Candida infections are, in some hospital and clinic populations, now the most common infestations of the vagina and female external genitals. These infections are more frequent with diabetes, pregnancy, and the use of oral contraceptives. Occasionally, the use of broad-spectrum antibiotics allows for growth of yeast in the intestine with subsequent spread to the vagina. (In rural areas and probably in most of suburban sprawl, *Trichomonas vaginalis* remains the most common infection.)

Diagnosis of *Candida* infections depends on careful examination of the typical cottage cheese-like discharge adherent to the walls of the vagina or labia minora ("inner lips"). Occasionally a smear for a microscopic exam or culture is necessary.

Treatment with nystatin is usually effective, using one vaginal "tablet" at bedtime. If used during the day, the "tablet" melts and tends to drip uncomfortably down the upper leg. If vaginal "tablets" alone do not clear up the infection, oral nystatin should be given as well. Uncircumcised male partners of women with yeast infections must be treated to avoid spread of infection back and forth.

Nystatin is now available from two manufacturers,

Lederle (Nilstat®) and Squibb (Mycostatin®). Alternatives include a newer and more expensive drug, candicidin, and amphotericin B. Nystatin is the cheapest and most effective of the standard therapies. In cases where yeast infections are precipitated by the use of "the pill" or broad-spectrum antibiotics, discontinuation of these medications allows for improvement of the .yeast infection.

MYLANTA®

magnesium hydroxide	200 mg
aluminum hydroxide	200 mg
simethicone	20 mg
(per tablet or 5 ml liquid)	

See Maalox®.

The antacid ingredients in Mylanta® are the same as in Maalox® except that Mylanta® has something additional called simethicone, promoted as an "antiflatulent." No well-controlled studies to date have shown the effectiveness of simethicone in releasing gas or decreasing flatulence.

Antacids can be very helpful in stomach disorders and the combination of the hydroxides of magnesium and aluminium is a good one. However, the combination can be bought for less money if one shops around a bit and buys in bulk. No prescription is necessary, and one need not ask for it by brand name. (A prescription raises the retail price.)

While neither Maalox® nor Mylanta® are prescription items, both were among the 200 most-prescribed products in the United States in 1973.

For ways to economize, see Magnesium and Aluminum Hydroxide Suspension in the Price Lists.

MYSTECLIN-F®

tetracycline equivalent to Tetracycline Hydrochloride, U.S.P.	250 mg
amphotericin B	50 mg

See Mycostatin®.

The alleged rationale for this drug is as follows: tetracycline, a broad-spectrum antibiotic, often alters the normal bacteria in the intestine to allow for an "overgrowth" of yeast, *Candida albicans*. Since amphotericin B is effective against the yeast, it should prevent its overgrowth by being added to the tetracycline in "prophylactic amounts." The clinical value of this addition is dubious. The addition of amphotericin may be useful when a very old or debilitated person, or a cancer victim on powerful chemicals suppressing normal body defenses, develops a yeast infection. But, nystatin (see Mycostatin®) is preferred in such yeast infections because it has fewer side effects than amphotericin and is cheaper.

A struggle has been going on now for years between the FDA and Squibb. The FDA has ordered Squibb to provide evidence that Mysteclin-F® is effective; despite rather poor arguments made for its use by the manufacturer, the drug remained among the top 200 drugs prescribed in 1973. To highlight this struggle, the statement of the National Academy of Sciences—National Research Council on this product is excerpted from the *Physicians' Desk Reference,* 1974 edn., p. 1413, below:

Recently, a panel of the National Academy of Sciences–National Research Council has stated that in its informed judgment Mysteclin-F is ineffective as a fixed combination. Further, it stated, "The Panel is not aware of evidence of proved efficacy of this combination in the prevention of disease due to monilial (i.e., candida) organisms, although suppression of growth of monilia may be accomplished. It should be noted that the apparent reduction of organisms in the feces may be an artifact due to residual antibiotic activity and thus may not reflect the true state in the patient. It is preferable, in the Panel's opinion, to prescribe antifungal drugs when clinically indicated, rather than to use them indiscriminately as 'prophylaxis' against an uncommon clinical entity seen during therapy with tetracyclines and other antibiotics."

Despite testimony to the contrary made by the deans* of two famous medical schools on the East coast before federal hearings, Mysteclin-F® has just been ranked "ineffective" (June 1, 1975, *FDA Report*).

NALDECON®

phenylpropanolamine hydrochloride	40 mg
Phenylephrine Hydrochloride, U.S.P.	10 mg
phenyltoloxamine citrate	15 mg
Chlorpheniramine Maleate, U.S.P.	5 mg

(per sustained-action tablet or 2 tsps syrup)

See Antihistamines; Cough Remedies; Chlor-Trimeton®; Neo-Synephrine®.

This concoction in a "sustained-action" preparation is offered for symptomatic relief of colds, upper respiratory infections, sinus troubles, etc. But, combinations such as Naldecon® multiply the potential side effects without providing increased effectiveness over one or two of the components administered separately. An added disadvantage of this preparation is its "sustained action" tablet form.

No company can guarantee that a "sustained action" preparation is going to work in every case for 6 to 12 hours. If a person has diarrhea, mouth-to-anus transit time can easily be as brief as 2 hours, which would make 6 hours of "sustained action" impossible. Such preparations have not been acceptable to the *United States Pharmacopeia* or *National Formulary* for this reason. Even if reliable, such a

---

* These deans, one of the Harvard and the other of the Yale Medical School, were paid consultants of E. R. Squibb, manufacturers of Mysteclin-F®, and could hardly have been expected to be impartial observers.

preparation would still be little more than an expensive luxury. Doctors who care to give a little thought to the matter will recognize that lifesaving drugs are not commonly marketed in "sustained action" dose forms. The pharmaceutical manufacturers are too shrewd to make that mistake.

Naldecon® is an expensive and possibly harmful fixed-dose combination product. The symptoms of the common cold and other minor upper respiratory infections are as well treated with aspirin and phenylephrine nose drops (Neo-Synephrine®), which can be bought over-the-counter, and chlorpheniramine (Chlor-Trimeton®) is a fine antihistamine.

See Actifed®, Ambenyl®, Benylin® Expectorant, Dimetapp®, Drixoral®, Novahistine® Expectorant, and Phenergan® Expectorant for similar criticism.

NEMBUTAL®   Sodium Pentobarbital, U.S.P.
See Chloral Hydrate, U.S.P.; Dalmane®; Seconal®.

Pentobarbital, better known by the brand name Nembutal®, is a widely used barbiturate sleeping medication. It is most effective if swallowed on an empty stomach in a quiet setting.

Addiction to and overdosage with pentobarbital are not uncommon. In addition, barbiturates interact with other drugs, most importantly, warfarin anticoagulants. Even when used appropriately, the drug may give a morning "hangover." The elderly are sometimes said to have "paradoxical" excitement instead of sedation when given barbiturates, but this has not been borne out in good studies.

The patent on pentobarbital expired years ago. Abbott owns the name Nembutal® by trademark law, but several different firms sell it for a fraction of Abbott's price. See Sodium Pentobarbital, U.S.P., in the Price Lists. The barbiturates and chloral hydrate are the cheapest sleeping pills. (Only when the side effects mitigate against the use of pentobarbital, secobarbital, or chloral hydrate should the popular Dalmane® be considered the drug of choice.)

NEODECADRON®   Dexamethasone Sodium
                                      Phosphate, N.F.   1 mg
                                   Neomycin Sulfate,
                                      U.S.P.   5 mg
                                   (per g)
See Hydrocortisone Cream, U.S.P.; Mycolog®.

NeoDecadron® is a combination of dexamethasone
topical steroid and the broad-spectrum antibiotic
neomycin. Reasons for avoiding topical antibiotics
and neomycin in particular have been well discussed
under Mycolog®. There is little evidence to suggest
that this preparation or similar ones promote healing
or prevent infections of wounds.

If skin problems require the use of topical steroids,
hydrocortisone cream should be tried first. If antibiotics are required because of skin or wound infections, they should be given orally or by injection.
One exception in which topical antibiotics may be
useful is in the case of serious burns. But even in
this circumstance the antibiotic is probably going to
be more effective if given by injection or by mouth.

NEOSPORIN®   Polymixin B Sulfate,
                                      U.S.P.   5000 units
                                   Zinc Bacitracin,
                                      U.S.P.   400 units
                                   Neomycin Sulfate,
                                      U.S.P.   5 mg
                                   (per g)
See Mycolog®.

This ointment, also called triple antibiotic ointment, has a "broad spectrum" of antibiotic activity,
combining three different antibiotics in a single ointment used both for skin and eye problems.

The use of topical antibiotics for skin wounds and
infections is at best debatable. However, if one is
going to put antibiotics on the skin, it is better to do
so with a preparation that has antibiotics alone, like
Neosporin®, rather than one with antibiotics in com-

bination with steroids, like Cortisporin® or Mycolog®.
(See Mycolog® for a discussion of the use of topical
antibiotics.) In general, these topical antibiotics should
probably never be used on skin wounds and infections because of frequent skin reactions to neomycin
and because they have never been shown to promote
healing or prevent infections. If infections are present
in wounds, and antibiotics are needed, they should
probably be given orally or by injection. Wounds
usually do well by themselves. The one exception
here is serious burns, which are sometimes appropriately treated with topical antibiotics.

The ophthalmic preparation is used for the treatment of eye infections with bacteria sensitive to the
antibiotics contained in the preparation. Allergies to
antibiotics have been reported after their use in eye
preparations, but this has usually been the case only
with penicillin preparations for ophthalmic use.

NEO-SYNEPHRINE®   Phenylephrine Hydrochloride,
U.S.P.

Phenylephrine is a useful synthetic agent whose
structure is very similar to adrenaline, but the slight
difference makes it more stable chemically, causes it
to exaggerate certain of the effects of adrenaline (*e.g.,*
blood-pressure-raising effect), and makes it have a
longer-lived action. Thus, phenylephrine is given by
injection to certain hospitalized patients, but in office
practice it is prescribed mainly as nose drops. The
swollen, turgid nasal lining that causes the "stuffiness"
of the common cold readily shrinks and the passages
open up in response to phenylephrine. Occasionally,
a person with a chronically stuffy nose (usually due
to an allergy) takes phenylephrine regularly for two
weeks or more, and he is likely to suffer a paradoxical
effect. The lining may swell instead of shrinking in
response to phenylephrine, and there may ensue a
vicious cycle where the drug is applied more and
more frequently in an effort to overcome the stuffiness. This is a possible adverse effect of all or nearly

all nasal decongestants related to phenylephrine. Used not more often than every two to four hours, phenylephrine drops are not likely to be absorbed into the blood in sufficient amounts to raise the blood pressure.

Phenylephrine may be bought cheaply without a prescription in any pharmacy. The best-known over-the-counter brand is Neo-Synephrine®, which comes in 1-ounce dropper bottles. A ¼ or ½ percent solution usually suffices for adults. The patient ought not to buy more than an ounce at a time, because when he puts the dropper tip into his nose, he contaminates it with bacteria and molds. When the dropper cap is screwed back on the bottle, the organisms multiply in the fluid, and in a few days particulate material representing colonies of bacteria and molds can be seen when the bottle is held up to the light. At this point the bottle should be discarded. (It goes without saying that it is at least unaesthetic to use drops from a bottle previously used by someone else.) Phenylephrine drops always come in a brown glass bottle, for exposure to light can cause the drug to decompose. A yellow or pink tint to the fluid indicates decomposition.

See Phenylephrine Hydrochloride, U.S.P. in the Price Lists.

NICOTINIC ACID (NIACIN)
  See Atromid-S®.

Nicotinic acid, or niacin, is a vitamin most important in the treatment of pellagra, a rare deficiency seen in people who eat only corn, who are alcoholics, or food faddists, or who are seriously ill with cancer. In such patients multiple B vitamins in addition to niacin should be given.

As recently as 1970, nicotinic acid was used as a component in mood-altering combination products for older people. This use took advantage of the unusual side effects of the drug, including flushing, tingling, and a feeling of warmth. These preparations have since left the most frequently prescribed 200 drugs, including Antivert®, which was the most popular of them all for a long time. Antivert's® manufacturer quietly removed the nicotinic acid component but failed to draw much attention to it and failed to change the product's name. Most doctors do not know this.

Nicotinic acid is most often used as a second-line or backup drug in the treatment of "high cholesterol" and other "high lipid states." There are at least two kinds of fats that can be elevated in the bloodstream: cholesterol and triglycerides. On the basis of which lipid or fat component in the blood is elevated, the "fat diseases" have been classified as Types I through V. Niacin lowers serum cholesterol and triglycerides by inhibiting the synthesis (manufacturing) of certain fats. It has been useful as a backup drug for patients who cannot take clofibrate (Atromid-S®) in the hyperlipidemias Types II, III, IV, and V. Diet, weight control, curbing alcohol intake, and giving up smoking are the most important treatments for these disorders. While medications may alter the blood fat levels to a moderate extent, no evidence exists to indicate that this has any beneficial effect on the patient's health. The *Handbook* considers Atromid-S® an experimental drug with as yet unknown toxicity.

Side effects of nicotinic acid are frequent and include—besides the flushing and tingling sensations—worsening of gout and diabetes, liver damage, and ulcers of the stomach. (See Osol, Pratt, and Altschule, *U. S. Dispensatory,* 26th edn. [Philadelphia: Lippincott, 1967], p. 758.)

NITROFURANTOIN, U.S.P.
See Macrodantin®.

NITROGLYCERIN, U.S.P.
(GLYCERYL TRINITRATE)
See Isordil®; Peritrate®.

In 1867, Lauder Brunton, a physician in Edinburgh, poured a few drops of amyl nitrite into a cloth and held it to the nose of a patient with angina pectoris. Brunton had recently observed in the laboratory of a colleague that amyl nitrite can temporarily lower the blood pressure in animals. He had a (perhaps mistaken) notion that angina pectoris was caused by a transient rise in blood pressure, and therefore surmised that relief might be found with a drug which could quickly lower it. Amyl nitrite seemed to be effective.

In later years, nitroglycerin taken under the tongue displaced amyl nitrate, because the effect of nitroglycerin is the same and it is easier to self-administer. Also, amyl nitrite has a strong odor; its use embarrassed elderly ladies sitting at the symphony. Nitroglycerin is (next to amyl nitrite) the best-known immediate treatment for angina pectoris, the pain caused by decreased oxygen flow to the heart. In the absence of nitroglycerin 1 to 3 ounces of straight whiskey is also effective.

If a heart patient takes nitroglycerin under the tongue, the pain of angina is usually gone within one to three minutes. Often patients are appropriately advised to take a "nitro" under the tongue just before some strenuous exercise, such as mowing the lawn or climbing stairs, to avoid chest pain.

The "prophylactic" or preventive use of "long-acting" nitroglycerin preparations, such Isordil® or Peritrate®, when taken by mouth, is unproved. When used under the tongue, like plain nitroglycerin, Isordil® and Peritrate® provide the patient with a single difference from plain nitroglycerin: higher cost.

NOLUDAR®   Methyprylon, N.F.
  See Nembutal®; Seconal®.

A sedative usually used as a "sleeping pill." Advertisements have emphasized its non-barbiturate chemical structure. This is not necessarily a clinical advantage. Noludar® lends itself in excessive usage or dosage to the same abuses as barbiturates—habituation, addiction, and suicide. Noludar® overdosage is as grave a medical emergency as overdosage with barbiturates. "Tolerance" to Noludar® can occur as it does to barbiturates.

Three hundred milligrams of Noludar® has a sleep-causing effect indistinguishable from that of 200 milligrams of secobarbital. For economy's sake, doctors should prescribe inexpensive secobarbital, pentobarbital, or chloral hydrate. When abuse or overdose is a possibility—as in patients with depression or suicidal tendencies—all of these drugs should be avoided. See these drugs in the Price Lists.

NORGESIC®		
	orphenadrine citrate	25 mg
	Aspirin, U.S.P.	225 mg
	Phenacetin, U.S.P.	160 mg
	Caffeine, U.S.P.	30 mg

See Aspirin, U.S.P.

This sedative–pain reliever is recommended for "symptomatic relief of mild to moderate pain of acute musculo-skeletal disorders" (*Physicians' Desk Reference*, 1974 edn, p. 1191). Norgesic® is simply an APC tablet with orphenadrine added; orphenadrine has belladonna-like actions. Norgesic® is not necessarily more effective for this purpose than 2 or 3 aspirins—and, perhaps, a hot bath!

NORINYL® 1+80, 21-DAY
See Oral Contraceptives.

NORLESTRIN®
See Oral Contraceptives.

NOVAHISTINE® DH		
	Codeine Phosphate, U.S.P.	10 mg
	Phenylephrine Hydrochloride, U.S.P.	10 mg

Chlorpheniramine Male-
ate, U.S.P.   2 mg
Chloroform, N.F.   13.5 mg
alcohol 5%
(per tsp)

NOVAHISTINE®   Codeine Phosphate,
EXPECTORANT   U.S.P.   10 mg
Phenylephrine Hydro-
chloride, U.S.P.   10 mg
Chlorpheniramine Male-
ate, U.S.P.   2 mg
glyceryl guaiacolate   100 mg
Chloroform, N.F.   13.5 mg
alcohol 5%
(per tsp)

*See Antihistamines; Cough Remedies; Dextrome-
thorphan Hydrobromide, N.F.; Neo-Synephrine®.*

These two decongestant-antitussive preparations
have been among the most frequent prescribed drugs
for a long time. Yet these concoctions have already
been commented upon under several other preparations (see Actifed®, Ambenyl® Expectorant, etc.).

If cough is a problem, dextromethorphan hydrobromide or codeine in small doses is recommended
for cough suppression. If nasal congestion is a problem, either phenylephrine nose drops or any one of
the cheapest antihistamines is suggested. Finally, if
throat tickle or throat dryness is a problem, sugar
candies are recommended. Cold and cough preparations, such as Novahistine® and the numerous others
available both with and without prescription, are
among the biggest "rip-offs" brought to you by the
drug manufacturers. The prescribing of such poly-
pharmaceuticals is undesirable because unwanted
effects are compounded, as are costs.

NYSTATIN, U.S.P.
See Mycostatin®.

OMNIPEN®
  See Ampicillin, U.S.P.

ORACON®-28
  See Oral Contraceptives.

ORAL CONTRACEPTIVES

Many different products are used for oral contraception. A natural situation in which it is impossible for a woman to get pregnant is when she is already pregnant. This is because the abundant production in pregnancy of one of the female hormones, progesterone, inhibits the release of new eggs (ovulation) and has many other effects as well. Deliberate molecule manipulating of progesterone has resulted in a variety of compounds (progestogens) whose ability to inhibit ovulation remains intact while other effects are minimized. By combining a progestogen with estrogen, another female hormone, a state reminiscent of pregnancy is induced. This explains the transient morning nausea or vomiting, swelling of the breasts, and occasional pigmentation and oiliness of the face that can accompany the taking of these drugs.

Use of "the pill" also includes control of irregular menses. Side effects, in addition to the symptoms of pregnancy mentioned above, include clots in the legs, elevated blood pressure, changes in metabolism of fats and sugars, and gall bladder disease. Less serious adverse effects include headaches, weight gain because of fluid retention, nausea, vaginal itch and yeast infections, and hair changes.

Most of the side effects are related to the estrogen content in "the pill," and recent attempts have been made both by physicians and the manufacturers of these pills to provide the minimum estrogen dose possible. In fact, a new "mini-pill" has no estrogens (sold as Micronor®, Nor-Q.D.®, and Ovrette®); the problem with this "mini-pill" is that women are more likely to become pregnant as compared with the other pills.

Listed below is a table with the various more commonly prescribed birth-control pills and the amount of estrogen and progestin in each. Increased estrogens usually means increased side effects. Increased progestins usually means increased protection against pregnancy. The estrogen-progestin combinations are usually given for 21 days and stopped for 7; the "mini-pill" is given for 28 days straight.

The question "Does taking 'the pill' increase the risk of cancer?" remains to be definitively answered. The evidence *in,* thus far (at the time of publication of the *Handbook*), shows *no* association between oral contraceptives and cervix or breast cancers; an association between the "day after" pill, diethylstilbestrol, and vaginal cancers in the daughters born to these women *has* been shown. If a woman takes diethylstilbestrol (DES) within 72 hours of sexual intercourse, pregnancy can be prevented (assuming, of course, the patient was not already pregnant). DES is recommended for post-intercourse contraception, but if it is unsuccessful, an abortion must be carried out.

Intrauterine devices are recommended by some doctors before oral contraceptives are tried. However, some 20 percent of women cannot tolerate these devices because of bleeding, cramps, or infection. Other mechanical contraceptive devices are highly effective in preventing pregnancy, though "the pill" is certainly more dependable.

Because so little is yet known of the possible long-term side effects of "the pill," one of us, R. B., saw to it when he was in private practice that every woman asking for "the pill" was given a talk covering all other possible methods of contraception. If the patient insisted on having "the pill" she was given a copy of the most recent *Physicians' Desk Reference* and asked to sit in the waiting room (or elsewhere) to read very carefully the manufacturers' list of known adverse side effects. If there were questions as to terminology, they were answered. When the reading

Brand*	Progestin	Estrogen	Wholesale cost of six months' supply
Demulen-21®	ethynodiol diacetate 1 mg	ethinyl estradiol 50 mcg	$11.58
Demulen-28®	ethynodiol diacetate 1 mg	ethinyl estradiol 50 mcg	$11.64
Micronor® ("mini-pill")	norethindrone 0.35 mg		
Norinyl®-21 (1 + 50)	norethindrone 1 mg	mestranol 50 mcg	$14.40
Norinyl®-21 (1 + 80)	norethindrone 1 mg	mestranol 80 mcg	$10.50
Norinyl®-28 (1 + 50)	norethindrone 1 mg	mestranol 50 mcg	$10.50
Norlestrin®-21 (1 + 50)	norethindrone 1 mg	ethinyl estradiol 50 mcg	$11.70
Norlestrin®-21 (2.5 + 50)	norethindrone 2.5 mg	ethinyl estradiol 50 mcg	$11.88
Norlestrin®-28 (1 + 50)	norethindrone 1 mg	ethinyl estradiol 50 mcg	$11.70
Norlestrin® FE, 28 (1 + 50)	norethindrone 1 mg	ethinyl estradiol 50 mcg	$11.70
Norlestrin® FE, 28 (2.5 + 50)	norethindrone 2.5 mg	ethinyl estradiol 50 mcg	$11.88
Ortho-Novum® (1 + 50)	norethindrone 1 mg	mestranol 50 mcg	$11.69
Ortho-Novum® (1 + 80)	norethindrone 1 mg	mestranol 80 mcg	$11.69
Ovral® (21)	norgestrel 0.5 mg	ethinyl estradiol 50 mcg	$11.94
Ovral®-28	norgestrel 0.5 mg	ethinyl estradiol 50 mcg	$11.94
Ovulen®-21	ethynodiol diacetate 1 mg	mestranol 100 mcg	$11.58
Ovulen®-28	ethynodiol diacetate 1 mg	mestranol 100 mcg	$11.64

* These represent the most commonly prescribed oral contraceptives. If your brand is not listed in complete detail, look for it in the Price Lists.

had ended, the woman was asked to sign a form explaining that all this "trouble" was taken to educate her and, incidentally, to absolve me from any responsibility for future toxic effects associated with the use of "the pill." This procedure was developed and carried out on the suggestion of an important member of the staff of Wisconsin Senator Gaylord Nelson's Subcommittee on Monopoly.

ORINASE®   Tolbutamide, U.S.P.

Tolbutamide, the most widely prescribed oral drug that can lower blood sugar, was developed by a German corporation. Upjohn is the sole American licensee, and hence has a monopoly on the manufacture and sale of tolbutamide tablets. For many years tolbutamide has been one of Upjohn's most profitable items, since it is one of the most prescribed drugs for people of all ages and especially for those over 65. In 1974 it was the 47th most-prescribed drug for people of all ages.

Good evidence exists which reveals that it is 95 percent likely that tolbutamide is a fatal poison when taken regularly. No evidence exists to show that it prevents any severe complications of diabetes, and excellent evidence does exist to suggest that its use is causing 10,000 to 15,000 excess deaths per year from heart disease.*

Physicians usually treat older patients with "diabetes" with this drug. But several questions should be answered in detail before any patient is placed on any medication for diabetes: Does the patient *really* have diabetes? There is usually little doubt about the diagnosis in those in the less-than 30 group. They are thin, usually have a clear-cut family history of diabetes, and present other symptoms that lead the doctor to suspect the disease. These patients require *insulin*, regular exercise, and a healthy life free from cigarette smoking. "Diabetes" in older, overweight persons is often picked up on "routine" tests for sugar in the urine or for sugar level in

* *Journal of the American Medical Association,* 231: 583–608 (February 10, 1975). Also see "Upjohn and Orinase®," pages 106–109 above, and the Addenda.

the blood. Most often, these patients have no symptoms of diabetes and, therefore, have what should more properly be called "chemical diabetes," because it is doubtful that they are truly diabetic. The patient is usually obese, and if treatment is thought necessary he should start with weight reduction and an exercise program. If these fail, insulin should be used in small doses.

The recent confirmation* by world-famous statisticians of the internationally respected Biometric Society that the use of Orinase® causes so many deaths annually is a scandal worse than the Chloromycetin® one. Physicians who continue to prescribe Orinase® may very well be asking for a malpractice suit. Unnecessary prescribing is as serious a matter as unnecessary surgery.

ORNADE®

Chlorpheniramine Maleate, U.S.P.	8 mg
phenylpropanolamine hydrochloride	50 mg
isopropamide iodide	2.5 mg

See Antihistamines; Cough Remedies; Ephedrine Sulfate, U.S.P.; Neo-Synephrine®.

The comments made under similar concoctions of antihistamines, ephedrine-like drugs, and cough-cold-congestion preparations apply. The Ornade® combination is hardly a contribution to medicine. Spansules®, or long-acting capsules, are not acceptable to either the *U.S.P.* or *N.F.* because of their variable absorption and time course of action. Patients would do better with chlorpheniramine maleate alone for congestion and perhaps phenylephrine nose drops (see Chlor-Trimeton® and Neo-Synephrine®).

Despite the limited effectiveness of any of these concoctions to alter the course of the common cold or nasal-congestion problems, they remain among the most popular drugs on the market. Ornade® has been among the top 50 drugs prescribed in the U.S. for many years.

ORTHO-NOVUM®

* *Ibid.*

ORTHO-NOVUM® 1/50-21

ORTHO-NOVUM® 1/80-21
See Oral Contraceptives.

OVRAL®
See Oral Contraceptives.

OVULEN®
See Oral Contraceptives.

OXAZEPAM
See Serax®.

OXYGEN, U.S.P. (100 PERCENT OXYGEN)

Millions of people have chronic lung disease, usually the result of cigarette smoking. It is North America's number-one public and private health problem.

Shortness of breath is a universal symptom of this disease, and it can be so severe that even the mildest exertion is extremely unpleasant. One hundred percent oxygen is a powerful drug whose potential for good and bad requires clarification, since many patients are treated with it at home (where they self-administer it) and in hospitals. Too little thought has been given to dosage, although it is as critical a consideration as with any other drug in the pharmacopeia. On the other hand, too much has been made of intermittent positive pressure respirators, inhalation of agents to "liquefy" sputum, the taking of arterial blood samples for a measurement of acidity (pH), etc. Some physicians are under the mistaken impression that, by merely limiting the inflow of oxygen to about 1½ liters per minute through a nozzle placed in the nose, a properly low concentration of oxygen is being supplied to the patient. Under these circumstances he cannot know exactly what oxygen concentration the patient is breathing (how much "room" air the patient is simultaneously breathing through his mouth would affect the concentration considerably). This situation more frequently than not obtains even in some of our largest and supposedly "best" hospitals. The doctor is also likely—in fact, he probably *will*— leave orders for the artery in the patient's arm to be punctured 4 times a day and direct that the blood be examined for the partial pressure of dissolved oxygen and carbon dioxide with a very elaborate electronically wired instrument designed to carry out these measurements *to the second decimal point*. A third determination of hydrogen ion concentration (pH) will also be made *to the second decimal point*. The picture is ludicrous: the doctor has "adjusted" the concentration of inspired oxygen in an exceedingly imprecise way, and then he goes about trying to make measurements of blood gases to the hundredth of a decimal point. (These measurements are *very* expensive; they add considerably to the cost of the hospitalization).

It is a fact that recurrent turns for the worse in chronic lung disease are attended by a strong natural tendency to get well with simple treatment. The patient must be tided over what is most commonly an acute infection of the lung. When superimposed on a chronically deranged lung, an acute infection can cause critical worsening of ventilation/blood-flow mismatch and diminish blood oxygenation enough to make the patient turn dusky (cyanosis), or duskier than usual. Provided the patient is comfortable, at rest, and clear in his mind, cyanosis need not trigger a panic response. If he is given an antibiotic (tetracycline is the usual one), is encouraged to cough deeply and frequently, and *is given no sedative under any circumstances,* the patient is likely to weather the storm and avoid hospitalization. Sometimes a short course of prednisone is helpful if wheezing is a prominent symptom.

The two most common reasons for complication leading to hospitalization are:

1. administration of a sedative of any sort;
2. administration of 100 percent oxygen. Either can easily cause the patient to breathe less, resulting in accumulation of carbon dioxide in concentrations high enough to cause confusion or unconsciousness. *When this occurs, the situation is seriously compounded by suddenly "taking away" the 100 percent oxygen, a maneuver which will inevitably cause the blood suddenly to be even less well oxygenated than it was in the first place.*

It has been demonstrated well enough that use of 24 percent instead of 100 percent oxygen is far safer and almost always provides enough improvement of blood oxygenation for the resting patient. A simple way to "convert" 100 percent to 24 percent oxygen has been invented by Dr. E. J. M. Campbell (formerly of Hammersmith Hospital, London, and now Chairman of the Department of Medicine, McMaster University, Hamilton, Ontario). It is a simple, lightweight, clear plastic mask that costs only a dollar or two and should replace nasal catheters, oxygen tents, and other kinds of masks in caring for patients with acute or chronic lung disease. The Campbell invention makes use of the "Venturi principle": when 100 percent oxygen is directed into a nozzle at a rate of about 4 liters per minute, room air is sucked in through side holes in the correct proportion to dilute it to 24 percent. (Room air is 21 percent. A 3 percent increase is considerable—more than 20 millimeters mercury partial pressure.)

It may safely be predicted that use of the "Venturi mask" (and avoidance of sedatives) in patients with "chronic bronchitis and emphysema" will obviate much unnecessary complication and hospitalization. The mask is one of the most important contributions made to pharmacotherapeutics in recent years.

In North America the Ventimask® can be obtained from any reputable medical supply house. Although cost may vary from house to house, the Ventimask® is very inexpensive and may be used again and again by a single person. (There are also 28 and 35 percent Ventimasks®, but their routine use is not recommended.) Physicians interested in a detailed physiological analysis of "acute respiratory failure in chronic bronchitis and emphysema" and use of 24 percent oxygen are referred to Dr. Campbell's J. Burns Amberson Lecture, printed in the *American Review of Respiratory Diseases,* Volume 5 (October 1967), pages 626–639.

OXYPHENBUTAZONE, N.F.
See *Tandearil®.*

OXYTETRACYCLINE HYDROCHLORIDE
See *Terramycin®.*

PANMYCIN®   Tetracycline Hydrochloride, U.S.P.

This is Upjohn's brand of tetracycline. See Tetracycline Hydrochloride, U.S.P., for uses and actions of this drug.

PAPAVERINE HYDROCHLORIDE, N.F.
See *Pavabid®.*

PARAFON FORTE®   Acetaminophen, N.F.   300 mg
chlorzoxazone   50 mg

This product is a combination of the mild pain reliever acetaminophen and a so-called muscle relaxant, chlorzoxazone (Paraflex®). Chlorzoxazone has not convincingly been shown to be a "muscle relaxant," however. There is little use for this drug, although its name undoubtedly enhances its sales.

The National Academy of Sciences—National Research Council did eventually classify this drug as "probably effective." My guess is that the effectiveness is largely due to the acetaminophen content. In all probability, a couple of aspirin tablets and a hot bath will work as well. The *AMA Drug Evaluations,* 2nd ed., states: ". . . the rationale for use of the preparation is highly questionable" (p. 274).

Despite these statements, the drug ranked among the top 200 drugs prescribed in 1973, and its sales were improved from the year before.

PAREGORIC, U.S.P.
(CAMPHORATED TINCTURE OF OPIUM)

Paregoric is the most effective antidiarrhea agent for use in ambulatory patients. The fact that it is camphorated discourages excessive oral intake. Washed down or diluted with a little water, paregoric tastes strikingly like the apéritif Pernod. A teaspoonful or two every 4 to 6 hours almost always takes care of simple diarrheas.

Other preparations available for control of serious diarrhea include Lomotil®, kaolin mixture with pectin (Kaopectate®), and tincture of opium. Of these, Lomotil® is relatively more expensive than either paregoric or tincture of opium. Kaopectate® is of questionable usefulness despite its wide acceptance and sales. Tincture of opium is as effective as paregoric but must be administered in smaller amounts (*i.e.,* drops), which makes it more difficult to control dosage. Tincture of opium is also more subject to abuse and is more likely to cause the unwanted side effects of opiates.

For those who are traveling, diarrhea is a well-known problem. The *Handbook* recommends no antibiotics for prevention of such diarrhea (often Entero-Vioform®, which was found "ineffective" by the FDA, or tetracycline is used), but urges all travelers to take paregoric with them (a prescription is usually necessary abroad) and avoid uncooked foods and foods where contamination is likely.

PAVABID®   Papaverine Hydro-
                                                      chloride, N.F.   150 mg

This drug is a fascinating medication with little proved usefulness in patients. It is recommended for "the relief of cerebral and peripheral ischemia associated with arterial spasm" and for "myocardial ischemia complicated by arrhythmias" (*Physicians' Desk Reference*, 1974 edn., p. 952). This means that it is recommended for decreased blood flow around the brain and for angina pectoris (heart pain). The evidence for its usefulness in these situations is very poor at best.

The drug is a non-narcotic derived from opium, which, when given in the veins of dogs, relaxes blood vessels in spasm. Careful studies in humans, however, do not allow us to conclude that the drug has any real usefulness. Like Cyclospasmol®, Vasodilan®, and nicotinic acid (when used for "pepping up" older people), Pavabid® is not recommended for use at any time. As with these other medications, the physician is often forced to "do something" about senile, lethargic, or otherwise slowed older people. These pills are not the answer.

Pavabid® is provided in a gloriously named "Plateau CAP®," a form of longer-acting capsule preparation, we suppose. While the name may provide some nice thoughts and placebo effect, the side effects from this drug are real. In the most careful study using the drug, approximately 20 percent of people given the preparation developed abnormal liver tests. Other side effects include nausea, abdominal discomfort, constipation and/or diarrhea, and flushing of the face.

PEDIAMYCIN®   erythromycin ethylsuccinate
See E-Mycin®; Erythrocin® Stearate; Ilosone®.

This erythromycin product is prepared primarily for use in children. The liquid and drops are, indeed, the only convenient form to give infants and younger children; Abbott's Erythrocin® is also available in these more convenient vehicles.

Erythromycin should be restricted to use in children who are allergic to penicillin, although penicillin allergy is rare in children. The expense of erythromycin compared to penicillin is substantial and there are very few infections treated with erythromycin that cannot also be treated with simple penicillin.

Since erythromycin ethylsuccinate is a different salt of erythromycin than Erythrocin® Stearate or Ilosone®, the other erythromycins, it usually requires 400 milligrams of Pediamycin® to be equivalent to 250 milligrams of the others.

PENBRITIN®   Ampicillin, U.S.P.
  See Ampicillin, U.S.P.

Penicillin G is a narrow-spectrum antibiotic, but when it is given in massive doses intravenously (20 to 40 million units per day) it is an excellent broad-spectrum antibiotic. However, it is impossible to provide sufficient dosage by mouth to obtain this effect. Ampicillin, a variant of penicillin, is a drug developed by the British (hence "Penbritin®"), which when taken by mouth does provide the broad-spectrum effect.

While ampicillin is a useful drug in certain selected cases, there is little reason that it should be so widespread in its use or popularity. Ampicillin is the drug of choice for treatment of ear infections and meningitis when they occur in children and when they are caused by the bacterium *H. influenzae.* Ampicillin is also often useful in treating gastrointestinal infections with bacteria of the *Salmonella* family. For very rare kinds of urinary tract infections, ampicillin may be the drug of choice. *Ampicillin is not effective against staphylococcus that is resistant to penicillin G or V.*

In chronic chest infections (bronchitis) and acne, tetracycline is preferred and cheaper. In the most common urinary tract infections, sulfas are preferred and cheaper (see Gantrisin®). In infections such as streptococcal ("strep") sore throats, simple pneumonias, and others, penicillin G is preferred and considerably cheaper.

Recent uses of ampicillin include oral treatment

of gonorrhea; a dose of 3.5 grams is given 30 minutes after a 0.5 dose of probenecid. Alternative treatment for gonorrhea is a large dose of penicillin given in the buttocks.

Ampicillin is not non-toxic. It causes allergic reactions similar to those caused by penicillin. *No* person who is known to be penicillin-allergic should use ampicillin. Indeed, there is a higher incidence of allergic reactions to ampicillin than to penicillin G or V. Occasionally, stomach upset is associated with the drug.

Ordering expensive drugs to do certain jobs when other less costly drugs could produce the same desired effect is as wasteful of patients' money as prescribing costly brand equivalents of generic drugs. Casual prescribing of ampicillin is one of the best examples of this kind of practice, which is encouraged by advertisements in medical journals and by drug salesmen—sources that naturally avoid discussion of comparative cost.

Generic ampicillin is rising in popularity on physicians' prescription pads, and with good reason. Generic ampicillin, if used to fill a prescription, can cost patients substantially less than the more common brand-named products. It is an interesting coincidence that the five brand-named ampicillins that ranked among the top 200 drugs prescribed in 1973 were within pennies of each other when bought wholesale. (They included Amcill®, Omnipen®, Penbritin®, Polycillin®, and Principen®, all of which were approximately double the wholesale price of the least expensive generic product.) Price competition had begun by 1975.

PENICILLIN

The pioneer and still the antibiotic combining highest therapeutic effectiveness with greatest all-round safety is common penicillin G, the first of a series of substances produced naturally by various bacteria and fungi to be widely used in treating infections. Penicillin was introduced to clinical medicine in 1942, but its actual discovery harks back to 1929, when a British bacteriologist, Alexander Fleming, noticed that the common germ staphylococcus did not grow on a gelatinous, nutrient-impregnated "culture medium" in the immediate vicinity of colonies of common penicillium fungus. (Fungus colonies are common on the surface of such media because fungus spores, normally in the air everywhere, often settle on the surface of a culture plate if it is uncovered for a few moments.) Fleming appreciated the possible significance of his observation: that a growing colony of a common mold can inhibit growth of a germ that is often the cause of serious infection. Surmising that the fungus colony might be diffusing an antibacterial substance through the gelatin in a concentric ring around the colony, he purposely turned to growing the penicillium mold in large amounts. Making crude extracts of many combined colonies, he then attempted to treat skin wounds infected with staphylococcus by applying the extract to their surface.

Results of Fleming's experiments at Saint Mary's Hospital, London, were not encouraging; we now realize that his extraction process was faulty. However, he described his experience in a medical journal read internationally by all professional bacteriologists. Howard Florey, also a British medical researcher, read about Fleming's intriguing work and kept it in the back of his mind. Ten years later, Florey and some colleagues, chief among them a refugee chemist, Chain, succeeded in extracting from penicillium molds a crude material which regularly prevented death from experimentally induced pneumonia in mice. Chain's group came up with a small amount of material—"penicillin"—which was tried out on humans dying of widespread infection with staphylococcus.

This phase of the Florey–Chain studies is of anecdotal interest. I am indebted to Dr. Charles Fletcher, now of London's Hammersmith Hospital, for many of the details. As Florey and Chain looked on, the first crude penicillin was injected intravenously by Fletcher into a patient dying from multiple abscesses and bloodstream infection caused by staphylococcus.

Fletcher, then a young doctor in training, had been asked to make the injection by his mentor, Professor Witt, to whom Florey and Chain had applied for help in doing the tests on human beings. Within a few moments of the injection, the patient had a shaking chill followed by a high fever, a reaction attributed to impurities in the extracted drug. Chain's group returned to the laboratory to "clean up" the extract. Following that, four or five patients with severe staphylococcus disease tolerated the intravenous injections very well and recovered from their illness, until then nearly universally fatal. The last patient to be treated was a strapping policeman with multiple "metastatic" staphylococcus abscesses. After only one or two injections (which seemed to cause a definite initial improvement) the available supply of the drug was exhausted, but quite unexpectedly Chain's group was unable to replenish the supply; it could not reproduce its initial feat of extracting active penicillin from penicillium mold. This patient relapsed and died.

By now it was the early days of World War II, and England could not provide the necessary facilities for the development of reliable techniques of isolating penicillin. Chain was flown to the United States to enlist help. The Office of Scientific Research and Development arranged for United States government grants to be given to twenty different drug companies to research ways of extracting the important drug. The then head of the office is reported to have expressed disappointment over the companies' unwillingness to exchange experimental results[*] and the fact that the "firms were too busy trying to corner patents on various processes in the production of penicillin to produce much of it."[†] In the end, it was the publicly supported Northern Regional Research Laboratory of the United States Department of Agriculture in Peoria, Illinois, which found the means

[*] Morton Mintz, *By Prescription Only* (Boston: Houghton Mifflin Company, 1967), pp. 365, 366.

[†] Richard Harris, *The Real Voice* (New York: The Macmillan Company, 1964); *The New Yorker*, March 14, 21, and 28, 1964.

to produce penicillin cheaply and in massive quantities. The laboratory used penicillium mold from the surface of a cantaloupe purchased in a Peoria market. The first official announcement of the feat was on January 26, 1943.*

In keeping with policy, the government made details of the process available free to the twenty drug companies it had been subsidizing. Several began to manufacture and sell the drug at high prices. The British government had to pay them millions of pounds for it—a cause of ill-will that has not been forgotten. Many British physicians are still under the mistaken impression that the high prices resulted from an American firm taking out a patent on penicillin, something which their own top medical leaders considered doing at the time of the Florey–Chain discovery but rejected as unethical. As stated, there was actually no private patent protection in the United States, and since the production feat was eventually reproduced by several competitors, penicillin finally became available from a number of sources, price competition resulted, and its cost plummeted.

All penicillin G (the original and still most useful variety of penicillin) powder made in the United States comes at present from six corporations, who sell it to the scores of native "generic" manufacturers, where it is stamped into tablets, a process requiring the addition only of a binding gum and a disintegrant such as cornstarch. Every batch of tablets must by law meet the certification requirement of the Food and Drug Administration, including specifications as to pH, moisture content, heat stability, safety, and potency. The extremely high solubility of penicillin G practically eliminates the possibility that a tablet will not deliver its drug content to the bloodstream. Recently, an editorial in the *Journal of the American Medical Association* † raised questions for the practic-

* Research Achievement Sheet of the United States Department of Agriculture, Agricultural Research Administration, No. 52 (c), March 4, 1946.

† "Generic Drugs and Therapeutic Equivalence," *206*:1785 (November 18, 1968).

ing doctor about "the present method of handling penicillin" and stated that even a "pure" commercially available preparation of penicillin G might harbor "impurities capable of causing allergic reactions" —and "thus a cheaper, less pure penicillin may not be cheaper as far as the patient is concerned." The burden of the editorial was clearly to plant suspicion in doctors' minds about generic penicillin G tablets. The editorial failed to point out that the "impurities" it mentioned are analogues of penicillin introduced in the synthesis of the penicillin G powder,* not in the conversion of powder to tablets, and that the six American firms which make all of the powder are Abbott, Lilly, Merck, Pfizer, Squibb, and Upjohn. Surely the editorial did not mean to imply that any one of these is an unreliable manufacturer.

In the office, physicians should prescribe penicillin G tablets and the patient should buy the least expensive product available. The argument that doctors should use penicillin V (new and more expensive than penicillin G) because it is allegedly "more evenly absorbed" is entirely unconvincing. For the office and outpatient purposes to which penicillin G is put, it serves every bit as well. Since it is less expensive, penicillin G (generic) is preferable.

PENICILLIN G TABLETS (POTASSIUM PENICILLIN G TABLETS, U.S.P.) BUFFERED AND SOLUBLE

Penicillin is very useful for a wide spectrum of diseases and is most commonly given orally for mild infections caused by hemolytic streptococcus and pneumococcus. It is routinely taken daily for prevention of rheumatic fever. Rheumatic fever is a complication of throat infection with hemolytic streptococcus; such infections can be symptomless. Hemolytic streptococcus is as sensitive to penicillin G as it was thirty years ago; a routine oral daily dose prevents recurrence of rheu-

* G. T. Stewart, "Allergic Residues in Penicillins," *Lancet,* 1:1177–1183 (June 1967).

matic fever and further heart damage.* Oral penicillins are *not* suitable for treatment of very serious infections, such as severe pneumonias, and usually not for gonorrhea.

Penicillin G is the most important oral preparation. While readily absorbed from the gastrointestinal tract, it is subject to degradation by stomach acid and is not well absorbed if food is present. To avoid mixing the preparation with food, penicillin G should be taken 15 to 30 minutes before eating or 2 hours after eating. The usual dose is 125 milligrams (200,000 units) 3 or 4 times a day, although this is probably excessive. The major contraindication is allergy to penicillin, although it is a relative contraindication. In cases where penicillin could be lifesaving, the allergic person could be given it along with cortisone-like drugs to prevent any allergic symptoms.

Penicillin G is now somewhat less popular than in days gone by. The reason is that penicillin V has been extensively promoted and extolled as superior. It also costs considerably more. If the doctor asks himself, "Is this newer drug, penicillin V, so much more advantageous than penicillin G to be worth the increased cost?" the answer must be, "No."

Pentids®, Squibb's brand of penicillin G, should *not* be prescribed since it is so expensive. It costs more than penicillin V sold generically and even more than penicillin V sold under most of its brand names.

PENICILLIN V (POTASSIUM PHENOXYMETHYL PENICILLIN, U.S.P.)

See Penicillin G Tablets (Potassium Penicillin G Tablets, U.S.P.).

Only because of extensive promotion has penicillin V emerged in recent years as the oral penicillin that is most prescribed. The most common reason for

---

* "Prophylactic penicillin" is *not* capable, however, of preventing endocarditis, a serious infection that occasionally involves previously damaged heart valves.

giving penicillin is for streptococcus sore throats and
for streptococcus and pneumococcus middle-ear infections. The brand names are almost certainly best
avoided because of their greater cost. FDA controls
are a nearly 100 percent guarantee of the equivalence
of the various penicillin products marketed; claims of
both low cost and better efficacy for brand-name
products are unfounded. *Medical Letter* (*15*: 43,
[1973]), a reliable journal used by physicians who
wish to have unbiased information about drugs, states:
"There are no published reports establishing clinically
important differences between generic and brand name
penicillins." The brand-name products that have sold
the most, Pen-Vee® K and V-Cillin K®, are also
among the most expensive; perhaps this reflects the
added cost of advertising, which explains their
popularity.

In sum, penicillin G is the penicillin of choice
among the oral preparations, and to avoid great
expense it should be prescribed generically.

PENTAERYTHRITOL TETRANITRATE (PETN)
See Peritrate®.

PENTAZOCINE HYDROCHLORIDE
See Talwin®.

PENTIDS®   Potassium Penicillin G Tablets, U.S.P.
*See Penicillin; Penicillin G Tablets (Potassium Peni-
cillin G Tablets, U.S.P.); Penicillin V (Potassium
Phenoxymethyl Penicillin, U.S.P.).*

Pentids®, Squibb's brand name of penicillin G tablets, has continued to be widely prescribed by physicians even though it costs several times as much as
penicillin G marketed by numerous other firms.
One can calculate the cost to a patient with a history
of rheumatic fever if he takes two 200,000 unit
Pentids® daily for 20 years, and what it could cost

if purchased as generic penicillin G tablets. The difference may be well over $1000. Simply tell your physician to write penicillin G, not Pentids®, and then go to a big pharmacy chain if you don't know your local pharmacist, and insist that he *not* substitute Pentids® for it.

PENTOBARBITAL (SODIUM PENTOBARBITAL, U.S.P.)
See Nembutal®.

PEN-VEE® K
Potassium Phenoxymethyl Penicillin, U.S.P.

See Penicillin; Penicillin G Tablets (Potassium Penicillin G Tablets, U.S.P.); Penicillin V (Potassium Phenoxymethyl Penicillin, U.S.P.).

A brand name for penicillin V, Pen-Vee® K is among the most expensive.

PERCODAN®

oxycodone hydrochloride	4.5 mg
oxycodone terephthalate	0.38 mg
Aspirin, U.S.P.	224 mg
Phenacetin, U.S.P.	160 mg
Caffeine, U.S.P.	32 mg

See Aspirin, U.S.P.; Codeine Sulfate, N.F.; Codeine Phosphate, U.S.P.; Demerol®.

Percodan® is a pain reliever containing the narcotic oxycodone, which is related chemically to codeine but is stronger in both its pain-relieving and its addictive powers. The other ingredients are more familiarly known as APC, a combination of aspirin, phenacetin (similar to Tylenol®), and caffeine.

Along with Demerol®, Percodan® is the most popular strong pain reliever prescribed by physicians. Two or 3 Percodan® tablets are approximately equal in strength to 10 milligrams of morphine or 120 milligrams of codeine. Since morphine is only available for injection, it tends not to be prescribed for control of severe, chronic pain; furthermore, it is subject to much abuse by drug addicts. Codeine, on the other hand, is readily available at very little cost in pill form, and, if given in adequate doses, can be as effective as the more expensive meperidine (Demerol®) or Percodan®. When pain is so severe as to resist treatment with 120 milligram doses of codeine, methadone orally or morphine injections are the drugs of choice, both in efficacy and cost.

Physicians tend to be stingy with narcotic medications for pain, such as morphine and methadone. Studies have shown that in hospitalized patients with terminal cancer and other conditions where severe pain is a serious problem, about 75 percent of patients continued to have moderate to severe distress despite medication ordered by physicians. The reason for this pain was simple: doctors were unwilling to prescribe the strongest pain relievers (*i.e.*, methadone and morphine), and when drugs were prescribed they were given in too small doses and too infrequently.* In patients with terminal or very serious chronic illnesses, narcotics *should* be given in many cases despite the obvious addiction problem in order to control pain; there seems little point in worrying about addiction in a cancer patient destined to die within several months who also has excruciating bone pains. In patients with transient episodes of pain, such as pain following fractures, operations, and other situations, a one-week course of strong narcotics is unlikely to lead to addiction.

The *Handbook* recommends morphine injections or methadone pills rather than Percodan® or Demerol® by mouth for control of serious pain in cancer patients or patients with pain so severe as to preclude codeine therapy in 120 milligram doses. Patients who think Demerol®, Percodan®, or Talwin®

* R. M. Marks and E. D. Sachar, in *Annals of Internal Medicine*, 78:173 (1973).

are non-addicting are just dreaming. If their pain is so severe as to require large doses of these pills, they would do better with cheaper narcotics that effectively control their pain. Of course, a doctor's supervision is necessary.

PERIACTIN® cyproheptadine
See Antihistamines.

In pharmacology circles, there has been a recent resurgent interest in "biogenic amines," pharmacologically active substances occurring naturally in the body. The best known is histamine, which is present in almost all normal animal organs although its normal function is not known. Circumstantial evidence indicates that "release" of histamine from intracellular binding sites may cause some of the symptoms and signs of allergy. Another biogenic amine more recently the object of attention is 5-hydroxytryptamine, also known as "serotonin" and "5-HT." There has been nebulous speculation that 5-HT "release" may also play some role in allergy symptoms. Hence, chemists tried to come up with a drug which would at the same time act as antihistamine and anti-5-HT. Periactin® is such a drug when tested in the laboratory on isolated perfused rodent organs—a far cry from whole human beings. It has been promoted by Merck for "a wide range of acute and chronic allergic disorders and pruritic [itchy] dermatoses [skin abnormalities]," as well as everything that any other antihistamine has claimed for it. It seems that Merck would like to convey to the doctor the impression that the anti-5-HT property of Periactin® is likely to make it more effective than other antihistamines, but advertisements neglect to emphasize that 5-HT is *not present* in significant amounts in human skin.

Itch is caused by subliminal stimulation of the pain receptors in the skin. Severe itch, such as that associated with chicken pox, is, therefore, best treated with analgesics such as aspirin and codeine. Most other itches, except possibly "hives," which may sometimes be helped by an antihistamine, are best treated with an effective sedative, such as phenobarbital. Itching associated with eczematoid skin problems usually commands topical steroids (see Hydrocortisone Cream, U.S.P.). In poison ivy, oral steroids are given.

When an antihistamine is needed, either diphenhydramine hydrochloride (Benadryl®) or chlorpheniramine maleate (Chlor-Trimeton®) will suffice. (See pp. 156 and 164 and Antihistamines, p. 147.) Dermatologists are especially fond of Periactin®, Atarax®, and Vistaril® for control of itching; all are antihistamines that cost more but are no more effective in relieving itch.

PERI-COLACE®	Dioctyl Sodium	
	– Sulfosuccinate, N.F.	100 mg
	casanthrol	30 mg

Not content to have cornered the market on a common, useful, and potentially cheap non-prescription drug, Dioctyl Sodium Succinate, N.F., Mead Johnson uses a marketing device to insure against loss of any of the market to manufacturers who introduce price competition. They market Colace® with a laxative added and call it Peri-Colace® (Peristim® is the trademark name given to the laxative element). See Dioctyl Sodium Sulfosuccinate, N.F., in the Price Lists.

Casanthrol, as its name suggests, is one of the cascara anthraquinones. The combination of the two drugs is supposed to be useful because Colace® softens the stool and Peristim® stimulates activity (peristalsis) in the large bowel musculature to aid passage of stool.

There are at least two things to be said against this product:

1. The price is very high.
2. Fixed-dose combinations are not good generally, and here in particular.

Patients who take the drug habitually (as many elderly constipated persons might do with Peri-Colace®) can easily, without anyone's realizing it, be swallowing a component that either is not needed or could be harmful. The laxative habit is not one to encourage; it can result in chronic potassium depletion leading to kidney damage and a form of chronic muscle weakness. With dioctyl sodium succinate alone this is unlikely, since the effect of the drug is merely to moisten and soften the stool.

What should the doctor prescribe instead? What should the nursing home providing drugs paid for by Medicaid be buying instead? The answer is clear: dioctyl sodium sulfosuccinate, by that name and at low cost. Should there be reason temporarily to supplement its action with a laxative, one can use milk of magnesia.

PERITRATE®   pentaerythritol tetranitrate

PERITRATE® SA   pentaerythritol tetranitrate
   See Isordil®; Nitroglycerin, U.S.P. (Glyceryl Trinitrate).

This drug was devised by Swedish investigators many years ago and introduced then as a "long-acting" blood-vessel dilator possibly useful in angina pectoris. It fell out of favor until Warner/Chilcott promoted and marketed it.

Physicians disagree about the usefulness of this drug and similar preparations like Isordil® in preventing angina pectoris episodes. It has been "clinical impressions" that have supported their use, but careful clinical studies and experimentation fail to support the use of long-acting nitrates such as these.

Nitroglycerin taken under the tongue usually relieves the pain of angina pectoris within minutes. Long-acting preparations of nitroglycerin-related compounds, such as Peritrate®, have *not* been shown to prevent attacks of angina and should be avoided because of their expense and questionable efficacy. A clinical study has shown that by causing tolerance to nitrite drugs in general, pentaerythritol can make nitroglycerin, an old and usually reliable emergency drug for angina pectoris, less effective.*

PHENAPHEN®		
	Phenacetin, U.S.P.	194 mg
	Aspirin, U.S.P.	162 mg
	Phenobarbital, U.S.P.	15 mg

PHENAPHEN®		
WITH CODEINE	Phenacetin, U.S.P.	194 mg
	Aspirin, U.S.P.	162 mg
	Phenobarbital, U.S.P.	15 mg
	Codeine,	
	U.S.P.	15, 30, or 60 mg

See Aspirin, U.S.P.; Phenobarbital, U.S.P.; Tylenol®.

This is a variant of the nostrum which we have met before, a combination of too little aspirin and phenacetin and some phenobarbital for sedation, and sometimes codeine sprinkled in for added pain relief. One can buy one hundred 15 or 30 milligram phenobarbital tablets for the minimum cost of a prescription, and purchase inexpensive aspirin over the counter for very little. Two to 3 aspirin tablets and a tablet of phenobarbital should serve as well as Phenaphen® for most of the purposes for which this product is prescribed.

PHENAZOPYRIDINE HYDROCHLORIDE
See Pyridium®.

PHENFORMIN HYDROCHLORIDE
See DBI-TD®.

PHENERGAN®   Promethazine Hydrochloride, U.S.P.
See Antihistamines.

* J. L. Schelling, et al., *Clinical Pharmacology and Therapeutics,* 8:256 (1967).

Chemically a phenothiazine, promethazine is also similar to antihistamines in its effects. It has powerful sedative, antinausea, anti–motion sickness, and antihistamine properties. In suppository form it is useful in treating the patient who is miserable with acute nausea and vomiting. Promethazine is probably safer than some of the other phenothiazines—chlorpromazine (Thorazine®) and prochlorperazine (Compazine®)—since it is less likely to cause acute neurological symptoms, and jaundice due to small bile duct obstruction. Nausea caused by serious abdominal disease—for example, intestinal obstruction or appendicitis—is not an indication for the use of Phenergan®. Promethazine can cause drowsiness, low blood pressure, blood abnormalities, and skin rashes.

Promethazine is probably the best antinausea drug available. However, when combined with other drugs, it is not at all recommended. (See below.)

Phenergan® products can now be purchased by generic name at a considerable saving. As concerns suppositories, however, the number required is usually so small that shopping for generic ones can be a wild-goose chase.

PHENERGAN® EXPECTORANT	Promethazine Hydro-chloride, U.S.P.	5.00 mg
	fluid extract of ipecac	0.17 minims
	Potassium Guaiacol-sulfonate, U.S.P.	44.00 mg
	Chloroform, N.F.	0.25 minims
	Citric Acid, U.S.P.	60.00 mg
	Sodium Citrate, U.S.P.	197.00 mg
	alcohol 7%	
	(per 5 ml, or 1 tsp)	

| **PHENERGAN® EXPECTORANT WITH CODEINE** | Phenergan® Expectorant with Codeine Phos-phate, U.S.P. | 10 mg |
| | (per 5 ml, or 1 tsp) | |

PHENERGAN® VC EXPECTORANT

Phenergan® Expectorant
with Phenylephrine
Hydrochloride, U.S.P. 10 mg
(per 5 ml, or 1 tsp)

PHENERGAN® VC EXPECTORANT WITH CODEINE

Phenergan® VC Expec-
torant with Codeine
Phosphate, U.S.P. 10 mg
(per 5 ml, or 1 tsp)

See Antihistamines; Cough Remedies; Dextromethorphan Hydrobromide, N.F.; Neo-Synephrine®.

The four expectorant preparations above were each among the 200 most-prescribed drugs in the U.S. in 1973. All of the components excepting promethazine and codeine in these various expectorants are of questionable usefulness. Thus, physicians would do better by simply prescribing promethazine or another antihistamine for drying up secretions associated with colds, and codeine or dextromethorphan for cough suppression. The addition of systemic phenylephrine in the "VC" preparations (for vasoconstrictor, we presume) is less preferable than nose drops of the same drug (Neo-Synephrine®).

In sum, while promethazine is an excellent antihistamine-like drug with usefulness in nausea and drying up secretions, its combination in various concoctions is not justified. These third-rate blends benefit their manufacturers' pocketbooks, but not the good practice of medicine. It is better to take a single effective drug in preference to a hodgepodge; hodgepodges are more likely to cause side effects, and in practically every instance cost more.

PHENOBARBITAL, U.S.P.

Doctors and patients take this wonderful drug and all of its barbiturate cousins for granted. No one knows *how* they affect the brain, although the first barbiturate was described sixty-five years ago by two

German investigators, Emil Fischer and J. von Mering. The story behind their work is worth knowing.

Liebreich, another German, had introduced chloral hydrate (still a *U.S.P.* drug also) as a sleeping medication in 1869, and over the years molecule manipulation led to an appreciation that urethan, paraldehyde (also *U.S.P.*), and other related substances have similar effects. Fischer was a good organic chemist with an innate ability to conjure up the educated "hunch." He synthesized a variety of congeners, and he and his colleague tested each one on a dog. They struck on a molecular configuration that was able to put animals into stupefaction and sleep, followed by recovery hours later with no apparent aftereffects and with a good appetite. The most effective of the many compounds they tested was barbital, marketed in 1903 by the brand name Veronal®. Barbital is still available and is often useful. Its sedative effect is long-lasting, like that of phenobarbital, and because it is excreted from the body nearly exclusively by the kidneys* (whereas other barbiturates are more or less dependent on the liver for removal), barbital is a good sedative for persons whose liver function is impaired. (Barbital is not expensive, though it costs more than phenobarbital.)

One might ask why phenobarbital has so nearly replaced barbital in everyday practice. The answer probably is that phenobarbital was found to be peculiarly more effective as an anti-epilepsy drug, the sedative effect of barbital notwithstanding. Phenobarbital has been used to treat epilepsy since about 1912. (See also Dilantin® Sodium.)

It is encouraging to discover that doctors have not abandoned phenobarbital. The cost of an average phenobarbital prescription was well below the cost of the average brand-name prescription in 1973.

In addition to use as an anti-epilepsy drug, phenobarbital is most useful as a mild sedative similar to Valium®, Librium®, Tranxene®, and Serax® or sleep-

---

* Hence, barbital is not to be used where there is poor kidney function, lest accumulation and overdosage occur.

ing medication similar to the somewhat shorter-acting barbiturates, secobarbital (Seconal®) and pentobarbital (Nembutal®). The problems with phenobarbital include dependency and overdosage; it is best avoided in patients with "addictive" personalities or suicidal tendencies. As with any other sedative, the regular use of phenobarbital can cause a mentally depressed state. Its great advantage is low cost, only a fraction of that for drugs now most popular for sedation.

Rash is a not uncommon adverse effect of phenobarbital. It has a very characteristic appearance (once observed it is unlikely to be forgotten). This is not a serious matter, but is reason to discontinue taking phenobarbital.

**PHENOXYMETHYL PENICILLIN
(POTASSIUM PHENOXYMETHYL
PENICILLIN, U.S.P.)**
See Penicillin V.

PHENTERMINE RESIN
See Ionamin®.

PHENYLBUTAZONE, U.S.P.
See Butazolidin®; Butazolidin® Alka.

PHENYLEPHRINE HYDROCHLORIDE, U.S.P.
See Neo-Synephrine®.

"PILL, THE"
See Oral Contraceptives.

PILOCARPINE HYDROCHLORIDE, U.S.P.
See Isopto Carpine®.

PLACIDYL® ethchlorvynol
See Butisol®; Chloral Hydrate, U.S.P.; Nembutal®; Phenobarbital, U.S.P.; Seconal®.

Like Doriden® and Noludar®, Placidyl® has little medical advantage over secobarbital (Seconal®) or pentobarbital (Nembutal®), but it is far more costly than either of the latter. Habituation, poisoning, abuse, suicide—these can all happen as easily with Placidyl® as with any other. The usual bedtime dose is 500 milligrams. Its nice brand name and its availability in 100 and 200 milligram doses invite the doctor to prescribe it as a sedative ("tranquilizer") during the day, but this is an expensive way to provide sedation and is no more effective than phenobarbital or butabarbital (Butisol®).

POLARAMINE® Dexchlorpheniramine Maleate, N.F.
See Antihistamines; Chlor-Trimeton®.

Dexchlorpheniramine is a form of the antihistamine chlorpheniramine (Chlor-Trimeton®) from which the left-handed (levo-) molecules have been eliminated (see Dextroamphetamine Sulfate, U.S.P., for an explanation of this). It is clinically equivalent to chlorpheniramine, but only half the dose need be prescribed; of course, its cost is approximately twice that of chlorpheniramine on a milligram-for-milligram basis, but it has no clinical advantage whatever over chlorpheniramine. Polaramine® is a gimmick designed to extract a high price.

POLYCILLIN® Ampicillin, U.S.P.
See Ampicillin, U.S.P.

Of ampicillin preparations available, this one is the most expensive.

POTASSIUM CHLORIDE, U.S.P.

All of the diuretics used to treat high blood pressure and heart failure that cause excessive potassium loss in the urine often require potassium supplements either in diet or in medication form. The "thiazide" diuretics (Diupres®, Diuril®, Enduron®, Esidrix®, Hydrodiuril®, Hydropres®, Hygroton®, Lasix®, Metahydrin®, Rauzide®, Regroton®, Ser-Ap-Es®) are very frequently associated with this potassium loss. Other diuretics (Aldactazide®, Aldactone®, Dyazide®) are potassium-sparing and may even cause potassium accumulation in the bloodstream.

If potassium loss is a problem, diet intake of potassium should be increased by eating dried apricots, raisins, dates, dried peaches, dried figs, bananas, prune juice and orange juice. This not infrequently fails, and oral potassium itself must be given as an adjunct to diuretic therapy.

When oral potassium must be given, problems arise primarily because virtually all preparations taste horrible. The least expensive and probably worst-tasting is potassium chloride (elixir 10%), bought in quart or gallon jugs for very little. The most expensive are the "gimmick" preparations, including K-Lyte®, Kaon®, K-Lor®, Kaochlor®, and many many others. Most patients, however, *can* take the most awful-tasting stuff, either by sheer force or by hiding its taste in orange or cranberry juice or other liquids. Oral potassium should be taken in liquid form, never as *tablets,* since tablets can be very irritating to the stomach and intestine. *Very severe complications, including bowel perforation and serious bleeding, have been associated with enteric-coated potassium tablets.*

The best way to take potassium is in food form; if this is not adequate, elixir should be used and should be taken in as dilute a solution as possible just after meals.

**POTASSIUM PENICILLIN G
TABLETS, U.S.P.**
  See Penicillin G.

**POTASSIUM PHENOXYMETHYL
PENICILLIN, U.S.P.**
  See Penicillin V.

PREDNISOLONE, U.S.P.

  Prednisolone, U.S.P., a steroid drug, is equivalent
to Prednisone, U.S.P., in efficacy and actions. It is
more expensive, harder to find at low cost, and has
no advantage over prednisone for oral use.
  See the Price Lists for Steroid Drugs and for Prednisone, U.S.P.

PREDNISONE, U.S.P.

  Prednisone, U.S.P., is a steroid drug that is the
agent of choice for nearly every clinical situation
where an oral steroid is required.
  In the blood and tissues there is normally a plentiful amount of cholesterol. All of the important hormones—most of the female and male sex hormones
and the several made by the adrenal gland to control
salt, water, protein, and sugar metabolism—are derivatives of cholesterol. Cholesterol is one of a family
of chemicals called "sterols." All of the hormones
mentioned are sterol-like; hence the name "steroids."
However, when doctors use the word "steroids" in
everyday conversation, they usually are referring to
hormones made by the adrenal gland. It is too much
of a mouthful to always say "adrenocorticosteroids."
  The best-known and most useful orally administered steroid in office practice is prednisone. Hydrocortisone is best for *topical* application. The first
widely used adrenal steroid was cortisone, but cortisone must be converted to hydrocortisone in the

body in order to exert its activity. Oral steroids, more expensive for ordinary clinical use, include such brand-name items as Decadron® and Medrol®. Topical steroids, more expensive than hydrocortisone, abound as well.

For comparative prices of oral preparations, see Steroid Drugs and Prednisone, U.S.P., in the Price Lists. For topical preparations, see the Price Lists for Hydrocortisone Cream, U.S.P.

PREMARIN®   Conjugated Estrogens, U.S.P.
  See Diethylstilbestrol, U.S.P.

A mixture of naturally occurring hormones, often isolated from the urine of female horses, Premarin® is usually prescribed for menopausal symptoms. The advertisements for this product stress the need to "Keep her on Premarin®" and neglect to mention the substantial price. The product is available at large savings to the patient in its generic form, Conjugated Estrogens, U.S.P.; see Conjugated Estrogens, U.S.P., in the Price Lists.

Menopause is a natural phenomenon when the ovaries stop their normal functioning. The symptoms of flushing, sweats, and the drying of vaginal secretions that often lead to itching or pain with intercourse are effectively treated for a brief time with conjugated estrogens. Usually, these uncomfortable feelings pass within several days, and after several months the medication is often no longer needed. If decreased vaginal secretions are a problem after the menopause is over, vaginal creams or suppositories are very useful. While there is no scientific proof, most doctors who have treated large numbers of menopausal women with estrogenic substances are impressed by the alleviation of anxiety that accompanies treatment.

The side effects from Premarin® and other conjugated estrogen compounds can be serious, especially with therapy lasting more than several months or a year. The estrogens in the medication may cause vaginal bleeding, breast swelling and tenderness, and weight gain from fluid retention. Whether estrogens given in small amounts to menopausal women predispose the patients to cancer has not been demonstrated.

Before patients are placed on estrogens, they should be carefully examined for breast cancer and cancers of the female organs. While there is no clear evidence that estrogens *cause* breast cancer, they can aggravate an already existing one that has gone unnoticed. Further, most physicians would not prescribe estrogens for women whose family history is strong for breast cancer, since these women too are at increased risk for hidden breast cancers. Estrogens definitely increase in size already-existing fibroid tumors of the uterus.

The use of estrogens to avoid osteoporosis, or "thin bones," in menopausal women is inappropriate, since long-term treatment with these estrogens causes decreased bone formation.

Because of the risks of further cancer development and the worsening of bone problems that go along with aging, as well as because of expense, Premarin® and other conjugated estrogen compounds should be used only to tide women over the few months of menopause when flushing and sweats are a very serious problem. The recommendation of the manufacturer of Premarin®, to "Keep her on Premarin®", is unsafe. However, the advertising done by the firm undoubtedly explains why the drug ranked *5th* in the U.S. in 1972 and 1973 among most-prescribed drugs!

PRINCIPEN®   Ampicillin, U.S.P.
  See Ampicillin, U.S.P.

Because it is among the more expensive brandname ampicillins, Principen® should not be prescribed; generic ampicillin would save the patient money.

PRO-BANTHINE®   Propantheline Bromide, U.S.P.
  See Atropine Sulfate, U.S.P.; Tincture of Belladonna (Belladonna Tincture, U.S.P.)

Propantheline (Pro-Banthine®) and methantheline (Banthine®) are two similar compounds that are very popular in the treatment of patients with ulcers. They work in a fashion very similar to tincture of belladonna and atropine, the active component of belladonna. The effects of these drugs is to decrease the secretion of acid in the stomach and slow down movement of food through the stomach and intestine. Both are useful effects in patients with ulcers, since increased acid secretion and rapid exit of food from the stomach leave the stomach lining exposed to the acid and thus make ulcers worse.

Antacids are the first-line drugs in patients with ulcers and, when antacids do not help in alleviating pain, atropine or tincture of belladonna should be used. While somewhat more likely to produce side effects, including dryness of the mouth and blurred vision, atropine and tincture of belladonna are significantly cheaper than virtually all of the other "anti-cholinergic" preparations, including Pro-Banthine®. Although Banthine® is not a big-selling item, Pro-Banthine® is among the 200 most-prescribed drugs.

PROBENECID, U.S.P.
See Colchicine, U.S.P.; Zyloprim®.

Better known as Benemid®, this drug is used for treating gout. The usual dose is 500 milligrams twice daily.

When penicillin was scarce and expensive, there was a way to make a little go a long way. Probenecid interferes with the mechanism by which the kidneys excrete penicillin. Therefore, if probenecid tablets were given at the same time, very high blood levels of penicillin could be maintained when relatively small doses were injected. When penicillin became plentiful and was manufactured by several concerns, there was price competition and it became cheap. The need for probenecid would have disappeared had it not been noted that it exaggerates the excretion of uric acid by the kidneys. It was tried out in patients with gout, where there is an excess of uric acid in the blood and tissues. It was found to work well; deposits of uric acid in the tissues sometimes "melt" away and are excreted in the urine. Usually the blood level of uric acid eventually falls. If the drug continues to be taken, the new uric acid deposits in tissues do not occur.

Fortunately, probenecid is a quite safe drug; the incidence of serious toxicity is low. A serious unwanted effect—and it is rare—is on white blood cells, which should be counted at intervals. Since uric acid pours into the urine in high concentration after treatment is begun, it is important for the patient to drink a lot of water to offset the possibility of uric acid crystals settling out. *Aspirin should not regularly be taken with probenecid because it blocks probenecid's action.*

Anticipating that physicians might have a need to prescribe both colchicine and probenecid at the same time for people with chronic gout, Merck has marketed a fixed-dose combination tablet (Colbenemid®) —0.5 milligram of colchicine and 0.5 gram of probenecid—which costs $6.55/100. Mysteriously, the addition of 0.5 milligram of colchicine has pushed the price of probenecid from $5.62 to $6.55, hardly a bargain. The patent on probenecid has now expired. The drug is available inexpensively by its generic name as a glance at the Price Lists will show.

There is a concerted effort to deflect doctors away from the use of probenecid in the prophylactic treatment of gout in order to get them to use a newer product, Zyloprim® (allopurinol). Zyloprim® has the disadvantages of newness, possibly greater toxicity, high price, and a mechanism of action that the *Handbook* considers undesirable (see Zyloprim®).

PROCAINAMIDE HYDROCHLORIDE, U.S.P.
See Quinidine Sulfate, U.S.P.

All local anesthetics (procaine, cocaine, etc.) have the same potential effect on the irregularly beating heart. Procaine has been known for many years as a theoretically useful heart drug, but its derivative procainamide is better.

Procainamide's effects on the heart are very similar to those of quinidine. When first marketed, procainamide was given only intravenously to emergency cases of ventricular tachycardia, but later it was found to be effective when given by mouth to treat less severe forms of abnormal heart rhythm. There are no adequate comparative studies on the relative efficacy of procainamide and quinidine when taken orally, but it is very likely much the same. This is fortunate, since recently the price of quinidine suddenly shot up. (See Quinidine Sulfate, U.S.P., in the Price Lists.)

The usual dose of procainamide for ventricular extra heartbeats—the most common need for it in office practice—is 250 to 500 milligrams every 4 hours. Less commonly, the single dose is 1 gram. The need to take procainamide every 4 hours is its major drawback; quinidine, on the other hand, need to be taken only every 6 hours.

Procainamide is no longer patented. The generic drug is available at a reasonable price and can be taken with economic advantage by many who must take quinidine regularly. However, if procainamide is bought as Pronestyl®, the expense will be greater. See the Price Lists for Procainamide Hydrochloride, U.S.P., and Quinidine Sulfate, U.S.P.

PROCHLORPERAZINE MALEATE, U.S.P.
    See Compazine®.

PROLOID®   thyroglobulin
    See Thyroid, U.S.P.

This is Warner/Chilcott's brand name for thyroglobulin, which has no clinical superiority over plain desiccated thyroid. The price is much higher.

Thyroid hormones should be used only in patients with documented thyroid deficiency states and not for weight reduction or mood elevation in depressed individuals. However, incredibly enough, many people who are obviously not thyroid deficient have been placed on an expensive thyroid product and have been kept on it for years. Persons who are truly thyroid-deficient are rare. The reason why a normal person can be given thyroid hormone without his suffering ill effects from too much is that the moment 180 milligrams or less are given per day, the person's own thyroid gland will stop producing its own natural hormone. The average person produces about 180 milligrams of thyroid hormone daily. Thus, if less than this amount is given, the patient's metabolic status is unaffected. And, of course, he or she is now taking a "medicine" (taking *any* harmless tablet will make 60 percent or more of people "feel better").

PROMETHAZINE HYDROCHLORIDE, U.S.P.
See Phenergan®.

PROPANTHELINE BROMIDE, U.S.P.
See Pro-Banthine®.

PROPOXYPHENE(S)
See Darvocet-N® and other Darvon® preparations.

PROPRANOLOL HYDROCHLORIDE, U.S.P.
See Inderal®.

PROVERA®   Medroxyprogesterone Acetate, U.S.P.

Provera® is a progesterone female hormone used in gynecological disorders including absence of periods (*i.e.*, amenorrhea), and in abnormal bleeding. It should not be used in patients with active clots in the legs (thrombophlebitis) or a history of thrombophlebitis, severe liver disease, or suspected cancers of the breast or female organs.

The drug is also used frequently for threatening or habitual abortions in women who are pregnant; this use has *not* been well proved and physicians ought *not* to use it for these indications.

PSEUDOEPHEDRINE HYDROCHLORIDE
See Sudafed®.

PYRIDIUM®   phenazopyridine hydrochloride

Pyridium® is a dye, which, when given by mouth, colors the urine red-orange—an excellent placebo effect. It is claimed that it has mild urinary tract anesthetic qualities, but this is doubted by many doctors. The effect is dramatic, the cost is high, and the value is questionable. Its inclusion in combination with anti-infective agents used in urinary infections (*e.g.,* Azo Gantanol® or Azo Gantrisin®) adds very considerably to the price.

Unwanted side effects include stomach and intestinal discomfort, headaches, and occasionally serious blood disorders.

QUAALUDE®   methaqualone
See Chloral Hydrate, U.S.P.; Nembutal®; Seconal®.

The use of this sedative cannot be recommended. Quaalude® has no proved clinical advantage over other sedatives and sleeping medications known to be very effective and almost always less expensive.

Side effects are common and include minor stomach upset, headache, mouth dryness, and tingling and numbness in the hands and feet. Dependence on this drug—psychological and physical—are common, as is abuse of this and similar sedative preparations (Doriden®, Placidyl®).

See the Price Lists for Pentobarbital, Secobarbital, and Chloral Hydrate, U.S.P.

QUINAGLUTE®   quinidine gluconate
*See Quinidine Sulfate, U.S.P., and Procainamide
Sulfate, U.S.P.*

Quinaglute® is promoted as advantageous over
quinidine sulfate because of alleged extended action.
The amount of quinidine in 0.3 gram of quinidine
gluconate is equivalent to that in 0.2 gram of quinidine sulfate. It is claimed that the gluconate salt need
be taken only every 8 hours, as opposed to the sulfate
salt, which must be taken every 6 hours. For this
slight advantage, patients must pay a lot more.

Procainamide is less expensive but somewhat less
convenient than quinidine because it must be taken
every 4 hours.

See Quinidine Sulfate, U.S.P., and Procainamide
Hydrochloride, U.S.P., in the Price Lists.

QUINIDINE GLUCONATE
See Quinaglute®.

QUINIDINE SULFATE, U.S.P.
*See Procainamide Hydrochloride, ·U.S.P.; Quina-
glute®.*

This basic drug is used to treat certain abnormal
heart rhythms. Quinidine is a natural constituent of
the bark of the cinchona tree, as is quinine, whose
structure is a mirror image (stereoisomer) of quinidine (see also dextroamphetamine). Quinidine is believed to have more effect on heart function than
quinine.

A Dutch sea captain is credited with first having
drawn attention to the usefulness of quinine as a
heart drug. He was a frequent visitor to Dutch East
Indian ports, where malaria was rampant and where
cinchona bark was widely self-administered by the
population for fever from whatever cause. The popularity of cinchona bark was such that it had come to
be used indiscriminately for a wide variety of ills,

much as aspirin is today. The captain, who was subject to spells of irregular, rapid heartbeat, discovered that this condition was favorably affected by cinchona. He told his European doctor, Wenkebach, who described this observation in the medical literature in 1914. The greater efficacy of quinidine over quinine as a drug for heart disease was reported a few years later.

Until the mid-1960s, quinidine and quinine were inexpensive. In 1966 and again in 1973, the price suddenly rose sharply. The background is not entirely clear, but may be related to the control of all of the world's sources of supply of quinine by a single foreign cartel, largely Dutch and German.

Procainamide is often as effective as quinidine, if less convenient, and it is available at lower cost. There is an increased risk with patients taking procainamide that they will not be "covered" during the sleeping hours, since they must wake up at least once to take the capsule in the middle of the night. Yet low-priced quinidine is simply not available. Side effects from procainamide include unusual problems, such as "lupus erythematosus" syndrome—a syndrome affecting many organs with changes in blood vessels and other tissues. This is very rare, however.

See Quinidine Sulfate, U.S.P., and Procainamide Hydrochloride, U.S.P., in the Price Lists.

RAUWOLFIA SERPENTINA, N.F.
  See Reserpine, U.S.P.; Rauzide®.

RAUZIDE®	Rauwolfia Serpentina,	
	N.F.	50 mg
	bendroflumethiazide	4 mg

  See Potassium Chloride, U.S.P.; Reserpine, U.S.P.; Trichlormethiazide.

Rauzide® combines the high blood pressure medication of rauwolfia serpentina with a "thiazide" diuretic, bendroflumethiazide. The "thiazide" diuretic is

similar in effect to all the diuretics described thus
far in the thiazide category (Diuril®, Enduron®, Esi-
drix®, Hydrodiuril®, Hygroton®, Lasix®, Metahy-
drin®). The most significant of its effects is increased
urination and loss of potassium salts, requiring potassium supplementation either in food or medications.

The *Handbook* prefers reserpine (the purified active
principle in rauwolfia) over rauwolfia itself, and if a
thiazide is needed to potentiate its blood-pressure-lowering action, suggests that the patient procure a prescription written for hydrochlorothiazide. Pharmacies,
especially large ones, now usually carry inexpensive
generic hydrochlorothiazide. The patient must insist
that pharmacist not dispense Hydrodiuril®, an expensive
brand name for it.

REGROTON® Chlorthalidone, U.S.P. 50.0 mg
Reserpine, U.S.P. 0.125 mg
*See Potassium Chloride, U.S.P.; Reserpine, U.S.P.;
Trichlormethiazide.*

This medication is a combination product used to
treat high blood pressure. The combination offers no
advantage over its components taken separately.
Chlorthalidone (Hygroton®) offers no special advantage over less expensive thiazides; its longer action
may be viewed as a disadvantage, since side effects are
prolonged and patients are not infrequently bothered
by having to arise at night to urinate as a consequence. Rather than chlorthalidone, cheaper thiazides
should be used; *e.g.,* generic trichlormethiazide or
generic hydrochlorothiazide. As with all diuretics in
the chlorthalidone or "thiazide" classes, excessive
potassium losses may occur and may require potassium supplements either in the diet or by medications.

Reserpine is a good medication often used in association with thiazides, but it should be given separately
to ensure that dose adjustments can be made independently.

RESERPINE, U.S.P.
   See Rauzide®; Ser-Ap-Es®; Serpasil®.

Reserpine is the purified, most active compound of the Indian snakeroot plant, Rauwolfia serpentina. It is a good drug for treating mild high blood pressure. An interesting drug, it acts by depleting the body's store of an important nerve-transmitter chemical, and its effect is cumulative and very long-lasting. It is rarely ever necessary to take more than 0.25 milligram a day as treatment for high blood pressure, and in most cases 0.1 milligram is an adequate dose. Reserpine is not without side effects, and the cumulative effect of *large* doses has been known to cause severe mental depression. However, it is relatively safe in small doses.

Reserpine is more effective at lowering blood pressure when the patient takes a diuresis-causing drug at the same time. There are many combinations of reserpine with a thiazide on the market, but the doctor would be better advised to write individual prescriptions for reserpine and the least expensive thiazide (hydrochlorothiazide is the one of choice). This constitutes better therapeutic technique, and usually costs the patient less.

RITALIN®   Methylphenidate Hydrochloride, N.F.
   See Dextroamphetamine Sulfate, U.S.P.; Elavil®; Tofranil®.

This drug was developed in an effort to find a substance with the "mood-elevating" effects of amphetamines and tricyclic antidepressants (Elavil®, Tofranil®) minus their drawbacks. Ritalin® is limited in its effectiveness as a mood elevator. It probably should not be used for depression, since the tricyclic drugs are preferred if a drug is needed at all. Mild and temporary depressions are often self-limiting and do not require drug therapy. Use of Ritalin® can cause depression when levels reach a plateau or when the drug is discontinued.

Recent controversy abounds about the use of Ritalin® in hyperactive children. The *Handbook* defers judgment and recommendation for usage. The drug, as well as amphetamines, acts differently on children than on adults and *may* be of use in preadolescent "hyperkinetic" children.

The most serious side effect of Ritalin® is social: the drug is among the most commonly abused pills. At least one country, Sweden, has banned its sale.

ROMILAR®
See Dextromethorphan Hydrobromide, N.F.

SECONAL®   Sodium Secobarbital, U.S.P.

This drug is available at less cost by generic name. It is a good, effective sleeping medication and relatively safe when used in recommended doses. (There should be a rule: never more than 300 milligrams in any 24-hour period.) For best effect, the drug should be taken on an empty stomach.

Both secobarbital and pentobarbital are good sleeping pills. It is generally taught, and perhaps, it is true, that pentobarbital "hangs around" the body a little longer than secobarbital and may be more likely to cause hangover, but this is uncommon with either drug if the dose does not exceed 1 or 2 capsules (100–200 milligrams) at bedtime.

The patent on secobarbital expired many years ago, but most doctors are still writing for Seconal® and causing unnecessary expense. One way Lilly encourages the continued prescribing of Seconal® is by putting it up in bullet-shaped capsules which they have copyrighted and trademarked as "Pulvule®." The bullet shape has no medical advantage. If the doctor writes "Pulvule®" on the prescription, the antisubstitution law that aids the drug industry in many states locks patient and pharmacist into a transaction where the Lilly product must be dispensed. Thus, writing "secobarbital pulvules" makes the patient have to pay more.

For most lay people there is mystery, even a little magic, connected with drugs. Some who have been buying Seconal® for years and know that it works might be suspicious of a preparation which was not bullet-shaped and, therefore, resist buying it. Such people are allowing a psychological barrier to interfere with a sensible economic measure.

For what prices need be, see Sodium Secobarbital, U.S.P., in the Price Lists.

SER-AP-ES®

Reserpine, U.S.P.	0.1 mg
Hydralazine Hydrochloride, N.F.	25 mg
Hydrochlorothiazide, U.S.P.	15 mg

This cocktail of high blood pressure medications is a CIBA product that is among the best-selling of the bad drugs on the market. It should be avoided because it combines three separate medications in a single pill. Ser-Ap-Es® has the drawbacks of any such multiple-combination product: first, the dosage of individual components cannot be adjusted independently; second, one or more components might be unnecessary in different patients; third, the likelihood of unwanted side effects increases proportionately with the number of drugs a person takes.

Any one of the components in Ser-Ap-Es®, when given separately, is a good medication for high blood pressure. Economy and rational prescribing demand, however, that they be given separately, each in its properly adjusted dose. An alternative to Ser-Ap-Es® might be 5 milligrams of generic hydrochlorothiazide and 0.1 milligram of reserpine daily. Alternatively, hydralazine and a thiazide may be given together. But the combination of three makes for great expense and a higher likelihood of unwanted side effects.

SERAX®   oxazepam
See Phenobarbital, U.S.P.

Roche has made extraordinary profits on Librium®
and Valium®, sedatives or "tranquilizers." In the
body, Librium® is broken down into oxazepam and
it is probable that oxazepam is the chemical which
exerts the sedative effect. Wyeth has synthesized, patented, and marketed oxazepam under the brand name
Serax®.

A pharmacology professor at Emory University
Medical School in Atlanta told a Senate hearing of a
"funny experience" he had had. Wyeth was willing to
pay an investigator in Emory's dental school to test
the ability of Serax® to lessen the anxiety of patients
facing dental procedures. When the dental school
came up with a well-designed plan for a study that
would compare Serax® with phenobarbital and also
with a placebo, Wyeth refused to go along. They
would pay for the comparison of Serax® with the
placebo but not with phenobarbital.* According to
Dr. Harry Williams, who related this, "manufacturers
are not interested in comparing their drug with a
similar drug, unless they have evidence that their
drug is clearly superior to the similar drug."

While it is difficult to deny that in certain situations and with certain patients, Librium®, Serax®,
Tranxene®, or Valium® might be better than phenobarbital, it is hard to get away from the belief that
they are being prescribed unnecessarily in office practice. If phenobarbital had been synthesized only last
year and was being marketed enthusiastically today as
the "newest and best of tranquilizers," Librium®,
Serax®, Tranxene®, and Valium® would have some
stiff competition.

SERPASIL®   Reserpine, U.S.P.
See Reserpine, U.S.P.

Serpasil is CIBA's reserpine. The price is outrageous. Great savings can be offered the patient by

* *Competitive Problems in the Drug Industry*, Part 2, p. 461.

prescribing Reserpine, U.S.P., and instructing the patient to "shop around a little."

See Reserpine, U.S.P., in the Price List.

SILVER NITRATE, TOUGHENED
See Addenda.

SINEQUAN®   doxepin hydrochloride
See Elavil®; Tofranil®.

Sinequan® is a tricyclic antidepressant drug very close to Tofranil® and Elavil® chemically but advertised as a sedative and antidepressant. While as effective as the other tricyclics, its advantages over them are unclear.

Side effects with doxepin are similar to those with imipramine (Tofranil®) and amitriptyline (Elavil®), including heart rhythm changes, confusion or disturbed thinking processes, allergic rashes, dryness of the mouth, nausea and some gastrointestinal upset, and, rarely, blood disorders. Overdose with doxepin and the other tricyclic antidepressants is dangerous because of the possibility of death caused by sudden onset of very rapid or irregular heartbeat. A normally beating heart is a *sine qua non* for staying alive.

SPIRONOLACTONE, U.S.P.
See Aldactone®.

STELAZINE®   trifluoperazine
See Thorazine®.

One of the "mind drugs," a phenothiazine, Stelazine® is much prescribed by psychiatrists and is no doubt useful, but whether it has any advantage over Thorazine® or certain other phenothiazines is debatable. It is only the rare patient seen by the internist or general practitioner in office practice who must be given Stelazine®——or Thorazine® or any other pheno-

thiazine. Adverse side effects are not uncommonly
encountered with all phenothiazines, which should
therefore be reserved for situations serious enough
to warrant their use (usually, frank psychosis).

It is difficult not to believe that a good deal of
Stelazine® is being prescribed unnecessarily, since it
is among the 100 top drugs. A lot of it is going to
elderly people.

STERAZOLIDIN®	Prednisone, U.S.P.	125 mg
	Phenylbutazone,	
	U.S.P.	50 mg
	Dried Aluminum	
	Hydroxide Gel,	
	U.S.P.	100 mg
	Magnesium Trisilicate,	
	U.S.P.	150 mg

See Butazolidin®; Prednisone, U.S.P.; Maalox®.

This fixed combination of two very potent drugs
with serious side effects, prednisone and phenylbutazone (Butazolidin®), and an antacid mixture is not
recommended by the *AMA Drug Evaluations,* 2nd
edn., nor by the *Handbook.* Prednisone dosage should
always be adjusted individually; the same is true of
phenylbutazone. Placing the two drugs in one capsule
is as irrational as putting salt and pepper in the same
shaker.

If we may cite the *AMA Drug Evaluations,* 2nd
edn., "Many fixed combinations of drugs are marketed for the treatment of arthritis. None represent
good therapy, since individualization of dosage of
antirheumatic agents is required and the doses must
be altered, when necessary, for maximal effectiveness"
(p. 304). The combination of steroids with other
drugs, of steroids with antacids because of altered
absorption of the steroids, and of steroids with other
potential toxic drugs like phenylbutazone because of
compounding of serious side effects is bad practice
and should be avoided.

Simply stated, this drug should never be used.

SUDAFED®   pseudoephedrine hydrochloride
See Ephedrine Sulfate, U.S.P.

Pseudoephedrine is very closely related chemically to ephedrine and has similar uses and side effects. Pseudoephedrine is promoted primarily for stuffy noses. Stuffy noses are stuffy because the blood vessels in their lining are dilated and engorged with blood (not, as many think, because the air passages are occluded by secretions). To dose a person's whole body with a blood vessel constrictor in order to constrict the blood vessels in the nose is senseless practice. "Nasal congestion" is best treated by the local application of nose drops. Phenylephrine nose drops (Neo-Synephrine® ½ %) is the medication of choice. Phenylephrine drops also have the advantage of requiring no prescription. Consult with your pharmacist about the use of the drops.

SULFAMETHOXAZOLE
See Gantanol®.

SULFISOXAZOLE, U.S.P.
See Gantrisin®.

SUMYCIN®   Tetracycline Hydrochloride, U.S.P.
See Tetracycline Hydrochloride, U.S.P.

Squibb changed this to a hydrochloride salt of tetracycline without most doctors' knowing it. Doctors had begun to prescribe Sumycin® after discovering its once relatively low price compared with other brand names. Wholesale cost, however, is still more than that of Tetracycline Hydrochloride, U.S.P., when bought as such and not as a brand. See Tetracycline Hydrochloride, U.S.P., in the Price Lists for comparative costs.

Sumycin® ranked 24th among the most prescribed drugs in 1973. However, there has been a recent surge in generic prescriptions for tetracycline and other antibiotics, including ampicillin, erythromycin, and penicillin, highlighting a fine trend: physicians are becoming more aware of the need to save their patients money when they prescribe.

SYNALAR® fluocinolone acetonide
See Hydrocortisone Cream, U.S.P.

Synalar® is a potent steroid useful in several skin problems. The *Handbook* recommends the use of hydrocortisone cream as a first-line drug, however, because of its low cost. When hydrocortisone fails, any one of the more potent fluorinated creams such as Synalar® might help. The cost of the more potent cream is high.

For effects and side effects of topical steroid creams and ointments, see Hydrocortisone Cream, U.S.P., (p. 216).

SYNTHROID® Sodium Levothyroxine, U.S.P.
See Proloid®; Thyroid, U.S.P.

See Thyroid, U.S.P., for a discussion of this drug. Thyroxine and desiccated or dried thyroid can be very inexpensive. Synthroid® is considerably more expensive.

The advantage of Synthroid® over desiccated thyroid is its greater precision of dosage. But this offers no advantage in terms of clinical effects. And despite a great reliance on blood tests that provide precise figures for blood levels of thyroid hormones in treating people with underactive thyroid glands, therapy with thyroid hormones is as well measured by clinical response to drugs rather than blood tests.

Like Proloid®, Synthroid® is not recommended because of its high cost compared with desiccated thyroid or thyroxine. For prices, see Thyroid, U.S.P., in the Price Lists.

TALWIN®   pentazocine hydrochloride
*See Codeine Sulfate, N.F., Codeine Phosphate,
U.S.P.; Demerol®; Percodan®.*

Talwin® is a pain-relief medication recently widely
advertised and widely used. Since it is not subject
to narcotic controls, it may be prescribed freely by
phone to pharmacies. The law may soon change.

In one of the most carefully done experiments
determining comparative effects of different pain relievers, Talwin® in its usual 50 milligram oral dose
was similar in effect to 650 milligrams of aspirin.*
The price is several times that for aspirin.

Side effects from Talwin® include dependence
(usually mild and infrequent), dizziness, and difficulty
in thinking. Patients have also noted both insomnia
and euphoria.

For short-term use, codeine or codeine and aspirin
is preferred in the treatment of mild to moderate pain.
When pain is so severe as to require very strong
medications for prolonged periods—as in terminal
cancer patients with bone pain—methadone is preferred. (See Percodan® for a discussion of methadone.)

The pain-relieving power of Talwin® is no better
than that of codeine on a milligram-for-milligram
basis, because codeine is better regulated and abuse
is thereby better documented. Also codeine is much
cheaper.

TANDEARIL®   Oxyphenbutazone, N.F.
See Butazolidin®.

Tandearil® is a breakdown product in the body
of phenylbutazone (Butazolidin®), with the same
actions and side effects. Since Tandearil® has no
known superiority over Butazolidin®, it is hard to
understand why the same two companies who market
phenylbutazone also market this product.

* C. G. Moertel et al., in *New England Journal of Medicine*,
286:813 (1972).

Both phenylbutazone or oxyphenbutazone are useful in very limited situations, including an unusual arthritis affecting the spine called ankylosing spondylitis and acute gouty attacks, although they are not the preferred or first-line drugs in either case.

Side effects are serious, including fatal blood disorders, ulcers, liver damage, and fluid retention. Because these side effects are more severe in older patients, the drugs should be used with great caution.

TEDRAL®
See Ephedrine Sulfate, U.S.P.

TELDRIN®   Chlorpheniramine Maleate, U.S.P.
See Chlor-Trimeton®; Antihistamines.

This Smith Kline & French preparation is entirely the same as generic chlorpheniramine maleate, or Chlor-Trimeton®, but the chemical is packaged in a "long-acting" Spansule®, the SK&F name for such a capsule. This product offers no advantage over other antihistamine preparations and provides for unpredictable absorption and added cost. The claimed advantages of less frequent administration are generally not accepted as outweighing disadvantages associated with "timed-release" products, and the *N.F.* and *U.S.P.* do not recognize such preparations as acceptable by their standards.

TENUATE®   Diethylpropion Hydrochloride, N.F.
See Dextroamphetamine Sulfate, U.S.P.

Less effective and more expensive in helping with weight reduction, Tenuate® offers no obvious advantages over dextroamphetamine. While appetite suppressants may be of some use in the short term, long-term weight reduction and maintenance require a new way of life rather than episodic use of pills. That new way of life includes dietary discretion, exercise, and psychological support.

TERRAMYCIN®   Oxytetracycline Hydrochloride, N.F.
See Tetracycline Hydrochloride, U.S.P.

One of the early tetracycline-type antibiotics, Terramycin® has no clinical advantage over simple tetracycline. There are still physicians in practice whose sole hospital training experience with broad-spectrum antibiotics in the early 1950s was with Terramycin®. Some continue to write Terramycin® on the prescription blank because they know it works well. It does work well, but no better than the less expensive generic tetracyclines.

TETRACYCLINE HYDROCHLORIDE, U.S.P.

The tetracycline family was the second broad-spectrum antibiotic type to become available (1948). The first member of the family was chlortetracycline (Aureomycin®), the second was oxytetracycline (Terramycin®), and the third was tetracycline (Achromycin®, Achromycin® V, Panmycin®, Sumycin®, Tetrex®, and others). Other more recently developed tetracycline drugs include demethylchlortetracycline (Declomycin®), methacycline (Rondomycin®), doxycycline (Vibramycin®), and minocycline (Minocin®).

Simple tetracycline, as the hydrochloride salt, is the most popular and easiest to produce: It causes less gastrointestinal upset than the chlor- and oxy-derivatives. As for demethylchlortetracycline (Declomycin®), it sensitizes the skin to sunlight more severely than the others.

Of the entire family of tetracyclines, the one of choice is simple tetracycline, now widely available, and cheaply, as the hydrochloride salt. Squibb's Sumycin® was originally a phosphate salt, but the corporation converted to using the hydrochloride.* If the doctor writes "tetracycline," he leaves it to the patient and to the pharmacist as to which product is used to

* Despite the change, Squibb did not change the name of the product.

fill the prescription; patients must ask for the cheapest product on hand. Pharmacists must stock them! Generic prescriptions for tetracycline have become more popular recently, and in 1972 and 1973 generic tetracycline was among the two most frequently prescribed drugs for which generic names were used on the prescription blank.

Tetracycline is often overused. Its primary usefulness is in chronic bronchitis, when sputum changes in color from white to yellow or yellow-green and breathing becomes more difficult for patients with known chronic lung disease. It also has a place in the treatment of acne. Several unusual disorders are best treated with tetracycline, including cholera, rickettsial diseases, psittacosis (an unusual disease often contracted from parakeets), and others. The drug should *not* be used in simple viral respiratory infections or "colds."

Recently, the most expensive tetracycline preparations, Minocin®, Vibramycin®, and Declomycin®, have been extensively advertised and have grown in sales. These antibiotics offer no substantial advantages over plain tetracycline and in most cases have more severe side effects because of their slowed excretion.

Tetracycline should be prescribed and dispensed generically to ensure savings to patients. And·patients should be instructed by physicians to take the medication 15 to 30 minutes before eating and *never* to take it with milk or at the same time as any calcium-containing antacid. Calcium in milk forms an insoluble calcium tetracyclinate salt that greatly impedes absorption.

Tetracycline should not be prescribed to children under five or to women in the last half of pregnancy. (See Appendix A, Prescribing for Children.)

TETREX®   Tetracycline Hydrochloride, U.S.P.
See Tetracycline Hydrochloride, U.S.P.

Tetrex® is an expensive way to prescribe tetracycline. Physicians are undoubtedly more aware of the greater cost of Tetrex®, since it has fallen in sales recently, ranking 106th among prescribed drugs in 1972 and 153rd in 1973. During the same time, generic tetracycline prescriptions were up over 8 percent.

THEOPHYLLINE, N.F.
See Elixophyllin®.

"THE PILL."
See Oral Contraceptives.

THIORIDAZINE
See Mellaril®.

THORAZINE®   Chlorpromazine Hydrochloride, U.S.P.

Thorazine® is the prototype of phenothiazines. These drugs are used primarily in the treatment of psychoses. Thorazine® was discovered and synthesized by a French firm. It has little reason to be prescribed as frequently as it is in office practice; its major need is by psychiatrists for the treatment of otherwise unmanageable patients. For them Thorazine® is an indispensable, excellent form of treatment, so good that large, state-supported mental hospitals have been able to discharge many patients who, prior to the use of Thorazine® and related drugs, would have remained incarcerated for life. Mental hospitals are utterly dependent on it and its congeners, promazine (Sparine®), thioridazine (Mellaril®), fluphenazine (Prolixin®), perphenazine (Trilafon®), trifluoperazine (Stelazine®), thiothixene (Navane®), and others.

Thorazine® and Stelazine®, two of the most prescribed antipsychotic phenothiazines, are both marketed by Smith Kline & French. The company's net earnings in 1952 and 1953, immediately prior to Thorazine's® appearance on the market, were $4.3 and $5.0 million. In 1954 and 1955, with the marketing of Thorazine®, net earnings rose to $9.4 and

$16.0 million respectively. Despite these massive earnings increases, SK&F was immovable in price negotiations for the purchase of $2.5 million in drugs from them by New York State for use in mental hospitals in the mid-1960s.

Thorazine® can also be useful in preventing nausea and vomiting in conditions that are *not* short-lived or self-limiting, such as after radiation ("cobalt") therapy for cancer. However, Phenergan® is the first-choice medication for these problems, because it is less toxic and has more antihistamine-like effects.

Side effects with all of the phenothiazines include liver damage, rashes, unusual twitches and other body movements, drowsiness and lethargy, and occasional blood disorders.

In sum, Thorazine® is an excellent drug for psychotic patients, but it has little use outside the psychiatrist's hands. For serious nausea and vomiting, Phenergan® is recommended once correctable causes have been ruled out.

The patent on chlorpromazine has now expired and it is available generically at reasonable prices. See Thorazine® in the Price Lists.

THYROGLOBULIN
  See Proloid®.

THYROID, U.S.P.
  See Proloid®; Synthroid®.

Thyroid hormones are prescribed for patients with underactive thyroid glands. They should never be used as mood elevators or diet pills, since they can seriously affect the functioning of normal thyroid glands (if given in large-enough dose).

Various preparations are available, and all are either purified preparations of raw thyroid glands from animals or synthetic thyroid hormones. The synthetic preparations provide more accurate dosage, but the clinical effects are about the same whether the least accurate form—desiccated, or dried, thyroid—or the more accurate and purified forms—levothyroxine (Synthroid®) and others—are used. Cytomel®, liothyronine, once popular, is now less prescribed because it has a distinctly more rapid onset of action. Preparations that begin to act more slowly and are longer-acting are preferred.

The *Handbook* recommends the prescribing of either dried, or desiccated, thyroid, written as "Thyroid, U.S.P.," or levothyroxine. Sixty milligrams of thyroid is approximately equivalent to 0.1 milligram of levothyroxine. Liothyronine (Cytomel®) or liotrix (Euthroid®, Thyrolar®) products are considerably more expensive, with no advantage over Thyroid, U.S.P. or generic levothyroxine.

TIGAN®   trimethobenzamide hydrochloride
See Antihistamines; Phenergan®.

Many doctors prescribe Tigan® for nausea, but its effectiveness has been questioned. Its ability to affect nausea and vomiting any more effectively than a placebo has not been shown consistently.

There is less widespread doubt about the anti-nausea effect of diphenhydramine (Benadryl®) and of suppositories of promethazine (Phenergan®). For the acutely nauseated or vomiting patient (except when it is a sign of early pregnancy or related to correctable causes), the *Handbook* recommends Phenergan® suppositories.

TINACTIN®
See Addenda.

**TINCTURE OF BELLADONNA
(BELLADONNA TINCTURE, U.S.P.)**
See Atropine Sulfate, U.S.P.

In order to make this highly effective drug, 10 grams of the powdered leaves of the deadly nightshade plant are extracted into 100 milliliters (about 3 ounces) of a water–alcohol mixture. This drug is very inexpensive, which is fortunate, for it is the drug of choice to reduce hydrochloric acid secretion in the stomach and to cause considerable muscular relaxation within the gastrointestinal tract. A big advantage is that it lends itself to flexibility of dosage. To find the proper dose for any person is easy; he simply increases the number of drops taken from day to day until he develops either a dry mouth or trouble focusing his eyes on near objects. One or two drops less than the maximum tolerated dose is the best; it produces a good effect on the gastrointestinal tract, with a minimum of side effects. The disadvantages of belladonna are minor: because the tincture is a partially alcoholic solution, the bottle must be kept capped lest the vehicle evaporate and cause the active substance (atropine) to increase in concentration; also, a small dropper bottle may be inconvenient to carry on the person.

For more about the cost of Belladonna Tincture, U.S.P., see the Price Lists.

For those who prefer a tablet to the tincture, the active component of belladonna, atropine sulfate, should be prescribed. The usual dose is 0.4 milligram 3 or 4 times a day. See Atropine Sulfate, U.S.P., in the Price Lists.

TINCTURE OF OPIUM, CAMPHORATED
See Paregoric, U.S.P.

TOFRANIL®   Imipramine Hydrochloride, U.S.P.
See Elavil®.

Tofranil® belongs to the class of drugs known as tricyclic antidepressants. These drugs, including amitriptyline (Elavil®), have a three-ringed (or, tricyclic) chemical structure and are useful in the treatment of depression *not* directly associated with "tough" circumstances in life.

When antidepressant medications are indicated, either Tofranil® or Elavil® may be effective. They are usually given in several doses a day and require a week or more before their effects on behavior and depression are noted.

Side effects, when they occur, are serious with these drugs, with some reactions in 15 percent of all users and severe reactions in 5 percent *: dry mouth, palpitations, constipation, blurred vision, precipitation of glaucoma, sweating, dizziness, weight gain, urinary retention, nausea, vomiting, tremors, confusion, agitation, hallucinations, seizures, low blood pressure with standing, bleeding into the skin, jaundice, blood disorders, rashes, photosensitization, decreased libido, and impotence.

Tofranil® has been used for youngsters with enuresis, or bed-wetting. Its usefulness is debated.

Tofranil® and the other tricyclics are expensive. A recently released new form, Tofranil-PM®, a pamoate salt, offers little advantage. (Except, of course, to the manufacturer who charges more for it.) Tofranil-PM® comes in 150 milligram capsules, and at present is unavailable less expensively as a generic drug.

TOLAZAMIDE, U.S.P.
   See Tolinase®.

TOLBUTAMIDE, U.S.P.
   See Orinase®.

TOLINASE®   Tolazamide, U.S.P.
   See Orinase®.

Tolinase® is a sulfonylurea blood-sugar-lowering agent used in adult-onset diabetics. It is analogous to Orinase®, a slow poison, and should be removed

* Boston Collaborative Drug Surveillance Program, *Lancet,* 1:529 (1972).

from the market by the FDA. Diet, exercise, and insulin are the major tools for treating diabetes.

TRANXENE® chorazepate dipotassium
  See Phenobarbital, U.S.P.

Tranxene® is the most recent addition to the benzodiazepine sedatives, which include chlordiazepoxide (Librium®), oxazepam (Serax®), and diazepam (Valium®). It offers no advantages over these other benzodiazepines and, because it is the most recent on the market, may have side effects not yet discovered. The daily dose of chlorazepate is from 15 to 60 milligrams, which corresponds to approximately 10 to 40 milligrams of diazepam. Tranxene® offers no financial advantage over the other products; had Tranxene® been offered more cheaply than the others, arguments could be made for its being the benzodiazepine of choice, once side effects were determined over a several-year period.

The *Handbook* once again recommends the use of phenobarbital for mild sedation. When phenobarbital is not appropriate, as in patients who are suicidal, who take drugs that interact with phenobarbital (*e.g.,* warfarin), or who are made unduly sleepy with phenobarbital, the benzodiazepines chlordiazepoxide, diazepam, or the sedative meprobamate are the drugs of choice. In elderly people, a little wine is probably the best mild sedative of all.

TRIAMCINOLONE
  See Aristocort®; Kenalog®.

TRIAMTERENE
  See Dyazide®.

TRIAVIL® Perphenazine Hydrochloride, N.F. 2 or 4 mg

Amitriptyline Hydro-
chloride, U.S.P. 10 or 25 mg

See Elavil®; Thorazine®.

Triavil is a combination of "mind drugs": the antipsychotic or major tranquilizer perphenazine and the antidepressant amitriptyline (Elavil®). The drug is useful in psychotic patients whose illness is characterized by profound depression, but it should be prescribed only in very special cases, and always under close psychiatric care.

While fixed combinations are generally not sanctioned, this one is available in four dose combinations, making adjustment of dosages for each of the two components possible. The side effects of each of the two components are still compounded with this preparation, and the side effects of each drug are numerous and often serious. See Thorazine®, for the actions and side effects of perphenazine, a drug very similar to chlorpromazine; see Elavil®, for those of amitriptyline.

Triavil® is almost certainly overprescribed, ranking 39th in the nation among prescription drugs in 1973! It is also expensive, and much of the expense generated by prescriptions for Triavil® could be avoided if physicians prescribed one or the other component of the product rather than automatically prescribing the combination.

TRICHLORMETHIAZIDE

Trichlormethiazide is another "thiazide" diuretic. Despite the fact that it is not as popular as many of the thiazides, it is equal in effectiveness and somewhat less expensive than most others, though not significantly less costly than generic hydrochlorothiazide (p. 215).

"Thiazide" diuretics are used for two conditions: to lower high blood pressure and to rid the body of excess fluid. The ones most commonly used are Diuril®, Hydrodiuril®, Esidrix®, Enduron®, and Lasix®. Four milligrams of trichlormethiazide is approximately equal in effect to 500 milligrams of Diuril® and 50 milligrams of Hydrodiuril® or Esidrix®. Lasix® is probably a more powerful drug than the others.

Trichlormethiazide is available under two brand names: as Naqua®, an expensive Schering product, and as Metahydrin®, a slightly less costly Colgate-Palmolive (Lakeside Laboratories) product. It is also available in much less costly generic form. However, all of it is produced by either Lakeside or Schering. Significant savings would be had if generic trichlormethiazide were used instead of most of the other thiazides. An exception is generic hydrochlorothiazide, and the latter's advantage is its wider availability.

Trichlormethiazide can cause side effects similar to those caused by others. The most serious of these is potassium loss, which is combated both by the ingestion of potassium-rich foods and by the use of potassium chloride supplements.

By prescribing reserpine 0.1 milligram along with 4 milligrams of trichlormethiazide or 25 or 50 milligrams of hydrochlorothiazide, the doctor provides an excellent thiazide-reserpine combination. If it is necessary to gain greater control over the blood pressure, spironolactone (Aldactone®), methyldopa (Aldomet®), guanethidine (Ismelin®), and others may be added to obtain the desired effect.

TRIFLUOPERAZINE
See Stelazine®.

TRIHEXYPHENIDYL HYDROCHLORIDE, U.S.P.
See Artane®.

TRIMETHOBENZAMIDE HYDROCHLORIDE
See Tigan®.

TRIPLE SULFAS   Trisulfapyrimidines Tablets, U.S.P.

Sulfacetamide, Sulfadiazine,
and Sulfamerazine Tablets,
N.F.

One of the disadvantages of sulfonamide anti-infection drugs when they were introduced was their relative insolubility. Crystals could precipitate in the kidneys and cause blockage if the concentration of drug was too high in the urine and if the urine was acidic. One way to sharply minimize this possibility is by giving a mixture of three sulfonamide drugs, each representing one-third of the total dose. This way the total anti-infection effect is the same but the possibility of crystals precipitating is reduced by two-thirds. The *United States Pharmacopeia* and *National Formulary* each have an official triple sulfas preparation. The doctor need only write "Triple Sulfas 0.5 g tablet" and the patient can receive either the *U.S.P.* or the *N.F.* preparation, whichever the pharmacist has in stock. For prices, see Triple Sulfas in the Price Lists.

Triple sulfas were widely used for urinary infections in the late 1940s and early 1950s. Their place was taken by widely advertised sulfonamide, sulfisoxazole, a very soluble drug which when used alone is unlikely to cause crystal formation in the kidneys. It is doubtful that sulfisoxazole has any significant clinical advantage over triple sulfas, however. Sulfisoxazole is a Roche drug, marketed as Gantrisin® at a high price.

First choice for treating garden-variety urinary infection is triple sulfas for 7 to 14 days. The usual dose is two 0.5 gram tablets 4 times a day. The first day the dose should be twice this. The most important thing to be certain about in treating urinary infection is *that a bacterial culture demonstrates that the urine is free of bacteria 3 to 4 weeks after treatment has been discontinued.* For most infections seen in the office, this later culture is more important than one taken before treatment is started.

Advertising and promotion being what they are, Gantrisin® is one of the most prescribed drugs in the nation and triple sulfas is so little prescribed that no figures on its sales are available.

TRISULFAPYRIMIDINES TABLETS, U.S.P.
  See Triple Sulfas.

TUINAL®	Sodium Secobarbital,
	U.S.P. 25, 50, or 100 mg
	Sodium Amobarbital,
	U.S.P. 25, 50, or 100 mg

  See Nembutal®; Seconal®.

It is doubtful that Tuinal® is a significantly better "sleeping pill" than either secobarbital (Seconal®) or barbital (Nembutol®).

For comparative prices, see Sodium Secobarbital, U.S.P., and Sodium Pentobarbital, U.S.P., in the Price Lists.

TUSS-ORNADE®	caramiphen edisylate	20 mg
	Chlorpheniramine Ma-	
	leate, U.S.P.	8 mg
	phenylpropanolamine	
	hydrochloride	50 mg
	isopropamide iodide	2.5 mg
	(per 4 tsps approx)	

  See Cough Remedies; Actifed®; Actifed-C® Expectorant; Ambenyl® Expectorant; Benylin® Expectorant; Dimetapp®; Drixoral®; Naldecon®; Ornade®; Phenergan® Expectorant.

Tuss-Ornade®, like many others among the concoctions above, is an irrational combination of potentially toxic products offered as a cold remedy. The concoction offers little more than the chlorpheniramine maleate in it; this excellent component may be purchased generically as an antihistamine useful in drying up secretions generated by viral illnesses. If cough suppression is a problem, codeine or dextromethorphan is recommended.

TYLENOL®   Acetaminophen, N.F.

TYLENOL® WITH CODEINE

Acetaminophen, N.F. 300 mg
Codeine Phosphate, N.F.

7.5, 15, 30, or 60 mg

See Aspirin, U.S.P.; Codeine Sulfate, N.F.; Codeine Phosphate, U.S.P.

Acetaminophen, a non-prescription drug, is a pain reliever (analgesic) and antifever drug (antipyretic), like aspirin. It lacks the anti-inflammatory effects of aspirin, making it less useful in the treatment of arthritis disorders. Phenacetin, the "P" in APC tablets, owes its analgesic and antipyretic actions to its conversion within the body to acetaminophen.

The major advantage of acetaminophen is its infrequent ill effects on the stomach; it rarely causes stomach upset. Unfortunately, aspirin often does, although this effect may sometimes be avoided if ample water is taken with the aspirin. Acetaminophen is also less likely to prolong bleeding or interfere with anticoagulant drugs like warfarin than is aspirin. In patients with gout, acetaminophen is preferred to aspirin because aspirin interferes with the passage of uric acid out of the body through the kidneys, while acetaminophen does not.

Disadvantages of acetaminophen include the potential for serious kidney damage, *but only after very prolonged use.* If bought by its brand name, Tylenol®, acetaminophen can be expensive.

The combination of aspirin or acetaminophen with codeine is useful, since there is good evidence that the codeine adds an analgesic effect if doses of 30 or 60 milligrams are used. Smaller doses of codeine have minimal pain-relieving effects. While the addition of codeine to Tylenol® adds very little to the price of Tylenol®, savings ·may be had by buying generic acetaminophen "over-the-counter" and codeine by prescription; the two tablets could then be taken separately. The convenience would be somewhat less but the savings significant.

One reason for the popularity of Tylenol® with Codeine is that the combination is categorized as a Class III drug under the narcotics control laws.

Codeine alone, which is supposedly more subject to abuse, is more stringently controlled, as a Class II product. Class III products may be prescribed by the doctor over the telephone, but this privilege is not extended to Class II products.

VALISONE®   Betamethasone Valerate, N.F.
See Hydrocortisone Cream, U.S.P.

Valisone® is yet another of the topical steroid preparations used for skin problems of various descriptions. One of the fluorinated corticosteroids, betamethasone is similar to fluocinolone (Synalar®), flurandrenolide (Cordran®), and triamcinolone (Kenalog®) in power. Usually the less potent and far less costly topical steroid, hydrocortisone, will do as well. Only when hydrocortisone has failed (patients must be advised to rub it in very well) should Valisone® be used. Valisone® is slightly more expensive per ounce than the equivalent dose preparations of Kenalog® and Cordran®, and approximately equal in price to Synalar®.
See Topical Steroids in the Price Lists.

VALIUM®   diazepam
See Phenobarbital, U.S.P.

Valium® is a benzodiazepine sedative, best known as a "tranquilizer," and is *the* most prescribed drug in the U.S. for several years running. With Valium® and its chemical cousin, Librium®, Roche Laboratories has the bulk of the "tranquilizer" market; and that market is quite substantial, including the majority of adult Americans, who have at one time or another been given prescriptions for Valium® or Librium®.
Valium® and Librium®, as well as other benzodiazepines (Serax® and Tranxene®), are useful mild sedatives. They have some advantages over the barbiturates, which were the mainstay of sedative

drugs until the advent of meprobamate. Yet the vast market for "tranquilizers" that has developed in recent years seems disproportionate to the need. Indeed, the *Handbook* feels that this market developed largely in response to massive advertising on the part of Roche and others. There is some evidence that drug abuse problems in American young people are related to the propensity of their parents to "pop" pills.

Various claims made for the usefulness of oral Valium® as a muscle relaxant or in angina pectoris, irritable bowel, or ulcer disease are not supported with good evidence.

While side effects from Valium® are usually less severe than with the barbiturates, overdoses are not uncommon and have led to death. Drowsiness, nausea, blurred vision, headache, depression, hallucinations, and excitement, while unusual, do occur. Side effects are more common among the elderly.

Valium® is recommended as an excellent sedative in those for whom phenobarbital is contraindicated. Its extremely high cost is the major reason it should not be considered the drug of choice for tranquilization and sedation. Based on weight, Valium® is the most expensive drug on the American market. On a date (March 15, 1975) when the official value of gold was $35.00 an ounce, the same quantity of Valium® cost more than $1000 at the wholesale level—more than 25 times the cost of gold. (The factor is less, of course, if one uses as a value for gold the current European "floating" price for gold, which is about $150 for an ounce.)

VASODILAN®   isoxsuprine hydrochloride
   See Cyclospasmol®; Pavabid®.

Like cyclandelate (Cyclospasmol®) and papaverine (Pavabid®), Vasodilan® is recommended for decreased blood flow to the head and extremities. Its usefulness for these problems is dubious and the drug should probably never be prescribed.

The National Academy of Sciences–National Research Council has deemed the product only "possibly effective" for its advertised indications (*Physicians' Desk Reference,* 1974 edn., p. 991), and the *AMA Drug Evaluations,* 2nd edn., states: "Its alleged value in treating peripheral vascular disease and cerebral ischemic episodes has not been convincingly demonstrated" (p. 28).

Simply stated, as with Cyclospasmol® and Pavabid®, this drug should not be used.

V-CILLIN K®
Potassium Phenoxymethyl Penicillin, U.S.P.

See Penicillin V (Potassium Phenoxymethyl Penicillin, U.S.P.).

V-Cillin K® is another brand name for penicillin V. See Penicillin V for its uses, and for comparative prices see Penicillin V in the Price Lists.

VIBRAMYCIN®
doxycycline hyclate
See Tetracycline Hydrochloride, U.S.P.

Vibramycin® is a tetracycline with very few advantages and many disadvantages compared to plain tetracycline. Its advantages occur only rarely, in patients with poor kidney function who have very specific infections outside of the kidney for which tetracyclines are the drugs of first choice. Its disadvantages are great cost and also newness, making side effects less well understood. Vibramycin® has the same spectrum of antimicrobial activity as other tetracyclines. Claims of broader spectrum are not in accordance with available evidence, in the published opinion of the FDA and in the published admission of the manufacturer.*

* *Competitive Problems in the Drug Industry,* Part 9, pp. 3645-3647.

The recent marketing of Doxy II® by USV Pharmaceuticals is undoubtedly in response to the increasing market for tetracycline drugs like doxycycline (Vibramycin® and Doxy II®) and minocycline (Minocin®). With very special qualifications, these drugs offer few or no advantages over plain, cheap, generic tetracycline.

See Tetracycline Hydrochloride, U.S.P., in the Price Lists.

VIOFORM®-   iodochlorhydroxyquin   3%
HYDROCORTISONE   Hydrocortisone,
                        U.S.P.   0.5%, 1%
   See Hydrocortisone Cream, U.S.P.

Vioform®-Hydrocortisone is a combination of the antifungal antibacterial iodochlorhydroxyquin (Vioform®) with hydrocortisone to combat the inflammation and irritation that on occasion accompany dermatophyte or skin-fungus infections. Of course, this product should only be used when such fungal infections are documented with scrapings from the skin wounds and when inflammation and irritation are serious enough to warrant steroid therapy. Perhaps more appropriate therapy for dermatophyte infections would be griseofulvin orally and tolnaftate (Tinactin®) topically. If inflammation and irritation are very serious, topical hydrocortisone could be used.

VISTARIL®   hydroxyzine pamoate
   See Antihistamines; Atarax®.

This antihistamine drug is marketed primarily for sedation, tranquilization, and anti-itching effects. Atarax® and Vistaril® are marketed by the same parent company at identical prices. Neither is superior to a barbiturate for sedation nor to a cheaper antihistamine drug for anti-itching effects.

In 1972, Atarax® and Vistaril® ranked 165th and 151st, respectively, among the 200 most-prescribed drugs. In 1972, they were ranked 159th and 173rd, respectively. It would be of interest to know how many doctors have switched a patient from Vistaril® to Atarax® or vice versa in the belief that they were changing the nature of the medication. Vistaril®, a name with pleasant landscape overtones, very likely exerts a placebo effect.

VITAMIN B₁₂   Cyanocobalamin, U.S.P.

Discovery of the cure for pernicious anemia, once a universally fatal disease, is attributed to Drs. G. R. Minot and W. P. Murphy, who worked in the Thorndike Laboratory of the Boston City Hospital, a municipal facility. They received a Nobel Prize for demonstrating unequivocally, in 1926, that oral administration of crude raw liver restores pernicious anemia patients to health. Later came crude extracts of liver for injection. The identity of the active principle in liver extract remained unknown for many years; it was commonly called "extrinsic factor." Pernicious anemia is caused by inability of the stomach wall to make a substance ("intrinsic factor") whose presence is required if the "extrinsic (dietary) factor" is to be absorbed through the intestinal wall into the bloodstream (unless the dietary factor is given orally in enormous amounts, as in a pound or more of raw liver a day, which is impractical and expensive). "Extrinsic factor," once absorbed, is stored in the liver in high concentration, which is the reason for raw liver's effectiveness when taken by mouth. Many foods in a normal diet have sufficient "extrinsic factor" in them to keep one healthy, provided the stomach makes "intrinsic factor."

In a fascinating series of developments over the years, from 1926 to the present, much has been learned of the possible causes and effective treatment of pernicious anemia and certain closely related conditions. One important discovery is that the "extrinsic factor" is vitamin B₁₂. (This is an intentional simplification but close enough to the facts for our purposes here.) Vitamin B₁₂ is a complicated molecule, the only known pharmacologically active organic substance containing a cobalt atom. The cobalt accounts for the rich red color of the pure material.

Pernicious anemia, though not rare, is not a common disease. The diagnosis is not hard to make if the doctor thinks of it and takes a look at a well-made blood smear. Vitamin B_{12} (Cyanocobalamin, U.S.P.) administration is the specific treatment. The substance may be administered in either of two ways: by mouth or by injection. In oral administration, massive amounts must be given, around 1000 micrograms per week. (In the absence of "intrinsic factor" a small but effective percent of a massive dose gets through the gut wall into the blood by a diffusion process.) Administration by injection requires that only about 60 micrograms be given every 6 weeks (after initial treatment with larger amounts). Hence, it is wasteful and expensive to treat pernicious anemia by mouth, and may be less reliable. Since most patients can be taught to give themselves injections (insulin for diabetes), the most convenient and least expensive way to treat a reliable patient with uncomplicated pernicious anemia is to allow him to inject himself with 60 micrograms of B_{12} every 6 weeks. The injection should be deep subcutaneous. B_{12} is painless and non-irritating. It is not harmful if given in excess.

It is not suggested that patients with pernicious anemia be turned loose by the doctor with a vial of B_{12} and a syringe. A person being treated for uncomplicated pernicious anemia ought to see the doctor regularly, although once every 6 weeks seems a bit much if he feels well.*

As the person who really needs vitamin B_{12} will have to take it for the remainder of his days, cost is an important factor. Cyanocobalamin Injection, U.S.P., is available to the druggist for as little as $0.35 for a 10 cc vial containing 1000 micrograms per cc (see Vitamin B_{12} in the Price Lists for names and posted

---

* Economy can be maintained in medical practice by curtailing unnecessary visits to doctors' offices, unnecessary hospitalizations, and superfluous laboratory tests.

prices).* If the patient is armed with a 1 cc tuberculin syringe calibrated in tenths of a cc and injects himself with a generous tenth of a cc every 4 to 6 weeks, he can get a lot of mileage out of that vial at low cost. Cyanocobalamin is stable in neutral solution and at ordinary temperatures, but it is a good idea to keep it in the refrigerator or some other cool place.

There is no known medical indication for vitamin B_{12} administration except pernicious anemia. The enormous volume of this drug that is sold suggests that it is being used indiscriminately. Its red color, non-toxicity, and injectability make it an excellent placebo. It is impossible to gauge how much is being given by injection in doctors' offices, but a lot is prescribed to ambulatory patients, particularly in 2 oral preparations with the brand names Vi-Sorbin® and Trinsicon®.

VITAMINS

Medicine was revolutionized by Pasteur in the nineteenth century. He put the germ theory of disease on a solid footing. Physicians began to think habitually in terms of an external agent as the cause of all disease. That the *lack* of an external agent might cause disease was, therefore, a notion accepted with some skepticism by the medical profession.

A Dutch doctor in Java observed in 1897 that persons who ate polished rice were more likely to suffer from beriberi than those who ate unhusked rice. About twenty years later a scientist isolated a pure material from rice husks (polishings) which, on administration to individuals with beriberi, cured them. This material was the first vitamin isolated. It is called thiamine, and its usefulness is limited to conditions caused by its deficiency, including inflammation of peripheral nerves, certain brain abnormalities (especially in alcoholics), and a special kind of heart fail-

* Some common brands that cost more are Berubigen®, Betalin 12®, Dodecavite®, Redisol®, and Sytobex®.

326 The New Handbook of Prescription Drugs

ure. Yet thiamine is given for all kinds of peripheral
nerve inflammations which are not due to thiamine
deficiency. Likewise, vitamin C is given for certain
blood disorders where there is bleeding into the skin
and taken by the great masses for the common
cold although its proved efficacy is in doubt, and
vitamin B_{12} is injected for everything from anemia,
not remotely due to its lack, to psychoneurosis.

There is probably more indiscriminate prescribing
and self-dosing with vitamin preparations than with
any other drug or combination of drugs available
in pharmacies today. The immense lucrativeness of
the market is evidenced by the inclusion in one commonly used advertising source for doctors, *Physicians'
Desk Reference,* of several hundred different combinations of vitamins, and combinations of vitamins with
minerals. Without entering into a discussion of the
pros and cons of whether supplemental intake of vitamins is desirable or necessary for the average North
American, doctors and patients should be made aware
that there are only two *official* multivitamin preparations, one in the *United States Pharmacopeia* (Decavitamin) and one in the *National Formulary* (Hexavitamin). Each is potentially available at low cost,
but not many companies, large or small, seem anxious
to market them.

WARFARIN (SODIUM WARFARIN, U.S.P.)
See Coumadin®.

ZYLOPRIM®   allopurinol
See Colchicine, U.S.P.; Probenecid, U.S.P.

Allopurinol provides a rational but probably more
dangerous and certainly more expensive alternative
to probenecid, a reliable drug that has been used
for years to treat gout.

Allopurinol has a molecular configuration similar
to that of hypoxanthine, a naturally occurring body
substance. Hypoxanthine is converted to uric acid,

the culprit in gout. Because of an inherited "inborn error of metabolism," persons with gout make too much uric acid. If and when uric acid crystals precipitate in the joints or the kidneys, patients with gout suffer severe pain and other symptoms. Allopurinol interferes with the production of uric acid from hypoxanthine and lowers the uric acid levels. However, it can also raise the level of hypoxanthine dangerously.* Because the drug has an effect on the day-to-day metabolism of chemicals that lead to uric acid, it has little influence on the acute gouty attack once it has occurred. In such cases, colchicine is the agent of choice.

Rashes and fevers in approximately 3 percent of users comprise the major known side effects. Since the medication has come into common use only in the last few years, other side effects may yet be discovered.

* The *Handbook* views pharmacological agents that interfere with a chain of biochemical events as "metabolic monkey-wrenches." Patients on allopurinol have had hypoxanthine crystals form in their kidneys. Well aware of the tragic history of another "metabolic monkey-wrench," MER-29®, the *Handbook* advises caution with allopurinol and at present withholds recommedation for usage.

PART FOUR
Price Lists

With few exceptions, prices cited in the PDL are those current in April 1975, as listed in recent catalogues. Except where it says otherwise, *prices are those the druggist must pay.* In many cases he pays somewhat less than the stated price for generic drugs, either because he buys more than a minimum amount or because he pays cash. While all efforts have been made to ensure against error in listing prices, there is no guarantee. Variation in dates of issuance of catalogues could account for some discrepancies. Companies reserve the right to change prices without notice, and changes may have occurred during preparation of this book.

The druggist's markup is often 67 percent of the wholesale cost to show a profit of 40 percent of the retail price: this is standard retailing practice. Also, pharmacists are entitled to a professional fee for handling prescription items, keeping records, and checking for inadvertent prescription–writing errors by the doctor. At present the professional fee often takes the form of a minimum fee of about two dollars.

Price lists are not otherwise available to the general public. Patients are advised by the *Handbook* to ask their physicians to order and keep handy the catalogues of manufacturers of generic products.

In the lists which follow, drugs, both brand–name and generic, are generally found under the major brand–name product because it is the brand name which the physician will probably prescribe and with which he is most familiar. This arrangement of the list is for the reader's convenience in comparison. Of course, only the manufacturer expressly identified as such is the maker of the brand–name product. The other firms listed market the substance under its generic name or their own house names.

In the interest of saving space one drug manufacturing firm's name has been abbreviated: Interstate Drug Exchange has become IDE throughout. Also, the following definitions may be helpful to the lay reader:

> T.D. = Timed Disintegration
> mg = milligram
> g = gram
> gr = grain

Full names and addresses of cited sources of generic drugs can be found in Appendix C, page 429.

ACETAMINOPHEN, N.F.
See Tylenol®.

ACHROMYCIN®
See Achromycin® V.

ACHROMYCIN® V (Tetracycline Hydrochloride, U.S.P.)
See Lederle under Tetracycline and Tetracycline-Like Products.

ACTIFED®

Burroughs Wellcome (Actifed®)	tablets	$42.75/1000
	syrup	$4.30/pint
Darby (Allerfrin)	tablets	$26.90/1000
	syrup	$2.75/pint
Modern (Allerfrin)	tablets	$26.90/1000
	syrup	$2.75/pint
Wolins	tablets	$38.95/1000
	syrup	$3.90/pint

ACTIFED-C® EXPECTORANT

Burroughs Wellcome (Actifed-C® Expectorant)	syrup	$4.80/pint
Moore (Triacin)		$3.95/pint
Wolins		$4.35/pint

AFRIN® (Oxymetazoline Hydrochloride, N.F.)

Schering		drops	30 cc	$1.40
		spray	15 cc	$1.11

ALDACTAZIDE®

Searle   tablets $114.17/1000 ($53.21/500)

ALDACTONE® (Spironolactone, U.S.P.)

Searle   25 mg tabs $102.85/1000 ($47.32/500)

ALDOMET® (Alpha Methyldopa, U.S.P.)

Merck, Sharp &
  Dohme   250 mg tabs $61.69/1000

ALDORIL®

Merck, Sharp &
  Dohme   15 mg tabs $77.12/1000 ($7.95/100)
              25 mg $87.40/1000 ($9.00/100)

ALLERFRIN
See Darby and Modern under Actifed®.

ALLERNADE
See Modern under Ornade®

ALLOPURINOL
  See Zyloprim®.

ALUDROX®
Wyeth
  Many antacids are less costly and as effective. Ask your pharmacist.

AMBENYL® EXPECTORANT
Parke, Davis $5.09/pint

AMCILL®
See Parke, Davis under Ampicillin, U.S.P., and Ampicillin Syrups.

AMINOPHYLLINE, U.S.P.
Darby   100 mg tabs $1.90/1000

IDE	100 mg	$2.35/1000
Modern	100 mg	$1.55/1000
Searle	100 mg	$10.70/1000
Wolins	100 mg	$2.50/1000

AMINOSALICYLIC ACID, U.S.P. (PAS)

Lilly	0.5 g tabs	$12.40/500
Modern	0.5 g	$5.20/1000
Moore	0.5 g	$7.90/1000
Wolins	0.5 g	$7.85/1000

AMITRIPTYLINE HYDROCHLORIDE, U.S.P.
See Elavil®.

AMPICILLIN, U.S.P.
Brand names:
Ayerst

(Penbritin®)	250 mg caps	$60.81/500	($12.75/100)
	500 mg	$118.37/500	($12.46/50)
Bristol			
(Polycillin®)	250 mg	$143.43/1000	($15.33/100)
	500 mg	$145.74/500	($4.94/16)
Parke, Davis			
(Amcill®)	250 mg	$12.76/100	
Squibb			
(Principen®)	250 mg	$60.67/500	($12.67/100)
	500 mg	$118.95/500	($24.83/100)
Wyeth (Omnipen®)	250 mg	$45.61/500	($9.57/100)

Generics:

Darby	250 mg	$49.00/1000	($24.50/500)
	500 mg	$97.50/1000	(48.75/500)
IDE	250 mg	$48.00/1000	($24.00/500)
	500 mg	$92.00/1000	($46.00/500)
Modern	250 mg	$47.90/1000	
	500 mg	$91.00/1000	
Moore	250 mg	$50.50/1000	
	500 mg	$102.00/1000	
Schein	250 mg	$24.50/500	
	500 mg	$48.50/500	
Veratex	250 mg	$53.40/1000	
	500 mg	$102.60/1000	

| Wolins | 250 mg | $53.90/1000 |
| | 500 mg | $103.30/1000 |

AMPICILLIN SYRUPS
Brand names:
Ayerst (Penbritin®)

$2.60/200 cc (125 mg [200,000 Units]/tsp [5 cc])
($1.47/100 cc)
$4.00/200 cc (250 mg [400,000 Units]/tsp [5 cc])
($2.26/100 cc)

Bristol (Polycillin®)

$3.22/150 cc (125 mg [200,000 Units]/tsp [5 cc])
$4.67/150 cc (250 mg [400,000 Units]/tsp [5 cc])
($3.20/100 cc)

Parke, Davis (Amcill®)

$2.46/150 cc (125 mg [200,000 Units]/tsp [5 cc])
($1.48/80 cc)
$3.78/150 cc (250 mg [400,000 Units]/tsp [5 cc])
($2.26/80 cc)

Squibb (Principen®)

$3.80/150 cc (250 mg [400,000 Units]/tsp [5 cc])
($2.20/80 cc)

Wyeth (Omnipen®)

$1.83/150 cc (125 mg [200,000 Units]/tsp [5 cc])
($1.30/100 cc)
$3.80/150 cc (250 mg[400,000 Units]/tsp [5 cc])
($1.93/100 cc)

Generics:

Darby	$2.15/150 cc (125 mg [200,000 U]/tsp [5 cc])
	$3.30/150 cc (250 mg [400,000 U]/tsp [5 cc])
IDE	$1.55/150 cc (125 mg [200,000 U]/tsp [5 cc])
	$2.25/150 cc (250 mg [400,000 U]/tsp [5 cc])
Modern	$1.80/150 cc (125 mg [200,000 U]/tsp [5 cc])
	$2.85/150 cc (250 mg [400,000 U]/tsp [5 cc])
Moore	$1.50/150 cc (125 mg [200,000 U]/tsp [5 cc])
	($.99/100 cc)
	$2.40/150 cc (250 mg [400,000 U]/tsp [5 cc])
	($1.60/100 cc)
Schein	$1.35/150 cc (125 mg [200,000 U]/tsp [5 cc])
	$2.10/150 cc (250 mg [400,000 U]/tsp [5 cc])
Veratex	$1.60/150 cc (125 mg [200,000 U]/tsp [5 cc])
	$2.40/150 cc (250 mg [400,000 U]/tsp [5 cc])

Wolins $1.65/150 cc (125 mg [200,000 U]/tsp [5 cc])
                     $2.45/150 cc (250 mg [400,000 U]/tsp [5 cc])

ANHYDRON® (cyclothiazide)
See Lilly under "Thiazide" and "Thiazide"-Like Diuretics.

ANTIVERT® * (Meclizine Hydrochloride, U.S.P.)

Roerig (Antivert®)	12.5 mg tabs	$45.98/1000 ($22.99/500)
Darby	12.5 mg	$6.25/1000
	25.0 mg	$10.25/1000
IDE	12.5 mg	$6.00/1000
	25.0 mg	$8.00/1000
Modern	12.5 mg	$5.20/1000
	25.0 mg	$9.40/1000
Moore	12.5 mg	$6.15/1000
	25.0 mg	$10.95/1000
Schein	12.5 mg	$5.50/1000
	25.0 mg	$9.95/1000
Veratex	12.5 mg	$5.80/1000
	25.0 mg	$9.80/1000
Wolins	12.5 mg	$6.95/1000
	25.0 mg	$10.50/1000

APAP
See Modern, Schein, and Veratex under Tylenol®.

APRESOLINE® (Hydralazine Hydrochloride, N.F.)

CIBA (Apresoline®)	25 mg tabs	$41.70/1000 ($4.30/100)
	50 mg	$60.60/1000 ($6.25/100)
Darby	25 mg	$9.00/1000
	50 mg	$15.25/1000
IDE	50 mg	$11.50/1000
Modern	25 mg	$8.25/1000
	50 mg	$14.75/1000
Moore	25 mg	$8.30/1000
	50 mg	$13.95/1000
Schein	25 mg	$8.95/1000
	50 mg	$15.50/1000
Veratex	25 mg	$8.80/1000
	50 mg	$14.90/1000

*According to Volume V, June 1, 1975, FDA Interim Index to Evaluations for NAS-NRC Reviewed Drugs, page 9, Antivert® has been declared "Ineffective."

| Wolins | 25 mg | $9.75/1000 |
| | 50 mg | $15.95/1000 |

ARALEN®
See Chloroquine Phosphate, U.S.P.

ARISTOCORT® (Triamcinolone, U.S.P.)

Lederle (Aristocort®	2 mg tabs	$42.64/500	($8.95/100)
	4 mg	$76.34/500	($15.67/100)
	8 mg	$14.30/50	
	0.1% cream	$1.96/15 g tube	
	0.5%	$4.28/15 g tube	
Darby	2 mg tabs	$39.00/1000	($3.90/100)
	4 mg	$60.00/1000	($6.25/100)
	8 mg	$92.50/1000	($9.25/100)
IDE	4 mg	$42.00/1000	($21.00/500)
Modern	2 mg	$39.00/1000	($3.90/100)
	4 mg	$59.90/1000	
	8 mg	$92.50/1000	($9.25/100)
Moore	4 mg	$71.95/1000	
Schein	4 mg	$45.00/1000	($22.50/500)
Veratex	4 mg	$55.70/1000	
Wolins	4 mg	$62.60/1000	($31.30/500)

ARTANE®
See Lederle under Trihexyphenidyl Hydrochloride, U.S.P.

ASPIRIN, U.S.P.
300 mg tabs; gr V

Available from many manufacturers and/or distributors. Among corporations whose prices are higher than most are Norwich and Bayer. The patient should always buy the least expensive aspirin on the pharmacy shelf. Lilly markets aspirin with a trademarked name, A.S.A.® However, its wholesale price is not grossly out of line with that of non-branded aspirin.

ATARAX® (Hydroxyzine Hydrochloride, N. F.)

Roerig	10 mg tabs	$26.47/500
	25 mg	$42.65/500
	50 mg	$51.99/500
	100 mg	$13.40/100
	syrup	$6.10/pint

ATROMID-S® (clofibrate)
Ayerst   500 mg caps $7.10/100

ATROPINE SULFATE, U.S.P.
Darby	1/100 gr tabs	$1.85/1000
	1/200 gr	$1.90/1000
Lilly	0.4 mg	$.96/100
Modern	1/100 gr	$1.85/1000
	1/200 gr	$1.90/1000
Schein	1/100 gr	$1.85/1000
Veratex	1/200 gr	$2.20/1000
Wolins	1/100 gr	$1.85/1000
	1/200 gr	$1.90/1000

AUREOMYCIN® (Chlortetracycline Hydrochloride, N.F.)
See Lederle under Tetracycline and Tetracycline-Like Products.

AZO GANTRISIN®
Roche (Azo Gantrisin®)	tablets $18.35/500	($3.99/100)
Darby	0.5 mg tabs $15.50/1000	
Modern	tablets $41.00/1000	($20.50/500)
Moore	$17.95/1000	
Schein	$42.00/1000	($21.00/500)
Veratex	$14.60/1000	
Wolins	$18.90/1000	

AZULFIDINE® (salicylazosulfapyridine)
Pharmacia   0.5 g tabs $22.70/500 ($4.79/100)

BELLADONNA TINCTURE, U.S.P.
See Tincture of Belladonna.

BELLERGAL®
Dorsey (Bellergal®)	$57.00/1000 tablets	($5.70/1000)
	T.D tablets $11.10/100	
Schein	tablets $11.95/1000	

BENADRYL® (Diphenhydramine Hydrochloride, U.S.P.)
Parke, Davis (Benadryl®)	25 mg caps	$18.00/1000
	50 mg	$26.75/1000
Darby	25 mg	$5.50/1000
	50 mg	$5.75/1000

IDE	25 mg	$5.00/1000
	50 mg	$5.75/1000
Modern	25 mg	$5.50/1000
	50 mg	$5.75/1000
Moore	25 mg	$6.40/1000
	50 mg	$6.45/1000
Schein	25 mg	$4.50/1000
	50 mg	$4.60/1000
Veratex	25 mg	$5.20/1000
	50 mg	$5.40/1000
Wolins	25 mg	$5.95/1000
	50 mg	$6.90/1000

BENDECTIN®
Merrell-National   tablets $11.00/100

BENDOPA®
See ICN Pharma. under Dopa.

BENEMID® (Probenecid, U.S.P.)
Merck, Sharp & Dohme

(Benemid®)	0.5 g tabs	$53.35/1000 ($5.62/100)
Darby	0.5 g	$42.60/1000
IDE	0.5 g	$39.00/1000
Modern	0.5 g	$42.25/1000
Moore	0.5 g	$41.90/1000
Schein	0.5 g	$42.50/1000
Veratex	0.5 g	$42.80/1000
Wolins	0.5 g	$41.50/1000

BENTYL® (Dicyclomine Hydrochloride, N.F.)
Merrell-National

(Bentyl®)	10 mg caps	$40.60/1000 ($20.85/500)
	20 mg tabs	$57.90/1000 ($6.15/100)
Darby	10 mg caps	$9.75/1000
	20 mg tabs	$8.95/1000
IDE	10 mg caps	$8.50/1000
	20 mg tabs	$7.00/1000
Modern	10 mg caps	$9.75/1000
	20 mg tabs	$8.95/1000
Moore	10 mg caps	$9.95/1000
	20 mg tabs	$7.45/1000

Schein	10 mg caps	$8.95/1000
	20 mg tabs	$7.95/1000
Veratex	10 mg caps	$9.40/1000
	20 mg tabs	$7.90/1000
Wolins	10 mg caps	$9.95/1000
	20 mg tabs	$8.95/1000

BENTYL® WITH PHENOBARBITAL (Dicyclomine Hydrochloride, N.F., with phenobarbital)

Merrell-National (Bentyl® with Phenobarbital)	10 mg caps	$43.80/1000 ($22.55/500)
	20 mg tabs	$30.90/500 ($6.55/100)
Darby	10 mg caps	$9.95/1000
	20 mg tabs	$9.75/1000
IDE	10 mg caps	$8.75/1000
	20 mg tabs	$7.50/1000
Modern	10 mg caps	$9.95/1000
	20 mg tabs	$9.75/1000
Moore	10 mg caps	$10.50/1000
	20 mg tabs	$7.75/1000
Schein	10 mg caps	$9.75/1000
	20 mg tabs	$8.95/1000
Veratex	10 mg caps	$9.40/1000
	20 mg tabs	$9.30/1000
Wolins	10 mg caps	$10.70/1000
	20 mg tabs	$8.95/1000

BENYLIN® EXPECTORANT (diphenhydramine expectorant)

Parke, Davis (Benylin® Expectorant)	$4.00/pint
Darby	$1.65/pint
IDE	$1.75/pint
Modern	$1.40/pint
Moore	$2.05/pint
Schein	$1.85/pint
Veratex	$1.50/pint
Wolins	$2.10/pint

BENZTHIAZIDE, N.F.
See Exna®.

BERUBIGEN®
See Upjohn under Vitamin B₁₂ Injection, U.S.P.

BETALIN 12®
See Lilly under Vitamin B₁₂ Injection, U.S.P.

BIO/DOPA®
See DDR Pharma. under Dopa.

BRISTAMYCIN®
See Bristol under Erythromycin Stearate, U.S.P.

BROMPHENIRAMINE MALEATE, N.F.
See Dimetane®.

BUTABARBITAL (Sodium Butabarbital, U.S.P.)
See Butisol®.

BUTAZOLIDIN® (Phenylbutazone, N.F.)
Geigy   100 mg tabs $73.44/1000

BUTAZOLIDIN® ALKA
Geigy   100 mg caps $82.82/1000

BUTISOL® (Sodium Butabarbital, U.S.P.)

McNeil (Butisol®)	15 mg ¼ gr tabs	$20.00/1000	($2.00/100)
	30 mg ½ gr	$26.00/1000	($2.60/100)
	100 mg 1½ gr	$40.00/1000	($4.00/100)
Darby	¼ gr	$2.25/1000	
	½ gr	$3.20/1000	
IDE	¼ gr	$2.85/1000	
	½ gr	$3.25/1000	
Modern	¼ gr	$2.25/1000	
	½ gr	$3.20/1000	
Moore	¼ gr	$2.25/1000	
	½ gr	$2.95/1000	
Schein	¼ gr	$3.25/1000	
	½ gr	$3.65/1000	
Veratex	¼ gr	$3.00/1000	
	½ gr	$3.40/1000	
	1½ gr	$5.70/1000	

Wolins	¼ gr	$2.95/1000
	½ gr	$3.55/1000
	1½ gr	$3.95/1000

CAFERGOT®
See Sandoz under Ergonovine Maleate, U.S.P.; Ergotamine Tartrate, N.F.

CAMPHORATED TINCTURE OF OPIUM
See Paregoric.

CHLORAL HYDRATE, U.S.P.

Merck, Sharp & Dohme		
(Somnos®)	0.5 g caps	$3.40/100
Squibb (Noctec®)	0.5 g	$4.43/100
Darby	0.5 g	$10.30/1000 ($5.15/500)
IDE	0.5 g	$11.00/1000
Modern	0.5 g	$10.20/1000 ($5.10/500)
Moore	0.5 g	$11.75/1000
Schein	0.5 g	$12.95/1000
Veratex	0.5 g	$11.90/1000
Wolins	0.5 g	$12.75/1000

CHLORDIAZEPOXIDE HYDROCHLORIDE, N.F.
See Librium®.

CHLORMAL
See Darby under Chlor-Trimeton®.

CHLOROQUINE PHOSPHATE, U.S.P.

Moore	250 mg tabs	$93.75/5000	$19.95/1000 ($2.45/100)
Schein	250 mg enteric-coated tabs		$28.50/1000 ($3.00/100)
Wolins	250 mg tabs		$25.75/1000 ($2.85/100)
	250 mg enteric-coated tabs		$27.50/1000 ($2.90/100)

Winthrop (Aralen®) Winthrop has discontinued the distribution of this drug now that its patent has expired and other companies can manufacture it. Winthrop has altered the molecule to Hydroxychloroquine Sulfate, U.S.P., and sells it as Plaquenil® at a high price, but it has no clinical advantage over the original Chloroquine Phosphate, U.S.P. *See Plaquenil®.*

CHLOROTHIAZIDE, N.F.
See Diuril®.

CHLORPHENADE
See Wolins under Ornade®.

CHLORPHENIRAMINE MALEATE, U.S.P.
See Chlor-Trimeton®; Teldrin®.

CHLORPROMAZINE HYDROCHLORIDE, U.S.P.
See Thorazine®.

CHLORTETRACYCLINE
See Lederle under Tetracycline and Tetracycline-Like Products.

CHLORTHALIDONE, U.S.P.
See Hygroton®.

CHLOR-TRIMETON® (Chlorpheniramine Maleate, U.S.P.)
Schering

(Chlor-Trimeton®)	8 mg Repetabs®	$39.65/1000
	12 mg Repetabs®	$54.35/1000
	syrup	$16.83/gallon
Darby	4 mg tabs	$1.50/1000
	8 mg T.D. (Repetabs®)	$4.75/1000
	12 mg T.D. (Repetabs®)	$5.35/1000
	Chlor-Mal syrup	$1.95/pint
IDE	4 mg tabs	$2.00/1000
	8 mg T.D.	$5.25/1000
	12 mg T.D.	$5.75/1000
	Chlorpheniramine syrup	(2 mg/tsp) $1.70/pint
Modern	4 mg	$1.45/1000
	8 mg T.D.	$4.65/1000
	12 mg T.D.	$5.20/1000
	Chlorpheniramine syrup	(2 mg/tsp) $1.70/pint
Moore	4 mg tabs	$1.45/1000
	8 mg Delayed Action	$5.45/1000
	12 mg Delayed Action	$5.65/1000
	syrup	$1.70/pint

Schein	4 mg tabs	$1.20/1000
	8 mg timed tablet	$3.10/1000
	12 mg timed tablet	$3.75/1000
	syrup	$1.85/pint
Veratex	4 mg tabs	$1.40/1000
	8 mg T.D.	$4.80/1000
	12 mg T.D.	$6.00/1000
	syrup	$1.70/pint
Wolins	4 mg tabs	$1.45/1000
	(yellow) 8 mg D.A.	$4.95/1000
	(orange) 12 mg D.A.	$5.35/1000
	syrup	$1.75/pint

CLEOCIN® (clindamycin hydrochloride)

| Upjohn | 75 mg caps | $13.26/100 |
| | 150 mg | $23.49/100 |

CODEINE PHOSPHATE, U.S.P.

The *Handbook* recommends codeine sulfate because codeine phosphate, being more soluble, is more bitter to the taste. Prices for Codeine Phosphate, U.S.P., are practically identical with those of Codeine Sulfate, N.F.

CODEINE SULFATE, N.F.

IDE	15 mg tabs	$38.00/1000 ($19.00/500)
	30 mg	$35.00/1000
Lilly	15 mg	$29.77/1000 ($3.31/100)
	30 mg	$54.15/1000 ($6.77/100)
	60 mg	$102.82/1000 ($11.42/100)
Wolins	30 mg	$46.50/1000
Wyeth	15 mg	$4.36/100
	30 mg	$5.76/100
	60 mg	$9.56/1000

COLACE® (Dioctyl Sodium Sulfosuccinate, N.F. [DSS])

The two most advertised brand names are the most prescribed and command the greatest cost.

Hoechst (Doxinate®)	60 mg gelatin caps	$31.00/1000
Mead Johnson (Colace®)	100 mg gelatin	$76.81/1000
Darby	100 mg tabs	$6.45/1000
IDE	100 mg gelatin caps	$7.75/1000
Modern	100 mg gelatin	$9.55/1000

Moore	100 mg gelatin	$7.80/1000
Schein	100 mg gelatin	$8.95/1000
Veratex	100 mg gelatin	$8.80/1000
Wolins	100 mg gelatin	$7.75/1000

COLCHICINE, U.S.P.

Abbott	0.6 mg tabs	$3.59/100
Darby	0.6 mg	$3.35/1000
IDE	0.6 mg	$3.25/1000
Lilly	0.6 mg	$16.95/1000 ($1.99/100)
Modern	0.6 mg	$3.20/1000
Moore	0.6 mg	$3.75/1000
Schein	0.6 mg	$3.75/1000
Veratex	0.6 mg	$3.30/1000
Wolins	0.6 mg	$3.55/1000

COMBID® SPANSULES® (Prochlorperazine Maleate, U.S.P.)

| Smith Kline & French | | $76.00/500 |

COMPAZINE® (Prochlorperazine Maleate, U.S.P.)

Smith Kline & French	5 mg tabs	$8.35/100
	10 mg	$10.85/100
	Spansules® 10 mg	$7.90/50
	15 mg	$10.25/50
	suppositories 2½ mg	$2.95/12
	5 mg	$3.30/12
	25 mg	$4.15/12

COMPOUND-65
See Darvon® Compound-65.

CONJUGATED ESTROGENS, U.S.P.
See Premarin®.

CORDRAN® (Flurandrenolide, N.F.)

Dista (Cordran®)	0.05% cream $2.18/15 g	$6.60/50 g
IDE	0.025%	$2.00/30 g	$3.05/60 g
	0.05%	$2.00/15 g	$5.70/60 g
Modern	0.05%	$1.90/15 g	$5.60/60 g
Moore	0.05%	$2.02/15 g	$6.11/60 g

Schein	0.05%	$2.20/15 g	$6.50/60 g
Veratex	0.05%	$2.10/15 g	$6.30/60 g
Wolins	0.025%	$2.90/60 g	$10.50/225 g
	0.05%	$2.15/15 g	$6.20/60 g

CORT-DOME®
See Dome under Hydrocortisone Cream, U.S.P.

CORTEF®
See Upjohn under Hydrocortisone Cream, U.S.P.

CORTISPORIN®
| Burroughs Wellcome | ointment ½ oz $2.40 |
| | ophthalmic ⅛ oz $1.15 |

CORTRIL®
See Pfipharmecs under Hydrocortisone Cream, U.S.P.

COUMADIN® (Sodium Warfarin, U.S.P.)
Endo	2.0 mg tabs	$4.30/100
	2.5 mg	$4.30/100
	5.0 mg	$4.80/100
	7.5 mg	$5.80/100
	10.0 mg	$6.95/100

CRYSTODIGIN®
See Lilly under Digitoxin, U.S.P.

CYCLANDELATE
See Cyclospasmol®.

CYCLOSPASMOL® (cyclandelate)
Ives (Cyclospasmol®)	100 mg tabs	$19.95/500	($4.20/100)
	200 mg	$78.46/1000	
Darby	200 mg	$30.90/1000	
IDE	200 mg	$24.00/1000	
Schein	200 mg	$27.50/1000	
Veratex	200 mg	$26.70/1000	
Wolins	200 mg	$31.95/1000	

CYPROHEPTADINE
See Periactin®.

DALMANE® (flurazepam hydrochloride)
| Roche | 15 mg caps $23.20/500 ($4.89/100) |
| | 30 mg $28.10/500 ($5.87/100) |

DARVOCET-N®
Lilly tablets $43.80/1000 ($20.94/500)

DARVOCET-N® 100
Lilly tablets $39.53/500

DARVON® (Propoxyphene Hydrochloride, U.S.P.)
Lilly
(Darvon® Pulvules®)	65 mg caps	$68.80/1000 ($33.35/500)
Darby	65 mg	$13.40/1000
IDE	65 mg	$11.50/1000 ($5.75/500)
Modern	65 mg	$13.50/1000 ($6.75/500)
Moore	65 mg	$14.50/1000
Schein	65 mg	$12.75/1000
Veratex	65 mg	$13.30/1000
Wolins	65 mg	$14.50/1000

DARVON® COMPOUND-65 (propoxyphene compound 65)
Lilly (Darvon®
Compound-65)	Pulvules® $34.77/500
Darby	capsules $13.50/1000
IDE	$11.50/1000 ($5.75/500)
Modern	$13.50/1000
Moore	$15.60/1000
Schein	$17.25/1000
Veratex	$14.70/1000
Wolins	$15.40/1000

DARVON-N® (propoxyphene napsylate)
Lilly tablets $73.80/1000 ($35.85/500)

DARVON-N® WITH A.S.A. (propoxyphene napsylate with aspirin)
Lilly tablets $74.60/1000 ($36.30/500)

DBI-TD® (phenformin hydrochloride)

Geigy   50 mg caps $106.07/1000
                            100 mg $103.41/500   ($21.21/100)

DECADRON® (Dexamethasone Sodium Phosphate, N.F.)
Merck, Sharp & Dohme
  (Decadron®)   0.75 mg tabs $112.07/1000 ($11.55/100)
Darby   0.75 mg $21.40/1000
IDE   0.75 mg $33.00/1000
Modern   0.75 mg $19.90/1000
                  1.5 mg $41.00/1000   ($4.10/100)
Moore   0.75 mg $30.50/1000
Schein   0.75 mg $25.00/1000   ($2.50/100)
Veratex   0.75 mg $16.80/1000
Wolins   0.75 mg $28.50/1000

DECLOMYCIN® (Demethylchlortetracycline Hydrochloride, U.S.P.)
See Lederle under Tetracycline and Tetracycline-Like Products.

DECONADE
See Moore under Ornade®.

DECONGEX
See IDE under Ornade®.

DELTASONE®
See Upjohn under Prednisone, U.S.P.

DEMECLOCYCLINE HYDROCHLORIDE
See Lederle under Tetracycline and Tetracycline-Like Products.

DEMEROL® (Meperidine Hydrochloride, U.S.P.)
Winthrop   50 mg tabs $24.79/500   ($5.45/100)
              100 mg $48.64/500   ($10.29/100)

DEMETHYLCHLORTETRACYCLINE HYDRO-CHLORIDE, U.S.P.
See Lederle under Tetracycline and Tetracycline-Like Products.

DEMULEN-21®
Searle   tablets 6 x 21 $11.58
                     Triopak tabs 10 x 63 $56.10

DEMULEN-28®
Searle
                 tablets 6 x 28 $11.64
                         12 x 18 refills $22.68

DEXAMETHASONE SODIUM PHOSPHATE, N.F.
See Decadron®.

DEXEDRINE®
See Smith Kline & French under Dextroamphetamine Sulfate,
U.S.P.

DEXTROAMPHETAMINE SULFATE, U.S.P.
Smith Kline & French

(Dexedrine®)	5 mg tabs	$22.60/1000
	10 mg Spansules®	$31.90/500
	15 mg Spansules®	$41.00/500
Darby	5 mg tabs	$8.75/500
	10 mg	$11.75/500
IDE	5 mg	$7.00/500
	10 mg	$11.00/500
	15 mg T.D. caps	$10.00/250
Modern	5 mg tabs	$22.85/1000
	5 mg capsules	$3.05/50
	10 mg	$3.80/50
	15 mg	$4.80/50
Schein	5 mg tabs	$15.00/1000
	10 mg	$12.50/500
	10 mg T.D. caps	$10.75/250
	15 mg T.D. caps	$13.25/250
Wolins	5 mg tabs	$17.95/1000
	10 mg	$11.95/500
	10 mg T.D. caps	$9.95/250
	15 mg T.D. caps	$12.95/250

DEXTROMETHORPHAN HYDROBROMIDE, N.F.
See the Prescription Drug List entry.

DIABINESE (Chlorpropamide, U.S.P.)
Pfizer
                   100 mg tabs $23.83/500   ($4.84/100)
                   250 mg $94.38/1000 ($10.23/100)

DICLOXACILLIN (sodium dicloxacillin)
See Dynapen®.

DICYCLOMINE HYDROCHLORIDE, N.F.
See Bentyl®; Bentyl® with Phenobarbital.

DIETHYLPROPION HYDROCHLORIDE, N.F.
See Tenuate®; Tepanil®.

DIETHYLSTILBESTROL, U.S.P. (Stilbestrol)

Darby	1 mg tabs	$4.15/1000	
	5 mg	$5.20/1000	
Lilly	1 mg	$6.94/1000	($.92/100)
	5 mg	$18.45/1000	($2.46/100)
Moore	1 mg	$4.25/1000	
	5 mg	$6.15/1000	
Schein	1 mg	$4.35/1000	
	5 mg	$6.50/1000	
Veratex	1 mg	$3.90/1000	
	5 mg	$5.20/1000	
Wolins	1 mg	$3.95/1000	
	5 mg	$5.20/1000	

DIGITALINE NATIVELLE®
See Savage under Digitoxin, U.S.P.

DIGITOXIN, U.S.P.
Brand Names:

Lilly (Crystodigin®)	0.1 mg tabs	$3.75/500	($1.04/100)
Savage (Digitaline Nativelle®)	0.1 mg	$11.80/1000	($1.65/100)
Wyeth (Purodigin®)	0.1 mg	$3.39/500	($.92/100)

Generics:

IDE	0.1 mg	$2.00/1000
Schein	0.1 mg	$2.00/1000
Wolins	0.1 mg	$1.70/1000

DIGOXIN, U.S.P.

Burroughs Wellcome (Lanoxin®)	0.25 mg tabs	$7.90/1000
Darby	0.25 mg	$4.45/1000
IDE	0.25 mg	$4.35/1000
Modern	0.25 mg	$4.15/1000
Moore	0.25 mg	$4.50/1000

Schein	0.25 mg	$3.35/1000
Veratex	0.25 mg	$4.80/1000
Wolins	0.25 mg	$4.75/1000

DIHISTINE
See Veratex under Novahistine®.

DIHYDROXYPHENYLALANINE
See Dopa.

DILANTIN® (Sodium Diphenylhydantoin, U.S.P.)
Parke, Davis (Dilantin®)	1½ gr caps	$16.45/1000
Darby	1½ gr	$6.50/1000
IDE	1½ gr	$6.95/1000
Modern	1½ gr	$6.40/1000
Moore	1½ gr	$7.90/1000
Schein	1½ gr	$5.25/1000
Veratex	1½ gr	$6.30/1000
Wolins	1½ gr	$6.90/1000

DIMENHYDRINATE, U.S.P.
This is the same active drug as diphenhydramine HCl (Benadryl®). However, no prescription is required to purchase dimenhydrinate as Dramamine®. This is senseless and confusing.

DIMETANE® (Brompheniramine Maleate, N.F.)
Robins
(Dimetane®)	8 mg Extentabs®	$22.10/500	($4.75/100)
	12 mg Extentabs®	$30.90/500	($6.60/100)
	elixir	$3.00/pint	
	expectorant	$4.50/pint	
Darby	4 mg tabs	$8.25/1000	
	8 mg T.D. caps	$17.50/1000	
	12 mg T.D. caps	$18.95/1000	
	expectorant	$2.20/pint	
	expectorant DC	$2.75/pint	
IDE	4 mg tabs	$9.00/1000	
	8 mg T.D. caps	$13.50/1000	
	12 mg T.D. caps	$15.50/1000	
	expectorant	$2.00/pint	
	expectorant DC	$3.25/pint	

Modern		
	4 mg tabs	$8.25/1000
	8 mg T.D. caps	$17.50/1000
	12 mg T.D. caps	$18.95/1000
	expectorant	$2.10/pint
	expectorant DC	$2.70/pint
Moore	4 mg tabs	$9.95/1000
	8 mg T.D. caps	$16.50/1000
	12 mg T.D. caps	$18.25/1000
	elixir	$2.05/pint
	expectorant #1	$2.80/pint
	expectorant DC	$3.75/pint
Schein	4 mg tabs	$8.75/1000
	8 mg T.D. caps	$14.50/1000
	12 mg T.D caps	$16.50/1000
	expectorant	$2.60/pint
	expectorant DC	$3.75/pint
Veratex	4 mg tabs	$8.20/1000
	8 mg T.D. caps	$17.40/1000
	12 mg T.D. caps	$18.70/1000
	expectorant	$2.10/pint
	expectorant DC	$3.20/pint
Wolins	4 mg tabs	$8.90/1000
	8 mg T.D caps	$17.95/1000
	12 mg T.D. caps	$19.90/1000
	elixir	$2.05/pint
	expectorant	$2.35/pint
	expectorant DC	$3.40/pint

DIMETAPP®

Robins (Dimetapp®)	elixir	$4.25/pint
Darby		$1.95/pint
Modern		$1.95/pint
Moore		$2.05/pint
Schein		$2.10/pint
Veratex		$1.90/pint
Wolins		$2.05/pint

DIOCTYL SODIUM SULFOSUCCINATE, N.F. (DSS)
See Colace®; Peri-Colace®.

DIPHENHYDRAMINE HYDROCHLORIDE, U.S.P.
See Benadryl®; Benylin® Expectorant.

DIPHENOXYLATE HYDROCHLORIDE
See Lomotil®.

DIPHENYLHYDANTOIN (Sodium Diphenylhydantoin, U.S.P.)
See Dilantin®.

DIUPRES® *
Merck, Sharp & Dohme	Diupres 250 $48.65/1000
	Diupres 500 $75.37/1000

DIURETIC AP-ES
See Moore under Ser-Ap-Es®.

DIURIL® (Chlorothiazide, N.F.)†
Merck, Sharp & Dohme

(Diuril®)	250 mg tabs	$31.03/1000
	500 mg	$48.45/1000
Darby	250 mg	$20.50/1000
	500 mg	$33.20/1000
IDE	500 mg	$37.50/1000 ($3.75/100)
Modern	250 mg	$20.50/1000
	500 mg	$33.20/1000
Schein	250 mg	$36.50/1000
	500 mg	$57.00/1000
Veratex	250 mg	$20.50/1000
	500 mg	$33.20/1000

DONNAGEL-PG® (kaopectolin with paregoric)
Robins (Donnagel-PG®)	$4.00/pint ($1.60 6 oz.)
Moore	$2.20/pint
Schein	$2.10/pint

DONNATAL®
Robins (Donnatal®)	tablets	$14.50/1000
Darby (Hyosophen)		$1.35/1000
IDE (Spastolate)		$1.50/1000

---

* There are very few generics for Diupres®; to save money, use Hydropres®, whose effect is the same.

† See also Merck, Sharp & Dohme under "Thiazide" and "Thiazide"-Like Diuretics.

Modern (Hyosophen)	$1.25/1000
Moore (Spasmolin)	$1.60/1000
Schein	$1.65/1000
Veratex (antispasmodic tablets)	$1.30/1000
Wolins	$1.50/1000

DOPA (L-Dopa [levodopa]; dihydroxyphenylalanine)
DDR Pharma.

(Bio/Dopa®)	250 mg caps	$3.53/100	
	500 mg	$6.08/100	
Eaton (Dopar®)	100 mg	$2.52/100	
	250 mg	$4.08/100	
	500 mg	$68.40/1000	($7.08/100)
ICN Pharma.			
(Bendopa®)	250 mg	$35.44/1000	($3.94/100)
	500 mg	$61.88/1000	($6.88/100)
Roche (Larodopa®)	250 mg	$16.75/500	($3.60/100)
	500 mg	$30.00/500	($6.25/100)
	100 mg tabs	$2.26/100	
	250 mg tabs	$16.75/500	($3.60/100)
	500 mg tabs	$30.00/500	($6.25/100)
IDE	250 mg caps	$3.40/100	
	500 mg	$6.25/100	

DOPAR®
See Eaton under Dopa.

DORIDEN® (Glutethimide, N.F.)

U.S. Vitamin (Doriden®)	0.5 g tabs	$68.56/1000
Darby	0.5 g	$26.50/1000
IDE	0.5 g	$24.00/1000
Modern	0.5 g	$28.90/1000
Moore	0.5 g	$26.95/1000
Schein	0.5 g	$27.50/1000
Veratex	0.5 g	$26.40/1000
Wolins	0.5 g	$28.95/1000

DORMETHAN®
See Dextromethorphan Hydrobromide, N.F., in the Prescription Drug List pages.

DOXINATE®
See Hoechst under Colace®.

DOXYCYCLINE HYCLATE
See Vibramycin®.

DRAMAMINE® (Dimenhydrinate, U.S.P.)

Searle (Dramamine®)	50 mg tabs	$39.60/1000
Darby	50 mg	$3.60/1000
	syrup	$2.10/pint
IDE	50 mg tabs	$3.00/1000
Modern	50 mg	$3.60/1000
Moore	50 mg	$4.05/1000
	syrup	$2.15/pint
Schein	50 mg tabs	$3.95/1000
Veratex	50 mg	$3.60/1000
	syrup	$2.10/pint
Wolins	50 mg tabs	$3.75/1000

DRIXORAL®
Schering   tablets $4.89/60

DSS
See Colace®.

DYAZIDE® (triamterene)
Smith Kline & French   capsules $68.25/1000

DYNAPEN® (sodium dicloxacillin)

Bristol	125 mg caps	$13.29/100 ($3.28/24)
	250 mg	$23.82/100 ($6.01/24)
suspension 62.5 mg/5 cc	$1.69/80 cc	

ELAVIL® (Amitriptyline Hydrochloride, U.S.P.)

Merck, Sharp & Dohme	10 mg tabs	$40.63/1000
	25 mg	$81.27/1000
	50 mg	$144.36/1000 ($15.21/100)

ELIXOPHYLLIN®
See Prescription Drug List entry.

EMPIRIN® COMPOUND WITH CODEINE PHOS-PHATE
Burroughs Wellcome
   (Empirin® Compound)   ¼ gr tabs $26.10/1000
                      ½ gr $45.45/1000

Darby	¼ gr	$24.30/1000 ($12.15/500)
	½ gr	$41.40/1000
IDE	¼ gr	$19.75/1000
	½ gr	$28.50/1000
Modern	¼ gr	$23.90/1000 ($11.95/500)
	½ gr	$41.00/1000 ($20.50/500)
Schein	¼ gr	$25.50/1000 ($12.75/500)
	½ gr	$44.50/1000 ($22.25/500)
Veratex	¼ gr	$19.80/1000
	½ gr	$38.70/1000
Wolins	¼ gr	$27.50/1000
	½ gr	$46.50/1000

E-MYCIN® (erythromycin base [enteric-coated])*
Upjohn   250 mg tabs $12.98/100

ENDURON® (methyclothiazide)
See Abbott under "Thiazide" and "Thiazide"-Like Diuretics.

EPHEDRINE SULFATE, U.S.P.

Darby	25 mg ⅜ gr caps $7.60/1000
	50 mg ¾ gr $8.95/1000
Lilly	25 mg ⅜ gr $16.80/1000
	50 mg ¾ gr $3.51/100
Modern	25 mg ⅜ gr $7.40/1000
	50 mg ¼ gr $9.20/1000
Moore	25 mg ⅜ gr $7.10/1000
	50 mg ¾ gr $7.90/1000
Shein	25 mg ⅜ gr $7.95/1000
	50 mg ¾ gr $8.75/1000
Wolins	25 mg ⅜ gr $6.85/1000
	50 mg ¾ gr $8.80/1000

EQUAGESIC®
Wyeth   tablets $4.09/50

EQUANIL®
See Wyeth under Meprobamate, U.S.P.

* See also Erythrocin® Stearate; Erythrocin® Stearate
Liquid; Erythromycin Stearate, U.S.P.

ERGONOVINE MALEATE, U.S.P.; ERGOTAMINE TARTRATE, N.F.

Usually mixed with 1 mg of caffeine and sold as Cafergot®. Both substances may be used in tablet form to treat migraine headache. The product most commonly used, and nearly universally available in pharmacies, is Cafergot®. Since only a few tablets are prescribed at a time, little is to be saved by an individual patient shopping for its generic counterpart. Cafergot®, a Sandoz product, costs the pharmacist $12.42 per 100 tablets. Suppositories cost $5.04 per 12. *In using this drug, never exceed the doctor's prescribed dosage. Overdosage is very dangerous, and there is no known antidote!*

Sandoz (Cafergot®)   tablets $118.02/1000 ($12.42/100)
                       suppositories $5.04/12

ERYTHROCIN®
See Erythromycin Stearate, U.S.P., and Erythromycin Ethyl Succinate.

ERYTHROMYCIN BASE
Brand names:

Dista (Ilotycin®)	250 mg tabs enteric-coated	$10.00/100
Robins * (Robimycin®)	250 mg	$10.00/100
Upjohn (E-Mycin®)	250 mg	$12.98/100

Generics:

Abbott	250 mg	$10.00/100
Modern	250 mg	$6.40/100
Moore	250 mg	$6.60/100
Schein	250 mg	$6.50/100
Wolins	250 mg	$7.25/100

ERYTHROMYCIN ETHYL SUCCINATE GRANULES FOR ORAL SUSPENSION
Abbott (Erythrocin® Liquid-200)

                200 mg/5 cc (tsp) $12.98/pint (16 oz)
      (Erythrocin® Liquid-400)

                400 mg/5 cc (tsp) $24.19/pint (16 oz)

---

* Robins has been reported to buy its erythromycin from a generic manufacturer, Mylan Laboratories of Morgantown, West Virginia; *Competitive Problems in the Drug Industry*, Part 24, p. 10,165.

Dista (Ilosone®)

liquid	125 mg/5 cc (tsp)	$1.82/60 cc	
		$12.90/pint (16 oz)	
liquid	250 mg/5 cc (tsp)	$3.27/60 cc	
		$23.22/pint (16 oz)	

ERYTHROMYCIN STEARATE, U.S.P.

Brand names:

Abbott

(Erythrocin® Stearate)	125 mg tabs	$8.98/100 ($4.49/50)
	250	$14.99/100
	500	$19.50/100
Bristol (Bristamycin®)	250	$12.04/100
Smith Kline & French *		
(SK-Erythromycin®)	250	$10.15/100
	500	$20.30/100
Squibb * (Ethril®)	250	$9.95/100
(Ethril®)	500	$9.45/100

Generics:

Darby	250	$5.95/100
Modern	250	$6.25/100
	500	$12.75/100
Moore	250	$6.90/100
	500	$13.25/100
Parke, Davis *	250	$13.60/100
Pfizer *	250	$8.90/100
	500	$17.80/100
Schein	250	$6.45/100
	500	$12.85/100
Wolins	250	$6.95/100
	500	$14.95/100
Wyeth *	250	$8.95/100
	500	$17.50/100

ESIDRIX® (Hydrochlorothiazide, U.S.P.)

See CIBA under "Thiazide" and "Thiazide"-Like Diuretics.

Because of the expense of Esidrix®, the *Handbook* recom-

* These firms allegedly purchase their erythromycin from a generic manufacturer, Mylan Laboratories of Morgantown, West Virginia; *Competitive Problems in the Drug Industry,* Part 24, pp. 10165, 10169, and 10171.

mends generic hydrochlorothiazide in its stead; *see Hydro-chlorothiazide, U.S.P., for generic drug company prices.*

ESTROGENS
See under Premarin®; Diethylstilbestrol, U.S.P.

ETHAMBUTOL
See Myambutol®.

ETHCHLORVYNOL
See Placidyl®.

ETHRIL®
See Squibb under Erythromycin Stearate, U.S.P.

ETRAFON®

Schering		
	2-10 tablets	$8.40/100
	2-25	$10.50/100
	4-10	$9.30/100
	4-25	$11.40/100

EXNA® (Benzthiazide, N.F.)*

Robins (Exna®)	50 mg tabs	$65.00/1000 ($6.50/100)
Darby	50 mg	$19.00/1000 ($9.50/500)
IDE	50 mg	$16.00/1000
Modern	50 mg	$18.85/1000
Moore	50 mg	$19.65/1000
Schein	50 mg	$18.95/1000
Veratex	50 mg	$18.90/1000
Wolins	50 mg	$18.95/1000

FEOSOL® (Ferrous Sulfate, U.S.P.)
See Smith Kline & French under Ferrous Sulfate, U.S.P.

FERGON®
See Ferrous Gluconate, N.F.

FERO-GRADUMET®
See Abbott under Ferrous Sulfate, U.S.P.

* See also Robins under "Thiazide" and "Thiazide"-Like Diuretics.

FERRO-SEQUELS®
See Lederle under Ferrous Sulfate, U.S.P.

FERROUS GLUCONATE, N.F.
The *Handbook* recommends the use of ferrous sulfate over either ferrous gluconate or Fergon®

FERROUS SULFATE, U.S.P.
Brand names:
Abbott (Fero-
　Gradumet®)
	525 mg T.D. caps *	$51.40/1000	($5.14/100)

Lederle (Ferro-
　Sequels®) 150 mg T.D. caps *†　$43.74/1000
Smith Kline &
　French　　150 mg T.D. caps *　$46.50/100 ($23.25/500)
(Peosol®)　5 gr sugar-coated tabs $12.00/1000
Generics:

Darby	150 mg T.D. caps *	$7.50/1000
	5 gr sugar-coated tabs	$1.95/1000
IDE	150 mg T.D. caps *	$6.00/1000
	5 gr sugar-coated tabs	$2.25/1000
Lilly	5 gr tabs	$6.70/1000
Modern	150 mg T.D. caps *	$6.60/1000
	5 gr sugar-coated tabs	$1.90/1000
Moore	150 mg T.D. caps *	$7.50/1000
	5 gr sugar-coated tabs	$1.95/1000
Parke, Davis	5 gr tabs	$8.38/1000
Schein	150 mg T.D. caps *	$8.00/1000
	5 gr sugar-coated tabs	$2.35/1000
Veratex	150 mg T.D. caps *	$6.80/1000
	5 gr sugar-coated tabs	$2.80/1000
Wolins	150 mg T.D. caps *	$7.75/1000
	5 gr sugar-coated tabs	$2.00/1000

FIORINAL®
Sandoz (Fiorinal®)　　　　tablets $38.22/1000
　　　　　　　　　　　　capsules $23.64/500　($4.98/100)

* Placing ferrous sulfate in a "timed disintegration" dosage form is preposterous. Iron can be absorbed into the bloodstream only in the first few inches of the small intestine.

† Each contains 150 mg of ferrous fumarate, plus 100 mg of dioctyl sodium sulfosuccinate.

Darby (Isollyl)	tablets $6.95/1000	
IDE (Idenal)	$6.00/1000	
Modern (Isollyl)	$6.75/1000	
Schein	$31.40/1000	
Veratex	$35.60/1000	
	capsules $45.00/1000	($4.50/100)
Wolins	tablets $32.75/1000	
	capsules $38.40/1000	($19.20/500)

FIORINAL® WITH CODEINE *
Sandoz   capsules with ¼ gr (15 mg) codeine $8.38/100
              capsules with ½ gr (30 mg) codeine $10.94/100

FLAGYL® ORAL (Metronidazole, U.S.P.)
Searle   250 mg tabs $143.34/1000
           (vaginal) 500 mg $3.38/10

FLUOCINOLONE ACETONIDE
See Synalar®.

FLURANDRENOLIDE, N.F.
See Cordran®.

FLURAZEPAM HYDROCHLORIDE
See Dalmane®.

FULVICIN-U/F®
See Griseofulvin, U.S.P.

FURADANTIN®
See Nitrofurantoin, U.S.P.

FUROSEMIDE, U.S.P.
See Lasix®.

GANTANOL® (sulfamethoxazole)
Roche   0.5 g tabs $29.30/500

GANTRISIN® (Sulfisoxazole, U.S.P.)
Roche (Gantrisin®)   0.5 g tabs $25.60/1000

* Generic companies make a Fiorinal® equivalent (see above), but none make it in combination with codeine.

Darby	0.5 g	$11.50/1000
IDE (Sofrazole)	0.5 g	$11.50/1000
Modern	0.5 g	$11.20/1000
Schein	0.5 g	$8.95/1000
Veratex	0.5 g	$11.20/1000
Wolins	0.5 g	$12.95/1000

GARAMYCIN® (Gentamicin Sulfate, U.S.P.)

Schering

	0.1% cream 15 g tube	$1.53
	0.1% ointment 15 g tube	$1.53
0.3% ophthalmic solution	5 cc	$1.40

GLUTETHIMIDE, N.F.
See Doriden®.

GRIFULVIN V®
See Griseofulvin, U.S.P.

GRISACTIN®
See Griseofulvin, U.S.P.

GRISEOFULVIN, U.S.P.

Ayerst (Grisactin®)	125 mg tabs	$29.54/500	($6.56/100)
	250 mg	$59.00/500	($12.60/100)
	500 mg	$14.69/60	
McNeil (Grifulvin V®)	125 mg	$30.00/500	($6.20/100)
	250 mg	$50.30/500	($12.10/100)
	500 mg	$111.40/500	($22.90/100)
Schering (Fulvicin-U/F®)	125 mg	$3.67/60	
	250 mg	$28.28/250	($7.14/60)
	500 mg	$53.81/250	($13.59/60)

GUANETHIDINE SULFATE, U.S.P.
See Ismelin®.

H-H-R
See Schein under Ser-Ap-Es®.

HYDERGINE®

| Sandoz | 0.5 mg tabs $85.50/1000 |

HYDRALAZINE HYDROCHLORIDE, N.F.
See Apresoline®.

HYDROCHLOROTHIAZIDE, U.S.P.
See Hydrodiuril®; Hydropres®; and CIBA and Merck, Sharp & Dohme under "Thiazide" and "Thiazide"-Like Diuretics.

HYDROCORTISONE CREAM (or Ointment), U.S.P.
Brand names:
Dome (Cort-Dome®)

30 g	(1 oz)	¼%	$1.71/tube
120 g	(4 oz)	¼%	$4.31/jar
1 lb	(16 oz)	¼%	$14.38/jar
30 g	(1 oz)	½%	$2.90/tube
120 g	(4 oz)	½%	$10.10/jar
1 lb	(16 oz)	½%	$38.86/jar
30 g	(1 oz)	1%	$5.19/tube
120 g	(4 oz)	1%	$17.89/jar

Pfipharmecs (Cortril®)

15 g	(½ oz)	1%	$1.34/tube

Upjohn (Cortef®)

5 g	1%	$1.31/tube
20 g	1%	$3.82/tube
5 g	2½%	$2.57/tube
20 g	2½%	$7.59/tube

Generics:

Darby	30 g	(1 oz)	¼%	$.60/tube	($5.50/10 tubes)
	120 g	(4 oz)	¼%	$1.75/jar	($16.90/10 jars)
	30 g	(1 oz)	½%	$.80/tube	($7.50/10 tubes)
	120 g	(4 oz)	½%	$2.15/jar	($20.50/10 jars)
	1 lb	(16 oz)	1%	$13.25/jar	
Modern	30 g	(1 oz)	¼%	$.55/tube	($5.00/10 tubes)
	120 g	(4 oz)	¼%	$1.50/jar	($14.50/10 jars)
	30 g	(1 oz)	½%	$.75/tube	($6.50/10 tubes)
	120 g	(4 oz)	½%	$2.10/jar	($20.00/10 jars)
Moore	30 g	(1 oz)	¼%	$.53/tube	($6.15/12 tubes)
	120 g	(4 oz)	¼%	$1.40/jar	($4.50/pound jar)
	30 g	(1 oz)	½%	$.76/tube	($7.90/12 tubes)
	120 g	(4 oz)	½%	$2.10/jar	($6.30/pound jar)
	20 g		1%	$.81/tube	($9.20/12 tubes)
	1 lb	(16 oz)	1%	$9.75/jar	

Schein	30 g (1 oz) ¼ %	$.55/tube ($5.95/12 tubes)
	1 lb (16 oz) ¼ %	$4.50/jar
	30 g (1 oz) ½ %	$.80/tube ($8.95/12 tubes)
	1 lb (16 oz) ½ %	$7.25/jar
	20 g 1%	$.75/tube ($8.75/12 tubes)
	120 g (4 oz) 1%	$3.50/jar
	1 lb (16 oz) 1%	$9.95/jar
	20 g 2½ %	$1.85/tube ($21.50/12 tubes)
Wolins	30 g 1 oz) ¼ %	$.59/tube ($6.00/12 tubes)
	120 g (4 oz) ¼ %	$1.39/jar
	1 lb (16 oz) ¼ %	$3.95/jar
	30 g (1 oz ½ %	$.89/tube ($9.60/12 tubes)
	120 g (4 oz) ½ %	$1.95/jar
	1 lb (16 oz) ½ %	$7.95/jar
	5 g 1%	.$.59/tube ($6.00/12 tubes)
	20 g 1%	$.95/tube ($10.56/12 tubes)
	120 g (4 oz) 1%	$3.25/jar
	1 lb (16 oz) 1%	$11.95/jar
	20 g 2½ %	$1.79/tube ($20.40/12 tubes)
	1 lb (16 oz) 2½ %	$21.95/jar

HYDRODIURIL® (Hydrochlorothiazide, U.S.P.)
Brand names:

Abbott (Oretic®)	25 mg tabs	$26.15/1000
	50 mg	$41.18/1000
CIBA (Esidrix®)	25 mg	$36.50/1000
	50 mg	$57.00/1000
Merck, Sharp & Dohme		
(Hydrodiuril®)	25 mg	$31.03/1000
Generics:	50 mg	$48.45/1000
Darby	25 mg	$5.90/1000
	50 mg	$7.30/1000
IDE	25 mg	$5.75/1000
	50 mg	$6.50/1000
Modern	25 mg	$5.60/1000
	50 mg	$6.55/1000
Moore	25 mg	$6.75/1000
	50 mg	$7.50/1000
Schein	25 mg	$5.95/1000
	50 mg	$8.50/1000
Veratex	25 mg	$5.50/1000
	50 mg	$6.70/1000

| Wolins | 25 mg | $6.50/1000 |
| | 50 mg | $8.95/1000 |

HYDROMOX® (quinethazone)
See Lederle under "Thiazide" and "Thiazide"-Like Diuretics.

HYDROPINE
See Wolins under Hydropres®.

HYDROPRES® (Hydrochlorothiazide, U.S.P., with Reserpine, U.S.P.)
Merck, Sharp & Dohme

(Hydropres®)		25 mg tabs	$48.65/1000
		50 mg	$75.37/1000
Darby			
(Hydroserpine)	#1	25 mg	$7.45/1000
	#2	50 mg	$10.50/1000
IDE (Hydro-Reserpine)		25 mg	$8.00/1000
		50 mg	$12.00/1000
Modern (Hydroserpine)		25 mg	$6.95/1000
		50 mg	$9.50/1000
Moore		25 mg	$8.20/1000
		50 mg	$9.25/1000
Schein		25 mg	$6.45/1000
		50 mg	$11.95/1000
Veratex (Hydroserp			
Tabs)		25 mg	$7.50/1000
		50 mg	$11.90/1000
Wolins (Hydropine)	#1	25 mg	$8.90/1000
	#2	50 mg	$12.95/1000

HYDRO-RESERPINE
See IDE under Hydropres®.

HYDROSERP
See Veratex under Hydropres®.

HYDROSERPINE
See Darby and Modern under Hydropres®.

HYDROXYCHLOROQUINE PHOSPHATE, U.S.P.
See Plaquenil®; Chloroquine Phosphate, U.S.P.

HYDROXYZINE HYDROCHLORIDE, N.F.
See Atarax®; Vistaril®.

HYGROTON® (Chlorthalidone, U.S.P.)*
Geigy (Hygroton®)   50 mg $68.25/1000
                          100 mg $83.50/1000
U.S. Vitamin
   (Hygroton®)   50 mg tabs $73.19/1000
                          100 mg $89.15/1000

HYOSOPHEN
See Darby and Modern under Donnatal®.

IDENAL
See IDE under Fiorinal®.

ILETIN®
See Lilly under Insulin Injection, U.S.P.

ILOSONE® (Erythromycin Estolate, N.F.)
Dista   125 mg chewable tabs $6.36/50
               125 mg caps $11.26/100
               250 mg caps $102.75/500 ($20.79/100)
               500 mg tabs $40.23/100 ($19.74/50)
               drops 10 cc $1.16
See also Erythromycin Ethyl Succinate Granules for Oral Suspension.

ILOTYCIN®
See Dista under Erythromycin Base.

IMIPRAMINE HYDROCHLORIDE, N.F.
See Tofranil®.

INDERAL (Propranolol Hydrochloride, U.S.P.)
Ayerst   10 mg tabs $34.87/1000
                      40 mg $58.76/1000

INDOCIN® (Indomethacin, N.F.)
Merck, Sharp & Dohme 25 mg caps $80.66/1000
                     50 mg $13.31/100

   * See also U.S. Vitamin under "Thiazide" and "Thiazide"-Like Diuretics.

INH
See Isoniazid, U.S.P.

INSULIN INJECTION, U.S.P.

Lilly (Iletin®)	10 cc Regular Insulin	U 40	$.92
		U 80	$1.82
		U 100	$2.27
	10 cc Lente Insulin	U 40	$1.09
		U 80	$2.08
		U 100	$2.59
	10 cc NPH Insulin	U 40	$1.09
		U 80	$2.08
		U 100	$2.59
	10 cc Protamine Zinc Insulin (PZI)	U 40	$1.09
		U 80	$2.08
		U 100	$2.59
	10 cc Semilente Insulin	U 40	$1.09
		U 80	$2.08
		U 100	$2.59
	10 cc Ultralente Insulin	U 40	$1.09
		U 80	$2.08
		U 100	$2.59
Squibb	10 cc Regular Insulin	U 40	$.97
		U 80	$1.90
		U 100	$2.39
	10 cc Lente Insulin	U 40	$1.14
		U 80	$2.18
		U 100	$2.73
	10 cc NPH Insulin	U 40	$1.14
		U 80	$2.18
		U 10	$2.73
	10 cc Protamine Zinc Insulin (PZI)	U 40	$1.14
		U 80	$2.18
		U 100	$2.73
	10 cc Semilente Insulin	U 40	$1.14
		U 80	$2.18
		U 100	$2.73
	10 cc Ultralente Insulin	U 40	$1.14
		U 80	$2.18
		U 100	$2.73

10 cc Globin Insulin
with Zinc   U 40 $1.31
              U 80 $2.51
              U 100 $3.11

IODO-HC
See Veratex and Wolins under Vioform®-Hydrocortisone.

IONAMIN® (phentermine)

Pennwalt (Ionamin®)	15 mg caps	$12.45/100
	30 mg	$13.73/100
IDE	8 mg T.D. tabs	$1.10/100
Modern	8 mg tabs	$7.75/1000
	15 mg T.D. caps	$14.90/1000
	30 mg T.D. caps	$20.50/1000
Moore	30 mg T.D. caps	$21.75/1000
Schein	8 mg tabs	$7.75/1000
Veratex	8 mg	$7.60/1000
Wolins	8 mg	$8.25/1000
	30 mg T.D. caps	$24.50/1000

ISMELIN® (Guanethidine Sulfate, U.S.P.)

CIBA	10 mg tabs	$85.35/1000	($8.80/100)
	25 mg	$119.80/1000	($12.35/100)

ISOLLYL
See Darby and Modern under Fiorinal®.

ISONIAZID, U.S.P. (INH, or Isonicotinic Acid Hydrazide)

Parke, Davis (Niconyl®)	100 mg tabs	$7.98/1000	($.99/100)
Darby	50 mg	$2.65/1000	
	100 mg	$2.70/1000	
	300 mg	$6.40/1000	
IDE	100 mg	$3.25/1000	
	300 mg	$6.00/1000	
Lilly	100 mg	$8.99/1000	($1.12/100)
	300 mg	$2.55/100	
Modern (as INH)	100 mg	$2.70/1000	
Moore (as INH)	100 mg	$3.10/1000	
	300 mg	$7.50/1000	

Schein	50 mg	$2.50/1000
	100 mg	$3.45/1000
	300 mg	$6.95/1000
Veratex	100 mg	$2.60/1000
	300 mg	$6.30/1000
Wolins	50 mg	$2.50/1000
	100 mg	$3.45/1000
	300 mg	$6.85/1000

ISONICOTINIC ACID HYDRAZIDE
See Isoniazid, U.S.P.

ISOPTO CARPINE® (Pilocarpine Hydrochloride, U.S.P.)

Alcon (Isopto Carpine®)	15 cc Drop Tainer 1%	$1.70
	2%	$1.80
	3%	$1.90
	4%	$2.00
	6%	$2.40
Darby (Pilocarpine)	ophthalmic 15 cc 1%	$.80
	2%	$.85
	3%	$.90
	4%	$1.00
	6%	$1.10
IDE (Pilocarpine)	ophthalmic 15 cc 1%	$.85
	2%	$.85
	4%	$1.00
Modern (Pilocarpine HCl)	15 cc 1%	$.80
	2%	$.85
	3%	$.90
	4%	$1.00
	6%	$1.10
Moore (Pilocarpine HCl)	15 cc 1%	$.71
	2%	$.78
	3%	$.90
	4%	$.92
	6%	$1.10
Schein (Pilocarpine HCl)	15 cc 1%	$.80
	2%	$.85
	3%	$1.00
	4%	$1.10
	6%	$1.20

Veratex (Pilocarpine)	15 cc 1%	$.80
	2%	$.90
	3%	$1.00
	4%	$1.00
	6%	$1.20
Wolins	15 cc 1%	$.80
	2%	$.90
	3%	$1.05
	4%	$1.05
	6%	$1.30

ISORDIL® (isosorbide dinitrate)
Ives-Cameron

(Isordil®)	5 mg tabs	$37.20/1000 ($18.91/500)
	10 mg	$42.86/1000 ($21.66/500)
	40 mg T.D. tabs	$95.81/1000 ($48.65/500)
	40 mg T.D. caps	$10.25/100
	2.5 mg sublingual	$3.70/100
	5 mg	$18.91/500 ($3.97/100)
Darby	5 mg tabs	$9.95/1000
	10 mg	$14.75/1000
	2.5 mg sublingual	$14.50/1000
IDE	5 mg tabs	$8.50/1000
	10 mg	$12.00/1000
	40 mg timed caps	$25.00/1000
	2.5 mg sublingual	$11.50/1000
	5 mg	$13.00/1000
Modern	5 mg	$9.75/1000
	10 mg	$13.25/1000
Moore	5 mg	$8.95/1000
	10 mg	$13.95/1000
Schein	5 mg	$9.75/1000
	10 mg	$14.75/1000
Veratex	5 mg	$9.50/1000
	10 mg	$14.90/1000
Wolins	5 mg	$9.95/1000
	10 mg	$14.90/1000
	40 mg T.D. caps	$37.80/1000 ($18.90/500)
	2.5 mg sublingual	$13.95/1000
	5 mg	$15.95/1000

ISOSORBIDE DINITRATE
See Isordil®.

ISOXSUPRINE HYDROCHLORIDE
See Vasodilan®.

ISUPREL® MISTOMETER® AEROSOL
VIAL (Isoproterenol Inhalation, U.S.P.)
Winthrop   15 cc vial 1:40 $3.00

KAON® (potassium gluconate)

Warren-Teed (Kaon®)	tablets $24.00/500	($4.93/100)
	elixir $4.96/pint	
Darby	5 mEq SC Tabs $13.25/1000	
IDE	tablets $12.00/1000	($6.00/500)
	elixir $2.25/pint	
Modern	tablets $27.00/1000	($13.50/500)
	elixir $4.40/pint	
Moore	tablets $34.82/1000	($17.41/500)
	elixir $2.70/pint	
Schein	tablets $12.50/1000	
	elixir $2.65/pint	
Veratex	elixir $2.50/pint	
Wolins	tablets $7.75/1000	
	elixir $2.95/pint	

KAOPECTOLIN WITH PAREGORIC
See Donnagel-PG®.

KEFLEX® (cephalexin monohydrate)

Lilly	250 mg caps	$28.42/100
	500 mg	$55.83/100
	125 mg/cc for oral susp. 100 cc	$3.30
	250 mg/cc for oral susp. 100 cc	$6.21
	125 mg/cc for oral susp. 200 cc	$6.54
	250 mg/cc for oral susp. 200 cc	$12.30

KENALOG® (triamcinolone)

Squibb	creams 0.025% $1.20/15 g
	0.1% $1.96/15 g; $4.60/60 g
	0.5% $5.25/20 g

   Kenalog® is also available as an *ointment* in the same concentrations at practically identical prices. (Note that Kenalog® is the same drug as Aristocort®.)

LANOXIN®
See Burroughs Wellcome under Digoxin, U.S.P.

LARODOPA®
See Roche under Dopa.

LASIX® (furosemide)
See Hoechst under "Thiazide" and "Thiazide"-Like Diuretics.

L-DOPA
See Dopa.

LEVODOPA
See Dopa.

LEVOTHYROXINE, SODIUM, U.S.P.
See Synthroid®.

LIBRAX®
Roche   capsules $30.95/500 ($6.44/100)

LIBRIUM® * **(Chlordiazepoxide Hydrochloride, N.F.)**
Roche   5 mg caps $22.25/500
                        10 mg $29.25/500
                        25 mg $42.50/500

LINCOCIN® (lincomycin hydrochloride)
Upjohn   500 mg caps $28.17/100
  Essentially the same as Cleocin®.

LOMOTIL® (diphenoxylate hydrochloride)
Searle   2.5 mg tabs $175.57/2500 ($39.00/500)

MAALOX®
Rorer
See buying tips in the Prescription Drug List entry.

MACRODANTIN®
See Eaton under Nitrofurantoin, U.S.P.

* Although the patent on Librium® is generally believed to
have expired, production of generic chlordiazepoxide has been
delayed.

MAGNESIUM HYDROXIDE
See Maalox® in the Prescription Drug List.

MARAX®
Roerig   syrup $4.26 pint
            tablets $25.28/500

MECLIZINE HYDROCHLORIDE, U.S.P.
See Antivert®.

MEDROL® (Methylprednisolone, N.F.)
Upjohn		
	2 mg tabs	$9.09/100
	4 mg	$17.22/100
	16 mg	$25.20/50
	4 mg caps	$17.59/100

MELLARIL® (thioridazine)
Sandoz		
	10 mg tabs	$66.72/1000
	25 mg	$90.66/1000
	50 mg	$98.64/1000
	100 mg	$116.28/1000
	200 mg	$175.02/1000
	concentrate 30 mg/cc 4 oz	$5.22

MEPROBAMATE, U.S.P.
Wallace (Miltown®)	200 mg tabs	$5.20/100	
	400 mg	$61.20/1000	($31.20/500)
Wyeth (Equanil®)	200 mg	$46.80/1000	($4.80/100)
	400 mg	$58.00/1000	($29.50/100)
	400 mg caps	$5.25/50	
Darby	200 mg tabs	$4.45/1000	
	400 mg	$4.75/1000	
IDE	400 mg	$4.90/1000	
Modern	400 mg	$4.50/1000	
Moore	200 mg	$4.75/1000	
	400 mg	$5.05/1000	
Schein	200 mg	$4.85/1000	
	400 mg	$4.95/1000	
Veratex	200 mg	$4.40/1000	
	400 mg	$4.60/1000	
Wolins	200 mg	$4.95/1000	
	400 mg	$5.95/1000	

METAHYDRIN® (trichlormethiazide)
See Lakeside under "Thiazide" and "Thiazide"-Like Diuretics.

METHAQUALONE (QUAALUDE®)
   The *Handbook* does not recommend use of this medication.
See the Prescription Drug List under Quaalude®.
Rorer   100 mg tabs $20.00/500 ($4.20/100)
                        300 mg $29.20/500 ($6.15/100)

METHYCLOTHIAZIDE
See Abbott under "Thiazide" and "Thiazide"-Like Diuretics.

METHYLDOPA, U.S.P.
See Aldomet®.

METHYLPHENIDATE HYDROCHLORIDE, N.F.
See Ritalin®.

METHYLPREDNISOLONE, N.F.
See Medrol®.

METHYPRYLON, N.F.
See Noludar®.

METICORTEN®
See Schering under Prednisone, U.S.P.

METRONIDAZOLE, U.S.P.
See Flagyl®.

MICRONOR®
*See Oral Contraceptives chart in the Prescription Drug List
pages.*

MILTOWN®
See Wallace under Meprobamate, U.S.P.

MINOCIN® (minocycline hydrochloride)
See Lederle under Tetracycline and Tetracycline-Like Products.

MYAMBUTOL® (ethambutol)
Lederle   100 mg tabs $49.14/1000 ($5.24/100)
                        400 mg $159.71/1000 ($20.25/100)

MYCOLOG®
Squibb
creams 15 g $3.20
30 g $5.89
60 g $10.24
ointments 15 g $3.20
30 g $5.89
60 g $10.24

MYCOSTATIN® (Nystatin, U.S.P.)
Squibb
cream $1.65/15 g
ointment $1.65/15 g
tablets $10.14/100
vaginal tablets $3.40/30

MYLANTA®
Stuart
tablets $2.25/100
liquid $2.18/10 oz

MYSTECLIN-F®
Squibb
250 mg caps $19.98/100
syrup $1.95/60 cc

NALDECON®
Bristol (Naldecon®)
syrup $4.89/pint
T.D. tablets $39.85/500 ($8.21/100)
IDE (Nechlorin)
T.D. tabs $9.00/500
syrup $2.35/pint
Schein
(Quadra-Hist) tablets $18.95/1000
Veratex
T.D. tabs $19.50/1000
Wolins (Phendecon)
T.D. tabs $11.50/500

NAQUA® (trichlormethiazide)
See Schering under "Thiazide" and "Thiazide"-Like Diuretics.

NATURETIN® (bendroflumethiazide)
See Squibb under "Thiazide" and "Thiazide"-Like Diuretics.

NECHLORIN
See IDE under Naldecon®.

NEMBUTAL® (Sodium Pentobarbital, U.S.P.)
Abbott (Nembutal®)
50 mg caps $16.10/1000
100 mg $23.73/1000

Darby	100 mg	$9.50/1000
IDE	50 mg	$5.90/1000
	100 mg	$10.50/1000
Modern	100 mg	$9.50/1000
Schein	50 mg	$7.50/1000
	100 mg	$10.95/1000
Wolins	50 mg	$7.95/1000
	100 mg	$10.50/1000

NEODECADRON®
Merck, Sharp & Dohme   0.1% cream $1.75/15 g tube
$2.62/30 g tube

NEOSPORIN®
Burroughs Wellcome

(Neosporin®)	ointments	15 g (½ oz)	$1.83
		30 g (1 oz)	$3.00
	ophthalmic ointment 3.75 g (⅛ oz)		$.70
IDE	ointments (½ oz)		$.60
	(1 oz)		$.75
	ophthalmic ointment (⅛ oz)		$.60
Modern	ointments 15 g (½ oz)		$.60
	30 g (1 oz)		$.90
Moore	ointments (½ oz)		$.60
	(1 oz)		$.80
	ophthalmic ointment (⅛ oz)		$.65
Schein	ointments (½ oz)		$.55
	(1 oz)		$.75
Veratex	ointments (½ oz)		$.60
	(1 oz)		$.90
	ophthalmic ointment (⅛ oz)		$.60
Wolins	ointments (½ oz)		$.59
	(1 oz)		$.85
	ophthalmic ointment (⅛ oz)		$.60

NEO-SYNEPHRINE®   (Phenylephrine   Hydrochloride, U.S.P.)
See Neo-Synephrine® in the Prescription Drug List pages.

NICOBID®
See Armour under Nicotinic Acid.

NICOTINIC ACID *

Armour		
(Nicobid®)	125 mg T.D. caps	$46.20/1000
	250 mg T.D. caps	$59.70/1000
Abbott	50 mg tabs	$3.74/1000
	100 mg	$5.11/1000
Darby	50 mg tabs	$2.50/1000
	100 mg	$3.35/1000
	500 mg	$7.95/1000
IDE	100 mg	$2.90/1000
	400 mg T.D. caps	$4.00/1000
Modern	50 mg tabs	$1.75/1000
	100 mg	$2.60/1000
	500 mg	$6.50/1000
Moore	50 mg	$1.90/1000
	100 mg	$2.25/1000
	500 mg	$8.75/1000
Parke, Davis	50 mg	$3.96/1000
	100 mg	$5.47/1000
Schein	250 mg T.D. caps	$13.95/1000
Squibb	50 mg tabs	$3.99/1000
	100 mg	$5.41/1000
Upjohn	50 mg	$4.07/1000
Veratex	50 mg tabs	$2.00/1000
	100 mg	$2.50/1000
	500 mg	$6.80/1000
Wolins	25 mg	$1.65/1000
	50 mg	$2.35/1000
	100 mg	$2.50/1000
	500 mg	$6.80/1000

NITROFURANTOIN, U.S.P.

Eaton (Macro-		
dantin®) †	50 mg caps	$112.00/1000 ($13.50/100)
	100 mg	$224.00/1000 ($27.00/100)
Darby	50 mg tabs	$5.75/1000
	100 mg	$8.50/1000
IDE	50 mg	$5.50/1000
	100 mg	$8.25/1000
Modern	50 mg	$5.25/1000
	100 mg	$7.65/1000

* Nicotinic acid is often called niacin.

† Eaton changed the crystal size, put the crystal in a capsule, and increased the price a bit.

Moore	50 mg	$9.50/1000
	100 mg	$18.95/1000
Schein	50 mg	$5.75/1000
	100 mg	$8.50/1000
Veratex	50 mg	$5.70/1000
	100 mg	$8.30/1000
Wolins	50 mg	$5.95/1000
	100 mg	$8.75/1000

NITROGLYCERIN, U.S.P. (sublingual [hypodermic] tabs)

Darby	tablets	$.65/100	
IDE		$.70/100	
Lilly		$.72/100 regardless of strength (grains 1/100, 1/150, 1/200, 1/400)	
Modern		$.70/100	
Moore		$.59/100	
Schein		$.80/100	
Wolins		$.70/100	

NOLUDAR® (Methyprylon, N.F.)

Roche	50 mg tabs	$1.65/100
	200 mg	$22.40/500 ($4.73/100)
	300 mg caps	$26.80/500

NORGESIC®

| Riker | tablets $43.80/500 |

NORINYL® 1+50, 21-DAY;

NORINYL® 1+80, 21-DAY

| Syntex | 3 x 21 | $5.65 |
| | 6 x 21 (refill) | $10.95 |

NORLESTRIN® 21

| Parke, Davis | 5 x 21 tabs | $10.40 |

NORLESTRIN® FE 28

| Parke, Davis | 5 x 28 tabs   FE 1 mg | $10.50 |

NOVAHISTINE®

Dow * (Novahistine®)	elixir $4.14/pint
	DH liquid $5.90/pint
	expectorant $6.50/pint
IDE	decongestant elixir $2.25/pint
	decongestant expectorant $3.50/pint
	decongestant expectorant DH $3.25/pint
Modern (Phenhist)	elixir $1.90/pint
Moore (Novamor)	elixir $1.60/pint
	expectorant $3.70/pint
	DH expectorant $3.10/pint
Schein	decongestant elixir $1.75/pint
	decongestant DH liquid $2.95/pint
	decongestant expectorant $3.10/pint
Veratex (Dihistine)	elixir $1.80/pint
	expectorant $3.20/pint
	DH $2.90/pint
Wolins	decongestant elixir $1.95/pint
	decongestant expectorant $3.50/pint

NOVAHISTINE® DH
See Dow under Novahistine®.

NOVAMOR
See Moore under Novahistine®.

NYSTATIN, U.S.P.
See Mycostatin® and/or Tetrastatin®.

OMNIPEN®
See Wyeth under Ampicillin, U.S.P., and Ampicillin Syrups.

ORACON®

Mead-Johnson	6 x 21 tabs $10.50
	6 x 28 $10.50

ORAL CONTRACEPTIVES
See under individual brand name or in the chart under Oral Contraceptives in the Prescription Drug List.

* Which recently bought out Pitman-Moore.

ORETIC®
See Hydrodiuril®.

ORINASE® (Tolbutamide, U.S.P.)
Upjohn   0.5 gr tabs $76.19/1000

ORNADE®
Smith Kline & French
   (Ornade®)   Spansules® $53.50/500   ($11.05/100)
IDE (Decongex)   T.D. caps $11.00/1000
Modern (Allernade)   T.D. caps $8.90/1000
Moore (Deconade)   T.D. caps $9.25/1000
Veratex (Ornatex)   T.D. caps $9.60/1000
Wolins (Chlorphenade)   T.D. caps $10.95/1000

ORNATEX
See Veratex under Ornade®.

ORTHO-NOVUM®
Ortho   1/50–21 (63 dialpak) $5.65
               1/50–28 Dialpak, 6 x 28 $11.64
               1/50–21 Dialpak, 3 x 63 $16.95
               1/50–21 Dialpak, 12 x 21 $23.28
               1/80–21 Dialpak, 3 x 63 $16.95
               1/80–21 Dialpak, 12 x 21 $23.28
               1/80–28 Dialpak, 6 x 28 $11.64
               2 mg Dialpak, 3 x 63 $18.33
               2 mg Dialpak, 12 x 21 $23.30
               10 mg Dialpak, 20 $3.85
               SQ Dialpak, 60 $5.78
               SQ Dialpak, 6 x 20 $11.88

ORTHO-NOVUM® 1/50–21
Ortho   Box of 12 $23.28

ORTHO-NOVUM® 1/80–21
Ortho   Box of 12 $23.28

OVRAL®
Wyeth   tablets 6 x 21 $11.94
                         3 pak (63/pak) $5.85

OVRAL® 28
Wyeth

	tablets 6 x 28	$11.94
	336's (12 x 28)	$22.68

OVRETTE®
Wyeth

	tablets 6 x 28	$11.94

OVULEN®-21
Searle

(1 mg Compack) 126	$11.58
630 Triopak (10 x 63)	$56.10
21 Compack Refills	$87.40

OVULEN®-28
Searle

28 tabs (6 x 28)	$11.64
28 Compack Refills (12 x 28)	$22.68

OXAZEPAM
See Serax®.

OXYPHENBUTAZONE, N.F.
See Tandearil®.

OXYTETRACYCLINE HYDROCHLORIDE, N.F.
See Pfizer (Terramycin®) under Tetracycline and Tetracycline-Like Products.

PANMYCIN® (Tetracycline Hydrochloride, U.S.P.)
See Upjohn under Tetracycline and Tetracycline-Like Products.

PAPAVERINE HYDROCHLORIDE, N.F.
See Pavabid®.

PARA-AMINOSALICYLIC ACID, U.S.P.
See Aminosalicylic Acid, U.S.P.

PARAFON FORTE®
McNeil tablets $42.40/500

PARCOTANE
See Wolins under Trihexyphenidyl Hydrochloride, U.S.P.

PAREGORIC, U.S.P. (Camphorated Tincture of Opium)

Darby	$1.85/pint
Lilly	$1.84/pint
Modern	$1.85/pint
Parke, Davis	$1.63/pint
Veratex	$1.80/pint
Wolins	$1.95/pint

PAS
See Aminosalicylic Acid, U.S.P.

PAVABID® (Papaverine Hydrochloride, N.F.)
Brand names:

Marion (Pavabid®)	150 mg T.D. caps	$98.57/1000
Generics:		
Darby (Pavagen)	150 mg T.D. caps	$16.75/1000
Wolins (Pava-Wol)	150 mg T.D. caps	$33.95/1000
IDE	150 mg T.D. caps	$15.00/1000
Modern	150 mg T.D. caps	$14.95/1000
Moore	150 mg T.D. caps	$15.65/1000
	100 mg tabs	$13.95/1000
Schein	150 mg T.D. caps	$13.95/1000
	100 mg tabs	$15.50/1000
Veratex	150 mg T.D. caps	$16.90/1000

PAVAGEN, N.F.®
See Darby under Pavabid®.

PAVA-WOL®
See Wolins under Pavabid®.

PEDIAMYCIN® (erythromycin ethylsuccinate)

Ross	chewable tablets	$9.00/50
	suspension	$2.01/60 cc
	drops	$1.39/30 cc
	liquid, 200 mg/5 cc	$12.98/pint
	liquid, 400 mg/5 cc	$24.19/pint

PENBRITIN®
See Ayerst under Ampicillin, U.S.P., and Ampicillin Syrups.

PENICILLIN G, POTASSIUM, U.S.P.
See Pentids® Tablets; Pentids® Oral Suspension.

PENICILLIN V
*See Darby, IDE, and Wolins under V-CillinK® and V-Cillin
K® Oral Liquid. See Wolins under V-Cillin K® Oral Liquid.*

PENICILLIN V (tablets and suspensions)
See V-Cillin K®; Pen-Vee® K; Pediamycin®.

PENICILLIN VK®
See V-Cillin K®.

PENICILLIN VK
*See Modern, Moore, Schein and Veratex under V-Cillin K®
and V-Cillin K® Oral Liquid.*

PENTAERYTHRITOL TETRANITRATE (PETN)
See Peritrate®.

PENTAZOCINE HYDROCHLORIDE
See Talwin®.

PENTIDS® TABLETS (Potassium Penicillin G, U.S.P.)
Squibb

(Pentids®)	400,000 Unit caps	$93.00/1000	($4.65/50)
	400,000 Unit tabs	$8.45/100	($1.60/16)
Darby	100,000 Units	$4.95/1000	
	200,000	$7.65/1000	
	250,000	$8.65/1000	
	400,000	$12.40/1000	
IDE	250,000	$9.25/1000	
	400,000	$14.00/1000	
Lilly	100,000	$3.31/100	
	250,000	$7.19/100	
Modern	200,000	$6.40/1000	
	250,000	$8.50/1000	
	400,000	$12.20/1000	
Moore	100,000	$7.50/1000	
	200,000	$7.65/1000	
	250,000	$8.95/1000	
	400,000	$12.95/1000	
Schein	200,000	$7.95/1000	
	250,000	$8.95/1000	
	400,000	$12.95/1000	

Veratex	200,000	$8.30/1000
	250,000	$9.50/1000
	400,000	$15.90/1000
Wolins	200,000	$8.50/1000
	250,000	$9.50/1000
	400,000	$13.50/1000

PENTIDS® (Potassium Penicillin G, U.S.P.) FOR ORAL SUSPENSION

Squibb		
(Pentids®)	100 cc (400,000 Units per tsp [5 cc])	$1.68/bottle
	200 cc (400,000 Units per tsp [5 cc])	$2.85/bottle
Darby	60 cc (250,000 Units per tsp [5 cc])	$.65/bottle
	75 cc (400,000 Units per tsp [5 cc])	.85/bottle
	150 cc (400,000 Units per tsp [5 cc])	$1.35/bottle
IDE	60 cc (250,000 Units per tsp [5 cc])	$.65/bottle
	80 cc (400,000 Units per tsp [5 cc])	$.90/bottle
Modern	60 cc (250,000 Units per tsp [5 cc])	$.50/bottle
	75 cc (400,000 Units per tsp [5 cc])	$.80/bottle
	150 cc (400,000 Units per tsp [5 cc])	$1.35/bottle
Schein	60 cc (250,000 Units per tsp [5 cc])	$.70/bottle
	80 cc (400,000 Units per tsp [5 cc])	$.95/bottle
Veratex	60 cc (250,000 Units per tsp [5 cc])	$.70/bottle
	80 cc (400,000 Units per tsp [5 cc])	$.90/bottle
Wolins	60 cc (250,000 Units per tsp [5 cc])	$.75/bottle
	80 cc (200,000 Units per tsp [5 cc])	$.85/bottle
	150 cc (200,000 Units per tsp [5 cc])	$1.25/bottle

PEN-VEE® K
See Wyeth under V-Cillin K®.

PERCODAN®
Endo　　　　　　　　5 mg tabs $67.45/1000 ($34.65/500)

PERIACTIN® (cyproheptadine)
Merck, Sharp & Dohme

PERI-COLACE® (dioctyl sodium sulfosuccinate [Colace®] with casanthrol)

Mead Johnson		
(Peri-Colace®)	100 mg caps	$77.76/1000
Darby	100 mg	$14.95/1000

IDE	100 mg	$17.50/1000
Modern	100 mg	$12.50/1000
	100 mg tabs	$8.75/1000
Moore	100 mg caps	$14.25/1000
Schein	100 mg	$12.25/1000
Veratex	100 mg	$11.70/1000
Wolins	100 mg	$13.50/1000

PERITRATE® (pentaerythritol tetranitrate [PETN])
Warner/Chilcott (Peritrate®)

	10 mg tabs	$29.30/1000
	20 mg	$39.05/1000
	10 mg tabs with 15 mg phenobarbital	$32.55/1000
	20 mg tabs with 15 mg phenobarbital	$43.70/1000
	80 mg S.A. (T.D. caps) with 45 mg phenobarbital	$91.50/1000
Darby	10 mg caps	$1.40/1000
	10 mg caps with 15 mg phenobarbital	$1.90/1000
	20 mg caps	$1.70/1000
	20 mg caps with 15 mg phenobarbital	$2.25/1000
IDE	10 mg tabs	$1.50/1000
	20 mg	$1.65/1000
	10 mg tabs with 15 mg (¼ gr) phenobarbital	$1.85/1000
	80 mg T.D. caps	$18.00/1000
Modern	10 mg tabs	$1.40/1000
	10 mg tabs with 15 mg phenobarbital	$1.90/1000
	20 mg tabs	$1.70/1000
	20 mg tabs with 15 mg phenobarbital	$2.20/1000
	30 mg T.D. caps	$9.90/1000
	80 mg T.D. caps	$17.90/1000
Moore	10 mg tabs	$8.25/1000
	20 mg	$12.90/1000
	10 mg tabs with 15 mg phenobarbital	$11.70/1000
	30 mg T.D. caps	$11.95/1000
	80 mg T.D. caps	$23.50/1000
	30 mg T.D. caps with 50 mg secobarbital	$13.50/1000
Schein	10 mg tabs	$1.85/1000
	20 mg	$2.10/1000
	10 mg tabs with 15 mg phenobarbital	$2.25/1000
	20 mg tabs with 15 mg phenobarbital	$2.60/1000

Veratex	10 mg tabs	$7.00/5000 ($1.50/1000)
	20 mg	$8.00/5000 ($1.70/1000)
	10 mg tabs with 15 mg phenobarbital	$1.80/1000
	20 mg tabs with 15 mg phenobarbital	$2.10/1000
Wolins	10 mg tabs	$1.65/1000
	20 mg	$1.85/1000
	10 mg tabs with 15 mg phenobarbital	$2.00/1000
	20 mg tabs with 15 mg phenobarbital	$2.50/1000
	30 mg T.D. caps	$8.90/1000
	80 mg T.D. caps	$22.90/1000
	30 mg T.D. caps with 50 mg secobarbital	$7.95/1000

PETN
See Peritrate®.

PHENACETOPHEN
See Moore under Phenaphen®.

PHENAPHEN®

Robins (Phenaphen®)	capsules $20.25/1000 ($10.40/500)
	tablets $17.15/1000
IDE	capsules $10.00/500
Moore (Phenacetophen)	$8.75/1000
Schein	$10.40/500
Veratex	$8.90/1000
Wolins	$10.90/500

PHENAPHEN® WITH CODEINE
Robins   capsules $33.85/500 ($7.20/100)

PHENAZOPYRIDINE HYDROCHLORIDE
See Pyridium®.

PHENDECON
See Wolins under Naldecon®.

PHENERGAN® (Promethazine Hydrochloride, U.S.P.)

Wyeth (Phenergan®)	12.5 mg tabs	$37.39/1000 ($3.95/100)
	25 mg	$66.58/1000 ($6.99/100)
	50 mg	$10.72/100
Darby	25 mg	$8.50/1000
	50 mg	$19.00/1000

IDE	12.5 mg	$4.95/1000
	25 mg	$7.75/1000
	50 mg	$12.00/1000
Modern	12.5 mg	$3.25/1000
	25 mg	$6.25/1000
	50 mg	$10.75/1000
Moore	12.5 mg	$6.80/1000
	25 mg	$8.25/1000
	50 mg	$12.50/1000
Schein	12.5 mg	$4.95/1000
	25 mg	$7.95/1000
	50 mg	$11.75/1000
Veratex	12.5 mg	$4.20/1000
	25 mg	$8.40/1000
	50 mg	$18.80/1000
Wolins	12.5 mg	$5.95/1000
	25 mg	$8.50/1000
	50 mg	$11.75/1000

PHENERGAN® EXPECTORANT

Wyeth (Phenergan® Expectorant)	$3.82/pint
Darby	$1.75/pint
Modern	$1.75/pint
Moore	$1.70/pint
Schein	$1.95/pint
Veratex	$1.70/pint
Wolins	$2.45/pint

PHENERGAN® EXPECTORANT WITH CODEINE
(promethazine with codeine)

Wyeth (Phenergan® Expectorant with Codeine)	$5.02/pint
Darby	$2.20/pint
IDE	$2.50/pint
Modern	$2.20/pint
Moore	$3.00/pint
Schein	$2.85/pint
Veratex	$2.20/pint
Wolins	$2.95/pint

PHENERGAN® VC EXPECTORANT

Wyeth (Phenergan® VC Expectorant)	$4.31/pint

Darby	$1.95/pint
IDE	$2.25/pint
Modern	$1.85/pint
Moore	$2.05/pint
Schein	$2.25/pint
Veratex	$1.90/pint
Wolins	$1.90/pint

PHENERGAN® VC EXPECTORANT WITH CODEINE

Wyeth (Phenergan® VC Expectorant with Codeine)	$5.42/pint
Darby	$2.95/pint
IDE	$2.75/pint
Modern	$2.85/pint
Moore	$3.10/pint
Schein	$3.10/pint
Veratex	$2.40/pint
Wolins	$3.20/pint

PHENERGAN® SUPPOSITORIES

Wyeth	25 mg	$2.63/12
	50 mg	$3.49/12

PHENHIST

See Modern under Novahistine®.

PHENOBARBITAL, U.S.P.

Robins (Stental®)*	¾ gr	$10.45/500 ($2.20/100)
Darby	¼ gr	$1.35/1000
	½ gr	$1.75/1000
IDE	¼ gr	$2.00/1000
	½ gr	$3.00/1000
Lilly	¼ gr (15 mg)	$6.43/5000 ($1.57/1000)
	½ gr (30 mg)	$10.90/5000 ($2.60/1000)
Modern	¼ gr	$1.35/1000
	½ gr	$1.75/1000
Moore	¼ gr	$1.65/1000
	½ gr	$1.95/1000

* There is positively no excuse for marketing this preparation, a long-acting dose form. For phenobarbital, overdose with Stental® will be especially dangerous. FDA, please note.

Schein	¼ gr	$1.35/1000
	½ gr	$1.60/1000
Veratex	¼ gr	$1.40/1000
	½ gr	$1.90/1000
Wolins	¼ gr	$1.50/1000
	½ gr	$2.25/1000

PHENOXYMETHYL PENICILLIN (Potassium Phenoxymethyl Penicillin, U.S.P.)
See V-Cillin K®; Pen-Vee® K.

PHENTERMINE ROSIN
See Ionamin®.

PHENYLBUTAZONE, U.S.P.
See Butazolidin®; Butazolidin® Alka.

PHENYLEPHRINE HYDROCHLORIDE, U.S.P.
See Neo-Synephrine® in the Prescription Drug List pages.

"PILL, THE"
See under individual brand names in the chart under Oral Contraceptives in the Prescription Drug List. If not there, see under brand name in the Price Lists.

PILOCARPINE HYDROCHLORIDE, U.S.P.
See Isopto Carpine®.

PLACIDYL® (ethchlorvynol)
Abbott	100 mg caps	$2.61/100
	200 mg	$4.06/100
	500 mg	$35.09/500
	750 mg	$9.79/100

PLAQUENIL®
Winthrop   200 mg tabs $9.80/100
See also Chloroquine Phosphate, U.S.P.

POLARAMINE® (Dexchlorpheniramine Maleate, N.F.)
Schering	20 mg tabs	$2.58/100
	4 mg Repetabs®	$3.81/100
	6 mg Repetabs®	$5.86/100

POLYCILLIN®
See Bristol under Ampicillin, U.S.P., and Ampicillin Syrups.

POLY-VI-FLOR®
A multivitamin preparation requiring no prescription.
Mead Johnson
(Poly-Vi-Flor®)	chewable tablets	$25.12/1000
Darby		$5.35/1000
Modern		$5.25/1000
Schein		$5.95/1000
Veratex		$6.80/1000
Wolins		$7.95/1000

POTASSIUM CHLORIDE, U.S.P.
See Prescription Drug List entry.

POTASSIUM GLUCONATE
See Kaon®.

POTASSIUM PENICILLIN G, U.S.P.
See Pentids® Tablets; Pentids® Oral Suspension.

POTASSIUM PHENOXYMETHYL PENICILLIN, U.S.P.
See V-Cillin K®; Pen-Vee® K.

PREDNISOLONE, U.S.P.
Manufacture of this drug has been discontinued in tablet form. Though still available from generic distributors, it holds no advantage over prednisone when taken orally. It has the disadvantages of higher cost and more difficult availability.
Darby	5 mg	$9.90/1000
IDE	5 mg	$10.50/1000
Modern	5 mg	$9.50/1000
Moore	5 mg	$9.75/1000
Schein	5 mg	$8.50/1000
Veratex	5 mg	$11.60/1000
Wolins	5 mg	$9.95/1000

PREDNISONE, U.S.P.
Schering
(Meticorten®)		5 mg tabs $15.90/1000 ($7.95/500)

Upjohn (Deltasone®)	5 mg	$9.99/500 ($2.80/100)
Darby	5 mg	$8.25/1000
IDE	5 mg	$9.50/1000
Modern	5 mg	$8.25/1000
Schein	5 mg	$4.00/1000
Veratex	5 mg	$9.30/1000
Wolins	5 mg	$8.75/1000

PREMARIN® (Conjugated Estrogens, U.S.P.)*

Ayerst (Premarin®)	0.625 mg tabs	$41.23/1000 ($4.34/100)
	1.25 mg	$68.39/1000 ($7.21/100)
Massengill (Menest®)	0.625 mg	$39.45/1000
	1.25 mg	$66.95/1000
Darby	.0625 mg tabs	$12.95/1000
	1.25 mg	$22.90/1000
IDE	0.625 mg	$10.50/1000
	1.25 mg	$19.75/1000
Modern	0.625 mg	$12.70/1000
	1.25 mg	$22.75/1000
Moore	0.625 mg	$16.25/1000
	1.25 mg	$27.90/1000
Schein	0.625 mg	$13.95/1000
	1.25 mg	$24.50/1000
Veratex	0.625 mg	$13.30/1000
	1.25 mg	$23.20/1000
Wolins	0.625 mg	$15.25/1000
	1.25 mg	$26.50/1000

PRINCIPEN®
See Squibb under Ampicillin, U.S.P., and Ampicillin Syrups.

PRO-BANTHINE® (Propantheline Bromide, U.S.P.)

Searle (Pro-Banthine®)	15 mg tabs	$45.91/1000
Darby	15 mg	$7.95/1000
IDE	15 mg	$7.00/1000
Modern	15 mg	$7.50/1000
Moore	15 mg	$9.95/1000
Schein	15 mg	$10.50/1000

* For treating menopausal symptoms, diethylstilbestrol (stilbestrol) is as effective as Premarin® and enormously less expensive. One mg per day (of stilbestrol) is the usual dose.

| Veratex | 15 mg | $8.50/1000 |
| Wolins | 15 mg | $10.40/1000 |

PROBENECID, U.S.P.
See Benemid®.

PROCAINAMIDE HYDROCHLORIDE, U.S.P.

Squibb (Pronestyl®)	250 mg caps	$45.64/1000 ($5.06/100)
	375 mg	$7.04/100
	500 mg	$86.96/1000 ($9.13/100)
Darby	250 mg	$21.00/1000
	500 mg	$32.90/1000
IDE	250 mg	$17.00/1000
	500 mg	$29.00/1000
Modern	250 mg	$20.75/1000
	500 mg	$32.90/1000
Moore	250 mg	$23.90/1000
	375 mg	$24.00/1000
Schein	250 mg	$22.50/1000
	375 mg	$26.50/1000
	500 mg	$34.50/1000
Veratex	250 mg	$19.90/1000
	375 mg	$22.40/1000
	500 mg	$28.00/1000
Wolins	250 mg	$20.50/1000
	375 mg	$22.75/1000
	500 mg	$32.90/1000

PROCHLORPERAZINE MALEATE, U.S.P.
See Combid® Spansules®; Compazine®.

PROLOID® (thyroglobulin)

Warner/Chilcott

(Proloid®)	¼ gr tabs	$9.30/1000 ($1.00/100)
	½ gr	$10.20/1000 ($1.10/100)
	1 gr	$12.05/1000 ($1.30/100)
	1½ gr	$15.30/1000 ($1.65/100)
	2 gr	$2.35/100
	3 gr	$29.75/1000 ($3.20/100)
	5 gr	$37.65/1000 ($4.05/100)
Darby	1 gr	$7.25/1000

IDE	½ gr	$10.00/1000
	2 gr	$23.00/1000 ($2.30/100)
	3 gr	$31.00/1000 ($3.10/100)
	1 gr	$11.40/1000
Modern	1 gr	$6.75/1000
Moore	1 gr	$11.69/1000
	1½ gr	$14.85/1000
	2 gr	$22.80/1000 ($2.28/100)
	3 gr	$28.86/1000
	5 gr	$36.52/1000
Schein	1 gr	$8.75/1000
Veratex	1 gr	$7.40/1000
Wolins	1 gr	$7.55/1000

PROMETHAZINE HYDROCHLORIDE, U.S.P.
See Phenergan® and its variations.

PRONESTYL®
See Squibb under Procainamide Hydrochloride, U.S.P.

PROPANTHELINE BROMIDE, U.S.P.
See Pro-Banthine®.

PROPOXYPHENE(S) (Propoxyphene Hydrochloride, U.S.P.)
See the various Darvon®, Darvon-N®, and Darvocet-N® preparations.

PROPRANOLOL HYDROCHLORIDE, U.S.P.
See Inderal®.

PROVERA® (Medroxyprogesterone Acetate, U.S.P.)
Upjohn	2.5 mg tabs	$2.05/25
	10 mg	$16.62/100 ($4.38/25)

PSEUDOEPHEDRINE HYDROCHLORIDE
See Sudafed®.

PURODIGIN®
See Wyeth under Digitoxin, U.S.P.

PYRIDIUM® (phenazopyridine hydrochloride)
Warner/Chilcott

(Pyridium®)	100 mg tabs	$54.85/1000 ($5.90/100)
Darby	100 mg	$5.90/1000
IDE	100 mg	$6.50/1000
Modern	100 mg	$5.35/1000
Moore	100 mg	$7.75/1000
Schein	100 mg	$8.50/1000
Veratex	100 mg	$7.10/1000
Wolins	100 mg	$7.90/1000

QUAALUDE® (methaqualone)
Rorer

The *Handbook* does not recommend use of this medication.
See the Prescription Drug List entry. See Methaqualone for prices.

QUADRA-HIST
See Schein under Naldecon®.

QUINAGLUTE® (quinidine gluconate)
Cooper

The Handbook recommends the use of quinidine sulfate in its stead. Five-grain T.D. tablets cost $22.74 per one hundred.

QUINIDINE GLUCONATE
See Quinaglute®.

QUINIDINE SULFATE, U.S.P.*

Darby	3 gr tabs	$8.50/100
IDE	3 gr	$80.00/1000
Lilly	3 gr	$7.85/100
Modern	3 gr	$79.00/1000 ($8.40/100)
Moore	3 gr	$84.50/1000
Parke, Davis	3 gr	$9.40/100
Schein	3 gr	$79.50/1000
Veratex	3 gr	$115.40/1000
Wolins	3 gr	$80.80/1000

* Prices of quinidine are subject to sudden variations. Availability is also a common problem.

RAUWOLFIA SERPENTINA, N.F.
See Reserpine, U.S.P.; Rauzide®.

RAUZIDE®
Squibb   tablets $80.67/1000 ($8.48/100)

REDISON®
See Merck, Sharp & Dohme under Vitamin B$_{12}$ Injection, U.S.P.

REGROTON®
U.S. Vitamin   tablets $105.91/1000

RENESE® (polythiazide)
See Pfizer under "Thiazide" and "Thiazide"-Like Diuretics.

RESERPINE, U.S.P.

CIBA (Serpasil®)	0.1 mg tabs	$23.50/1000	
	0.25 mg	$39.50/1000	
Upjohn (Reserpoid®)	0.1 mg	$2.97/500	($.63/100)
	0.25 mg	$7.69/1000	($1.05/100)
Darby	0.1 mg	$1.15/1000	
	0.25 mg	$1.20/1000	
IDE	0.1 mg	$1.30/1000	
	0.25 mg	$1.35/1000	
Lilly	0.1 mg	$.74/100	
	0.25 mg	$9.76/1000	($1.12/100)
Modern	0.1 mg	$1.10/1000	
	0.25 mg	$1.15/1000	
Moore	0.1 mg	$1.95/1000	
	0.25 mg	$1.55/1000	
Schein	0.1 mg	$1.20/1000	
	0.25 mg	$1.20/1000	
Veratex	0.1 mg	$1.30/1000	
	0.25 mg	$1.10/1000	
Wolins	0.1 mg	$1.25/1000	
	0.25 mg	$1.35/1000	

RESERPOID®
See Upjohn under Reserpine, U.S.P.

RITALIN® (Methylphenidate Hydrochloride, N.F.)
CIBA   5 mg tabs $46.55/1000
                                      10 mg $66.45/1000
                                      20 mg · $93.10/1000

ROBIMYCIN®
See Robins under Erythromycin Base.

ROBITUSSIN®-DM
See Dextromethorphan Hydrobromide, N.F. in the Prescription Drug List pages.

ROMILAR® CF
See Dextromethorphan Hydrobromide, N.F., in the Prescription Drug List pages.

RONDOMYCIN® (methacycline)
See Wallace under Tetracycline and Tetracycline-Like Products.

SALURON® (hydroflumethiazide)
See Bristol under "Thiazide" and "Thiazide"-Like Diuretics.

SALUTENSIN®
Bristol   tablets $107.25/1000

SANDRIL®
See Lilly under Reserpine, U.S.P.

SECONAL®
See Lilly under Sodium Secobarbital, U.S.P.

SER-AP-ES®
CIBA (Ser-Ap-Es®)   tablets $79.55/1000
Darby (Tri-hydroserpine) $16.45/1000
IDE (Serathide) $13.50/1000
Modern (Tri-hydroserpine) $13.25/1000
Moore (Diuretic Ap-Es) $18.95/1000
Schein (H-H-R) $19.50/1000
Veratex (hydrochlorothiazide with
   reserpine and hydralazine) $15.80/1000
Wolins (Serpazide) $19.90/1000

SERATHIDE
See IDE under Ser-Ap-Es®.

SERAX® (oxazepam)
Wyeth

10 mg caps	$24.74/500
15 mg	$30.85/500
30 mg	$43.67/500

SERPASIL®
See CIBA under Reserpine, U.S.P.

SERPAZIDE
See Wolins under Ser-Ap-Es®.

SINEQUAN® (doxepin hydrochloride)
Pfizer

10 mg caps	$9.21/100
25 mg	$11.88/100
50 mg	$16.42/100
100 mg	$28.42/100

SK-ERYTHROMYCIN®
See Smith Kline & French under Erythromycin Stearate, U.S.P.

SODIUM BUTABARBITAL, U.S.P.
See Butisol®.

SODIUM DICLOXACILLIN
See Dynapen®.

SODIUM DIPHENYLHYDANTOIN, U.S.P.
See Dilantin®.

SODIUM LEVOTHYROXINE, U.S.P.
See Synthroid®.

SODIUM PENTOBARBITAL, U.S.P.
See Nembutal®.

SODIUM SECOBARBITAL, U.S.P.
Lilly (Seconal®)

¾ gr caps	$7.46/500	($1.82/100)
1½ gr	$11.18/500	($2.64/100)
Darby	1½ gr	$11.70/1000

IDE	1½ gr	$12.50/1000
Modern	1½ gr	$11.70/1000
Schein	¾ gr	$7.65/1000
	1½ gr	$8.95/1000
Wolins	¾ gr	$7.95/1000
	1½ gr	$10.50/1000

SODIUM WARFARIN, U.S.P.
See Coumadin®.

SOFRAZOLE
See IDE under Gantrisin®.

SOMNOS®
See Merck, Sharp & Dohme under Chloral Hydrate, U.S.P.

SPASMOLIN
See Moore under Donnatal®.

SPIRONOLACTONE, U.S.P.
See Aldactone®.

SPASTOLATE
See IDE under Donnatal.

STELAZINE® (trifluoperazine)
Smith Kline & French

	1 mg tabs	$74.50/1000 ($7.85/100)
	2 mg	$95.50/1000
	5 mg	$101.75/1000

STENTAL®
See Robins under Phenobarbital, U.S.P.

STERAZOLIDIN®
Geigy   capsules $8.65/100

STILBESTROL®
See Diethylstilbestrol, U.S.P.

SUDAFED® (pseudoephedrine hydrochloride)
Burroughs Wellcome

(Sudafed®)	30 mg tabs	$22.35/1000 ($2.85/100)
	60 mg	$35.55/1000 ($3.95/100)
syrup (30 mg/5 cc)		$3.15/pint

IDE	60 mg tabs	$9.50/1000
Modern	60 mg	$35.55/1000
Moore	60 mg	$10.95/1000
Schein	60 mg	$11.95/1000
	syrup (30 mg/5 cc)	$2.25/pint
	syrup (30 mg/5 cc)	$2.45/pint
Veratex	60 mg tabs	$8.90/1000
	syrup (30 mg/tsp)	$2.00/pint
Wolins	60 mg tabs	$11.90/1000
	syrup (30 mg/tsp)	$1.85/pint

SULFISOXAZOLE, U.S.P.
See Gantrisin®.

SUMYCIN® (Tetracycline Hydrochloride, U.S.P.)
See Squibb under Tetracycline and Tetracycline-Like Products.

SYNALAR® (fluocinolone acetonide)

Syntex	creams 0.01%	$3.06/45 g	($5.75/120 g)
	0.025%	$2.28/15 g	($6.30/60 g)
	ointment 0.025%	$2.28/15 g	($6.30/60 g)
	solution 0.01%	$4.20/60 cc	

SYNTHROID® (Sodium Levothyroxine, U.S.P.)

Flint (Synthroid®)	0.1 mg tabs	$14.78/1000
	0.2 mg	$20.06/1000
	0.3 mg	$30.10/1000
Darby	0.1 mg	$2.60/1000
	0.2 mg	$3.45/1000
IDE	0.1 mg	$2.50/1000
	0.2 mg	$3.50/1000
Modern	0.1 mg	$2.45/1000
	0.2 mg	$3.20/1000
Moore	0.1 mg	$2.70/1000
	0.2 mg	$3.70/1000
Schein	0.1 mg	$2.85/1000
	0.2 mg	$3.45/1000
Veratex	0.1 mg	$2.60/1000
	0.2 mg	$3.30/1000
Wolins	0.1 mg	$2.90/1000
	0.2 mg	$3.65/1000

SYTOBEX®
See Parke, Davis under Vitamin B₁₂ Injection, U.S.P.

TALWIN® (pentazocine hydrochloride)
Winthrop   50 mg tabs $9.15/50

TANDEARIL® (Oxyphenbutazone, N.F.)
Geigy   tablets $86.62/1000

TEDRAL®
   Contains ⅛ grain phenobarbital, 2 grains theophylline, and
⅜ grain ephedrine hydrochloride.
Warner/Chilcott
   (Tedral®)   tablets $39.95/1000
Darby (Theodrine) $5.35/1000
IDE (Theofedral) $5.50/1000
Modern (Theodrine) $5.20/1000
Moore (Theophenyllin) $4.80/1000
Schein (T.E.P.) $5.15/1000
Veratex (Theofedral)   formula $4.70/1000
Wolins (Theofedral)   formula $5.10/1000

TELDRIN® (Chlorpheniramine Maleate, U.S.P.)
Smith Kline &
   French
   (Teldrin®)   8 mg spansules® $28.50/500 ($5.85/100)
                 12 mg $38.25/500 ($7.85/100)
Darby   8 mg $7.45/1000
                12 mg $8.20/1000
IDE   8 mg $5.25/1000
                12 mg $5.75/1000
Modern   8 mg $6.45/1000
                12 mg $7.20/1000
Moore   8 mg $7.30/1000
                12 mg $8.15/1000
Veratex   8 mg $6.20/1000
                12 mg $6.70/1000
Wolins   8 mg $6.90/1000
                12 mg $7.95/1000

TENUATE® (Diethylpropion Hydrochloride, N.F.)
Merrell-National
   (Tenuate®)   25 mg tabs $56.40/1000 ($5.95/100)

Darby	25 mg tabs	$18.50/1000
	75 mg T.D. tabs	$28.50/1000
IDE	25 mg tabs	$11.50/1000
	75 mg T.D. tabs	$25.00/1000
Modern	25 mg tabs	$13.50/1000
	75 mg T.D. tabs	$27.90/1000
	75 mg T.D. caps	$37.00/1000
Moore	25 mg tabs	$13.65/1000
	75 mg T.D. caps	$39.50/1000
Schein	25 mg tabs	$17.95/1000
	75 mg T.D. tabs	$34.50/1000
	75 mg T.D. caps	$39.50/1000
Veratex	25 mg tabs	$16.90/1000
	75 mg T.D. tabs	$27.90/1000
Wolins	25 mg tabs	$19.25/1000
	75 mg T.D. caps	$46.25/1000

TENUATE® DOSPAN
Merrell-National (Tenuate®
  Dospan)   75 mg T.D. tabs $37.75/250 ($15.55/100)

T.E.P. (TABS)
See Schein under Tedral®.

TEPANIL® (Diethylpropion Hydrochloride, N.F.)
Riker   25 mg tabs $53.16/1000 ($5.64/100)

TERFONYL®
See Squibb under Triple Sulfas.

TERRAMYCIN® (Oxytetracycline Hydrochloride, N.F.)
See Pfizer under Tetracycline and Tetracycline-Like Products.

TETRACYCLINE (Tetracycline Hydrochloride, U.S.P.) AND TETRACYCLINE-LIKE PRODUCTS
Brand names:
Bristol (Tetrex® [Tetracycline
  Phosphate, N.F.*])   250 mg caps $15.87/100
Lederle (Achromycin® V [Tetracycline
          Hydrochloride, U.S.P.])
                  250 mg $37.95/1000

* No generic available.

(Aureomycin® [Chlortetracycline
Hydrochloride, N.F.*])

250 mg	$14.86/100

(Declomycin® [Demethylchlortetracycline
Hydrochloride, U.S.P.*])

150 mg caps	$19.62/100
150 mg tabs	$19.62/100
300 mg	$35.68/100

(Minocin® [minocycline
hydrochloride *])

100 mg caps	$39.22/100	($19.82/50)

Pfipharmecs (Tetracyn® [Tetracycline
Phosphate, N.F.*])

250 mg	$27.60/1000	($3.08/100)

Pfizer (Terramycin® [Oxytetracycline
Hydrochloride, N.F.])

125 mg	$9.80/100	
250 mg	$81.43/500	($18.10/100)

(Vibramycin® [doxycycline
hyclate])

50 mg	$18.10/50

Squibb (Sumycin® [Tetracycline
Hydrochloride, U.S.P.])

250 mg tabs or caps	$4.25/100

Upjohn (Panmycin® [Tetracycline
Hydrochloride, U.S.P.])

250 mg	$28.73/1000	($3.63/100)

Wallace (Rondomycin®
[methacycline *])

150 mg	$19.20/100
300 mg	$19.20/50

Generics:

Darby	250 mg caps	$12.45/1000
IDE	250 mg	$13.00/1000
Modern	250 mg	$12.40/1000
Moore	250 mg	$13.50/1000
Schein	250 mg	$8.45/1000
Veratex	250 mg	$13.90/1000
Wolins	250 mg	$13.95/1000

* No generic available.

TETRACYN® (Tetracycline Phosphate, N.F.)
See Pfipharmecs under Tetracycline and Tetracycline-Like Products.

TETRASTATIN® (Nystatin, U.S.P.)
Pfipharmecs   250 mg caps $12.39/100

TETREX® (Tetracycline Phosphate, N.F.)
See Bristol under Tetracycline and Tetracycline-Like Products.

THEODRINE
See Darby and Modern under Tedral®.

THEOFEDRAL
See IDE, Veratex, and Wolins under Tedral®.

THEOPHENYLLIN
See Moore under Tedral®.

THEOPHYLLINE, N.F.
See Elixophyllin® in the Prescription Drug List pages.

"THIAZIDE" AND "THIAZIDE"-LIKE DIURETICS
(Single Entities)

Abbott (Enduron®	2.5 mg tabs	$48.73/1000	
[methyclothiazide *])	5 mg	$66.96/1000	
Bristol (Saluron® [hy-drofiumethiazide *])	50 mg	$2.63/50	
CIBA (Esidrix®† [Hydrochlorothiazide, U.S.P.])	50 mg	$57.00/1000	
Hoechst (Lasix®	20 mg	$6.60/100	
[furosemide *])	40 mg	$9.25/100	
Lakeside (Metahydrin® ††	2 mg	$33.75/1000	
[trichlormethiazide])	4 mg	$53.75/1000	
Lederle (Hydromox® [quinethazone *])	50 mg	$42.95/500	($9.85/100)

* No generic available.

† At this price, patients should switch to generic hydrochlorothiazide at once.

†† Trichlormethiazide is available generically at about $4.85/1000 for 2 mg tabs and $4.95/1000 for 4 mg tabs.

Lilly (Anhydron® [cyclothiazide *])	2 mg	$61.13/1000	($6.46/100)
Merck, Sharp & Dohme (Diuril® [Chlorothiazide, N.F.**])	250 mg	$24.50/1000	
	500 mg	$39.95/1000	
Merck, Sharp & Dohme (Hydrodiuril® [Hydrochlorothiazide, U.S.P.**])	25 mg	$31.03/1000	
	50 mg	$48.45/1000	
Pfizer (Renese® [polythiazide])	1 mg	$42.46/1000	($4.42/100)
	2 mg	$66.30/1000	($6.98/100)
	4 mg	$103.23/1000	($11.64/100)
Robins (Exna® [Benzthiazide, N.F.**])	50 mg	$41.60/500	($6.60/100)
Schering (Naqua® †† [trichlormethiazide])	2 mg	$30.19/1000	($3.49/100)
	4 mg	$48.08/1000	($5.44/100)
Squibb (Naturetin® † [bendroflumethiazide])	5 mg	$71.44/1000	($7.51/100)
	10 mg	$11.53/100	
U.S. Vitamin (Hygroton® [Chlorthalidone, U.S.P.**])	50 mg	$73.19/1000	
	100 mg	$89.15/1000	

THORAZINE® (Chlorpromazine Hydrochloride, U.S.P.)

Smith Kline & French (Thorazine®)	10 mg tabs	$30.50/1000
	25 mg	$36.00/1000
	50 mg	$41.75/1000
	100 mg	$51.25/1000
Darby	10 mg	$12.75/1000
	25 mg	$16.50/1000
	50 mg	$20.95/1000
	100 mg	$30.50/1000
IDE	25 mg	$15.00/1000
	50 mg	$17.50/1000
	100 mg	$27.00/1000

* No generic available.

† At this price, patients should switch to generic hydrochlorothiazide at once.

** See under the brand name for generic drug company prices.

†† Trichlormethiazide is available generically at about $4.85/1000 for 2 mg tabs and $4.95/1000 for 4 mg tabs.

Modern	10 mg	$12.70/1000
	25 mg	$16.40/1000
	50 mg	$20.90/1000
	100 mg	$28.40/1000
Moore	10 mg	$11.95/1000
	25 mg	$16.10/1000
	50 mg	$18.95/1000
	100 mg	$27.80/1000
Schein	10 mg	$18.25/1000
	25 mg	$21.50/1000
	50 mg	$25.00/1000
	100 mg	$31.50/1000
Veratex	10 mg	$11.60/1000
	25 mg	$14.50/1000
	50 mg	$18.50/1000
	100 mg	$29.80/1000
Wolins	10 mg	$11.95/1000
	25 mg	$15.95/1000
	50 mg	$18.95/1000
	100 mg	$27.95/1000

THREAMINE
See Moore under Triaminic®.

THYROGLOBULIN
See Proloid®.

THYROID, U.S.P.

Armour	1 gr tabs	$6.77/1000
	2 gr	$12.60/1000
	3 gr	$21.33/1000
Darby	1 gr	$1.45/1000
	2 gr	$2.50/1000
IDE	1 gr	$1.75/1000
	2 gr	$3.00/1000
Lilly	1 gr	$5.57/1000
	2 gr	$10.24/1000
Modern	1 gr	$1.45/1000
	2 gr	$2.35/1000
Moore	1 gr	$1.95/1000
	2 gr	$3.15/1000

Schein	1 gr	$1.45/1000
	2 gr	$2.60/1000
Upjohn	1 gr	$3.77/1000
Veratex	1 gr	$1.80/1000
	2 gr	$2.60/1000
Wolins	1 gr	$1.45/1000
	2 gr	$2.75/1000

TIGAN® (trimethobenzamide hydrochloride)
Beecham	100 mg caps	$7.02/100
	250 mg	$39.33/500 ($8.29/100)
	100 mg suppositories	$3.23/10

TINACTIN® (Tolnaftate, U.S.P.)
Schering	cream 1%	$3.80/15 g tube
	powder 1%	$1.98/45 g unit
	solution 1%	$3.30/10 cc plastic vial

TINCTURE OF BELLADONNA (Belladonna Tincture, U.S.P.)
For prices, ask your pharmacist. Little will be saved by comparative shopping. Atropine sulfate tablets may be more convenient to use.

TINCTURE OF OPIUM, CAMPHORATED
See Paregoric, U.S.P.

TOFRANIL® (Imipramine Hydrochloride, U.S.P.)
Geigy (Tofranil®)	10 mg tabs	$59.13/1000
	25 mg	$92.32/1000
	50 mg	$183.64/1000
Modern	10 mg	$1.85/100
	25 mg	$24.60/1000
	50 mg	$3.45/100
Schein	10 mg	$15.95/1000
	25 mg	$24.95/1000
	50 mg	$32.50/1000

TOLINASE® (Tolazamide, U.S.P.)
| Upjohn | 100 mg tabs | $5.16/100 |
| | 250 mg | $10.98 |

TOLAZAMIDE, U.S.P.
See Tolinase®.

TOLBUTAMIDE, U.S.P.
See Orinase®.

TRANXENE® (clorazepate dipotassium)
Abbott   0.75 mg caps $5.90/100
           7.5 mg $7.50/100
           15 mg $12.50/100

TRIACIN
See Moore under Actifed-C® Expectorant.

TRIAMCINOLONE, U.S.P.
See Aristocort®; Kenalog®.

TRI-AMINE
See Moore under Triaminic®.

TRIAMINIC®
Dorsey (Triaminic®)   T.D. tablets $21.51/250   ($8.83/100)
                  syrup $7.48/pint *
IDE (Trilion)   T.D. tablets $9.00/1000
                  syrup $4.60/pint *
Modern (Triphenyl)   T.D. tablets $10.35/1000
                  syrup $4.60/pint *
Moore (Tri-amine)   T.D. tablets $11.50/1000
   (Threamine DM)   syrup $2.60/pint *
Schein (Tri-Hist)   T.D. tablets $12.95/1000
   (Tri-Hist)   syrup $2.45/pint *
Veratex   syrup $2.60/pint *
Wolins (Triwol)   T.D. capsules $12.50/1000
   (Triwol)   syrup $2.65/pint *

* Each 5 cc contains 6.25 milligrams of pyrilamine maleate, 6.25 milligrams of pheniramine maleate, 12.5 milligrams of phenylpropanolamine hydrochloride, 15 milligrams of dextromethorphan hydrobromide, and 90 milligrams of ammonium chloride.

TRIAVIL®

Merck, Sharp & Dohme	2/10 tabs	$41.74/500
	2/25	$52.87/500
	4/10	$46.52/500
	4/25	$57.65/500

TRICHLORMETHIAZIDE
*See Lakeside and Schering under "Thiazide" and "Thiazide'
Like Diuretics.*

TRI-HEXANE
See Darby under Trihexyphenidyl Hydrochloride, U.S.P.

TRIHEXIDYL
See Schein under Trihexyphenidyl Hydrochloride, U.S.P.

TRIHEXYPHENIDYL HYDROCHLORIDE, U.S.P.

Lederle (Artane®)	2 mg tabs	$13.23/1000
	5 mg	$26.25/1000
Darby (Tri-hexane)	2 mg	$6.50/1000
	5 mg	$8.75/1000
IDE	2 mg	$5.75/1000
	5 mg	$8.00/1000
Modern	2 mg	$14.80/1000
	5 mg	$29.40/1000
Moore	2 mg	$6.40/1000
	5 mg	$9.65/1000
Schein (Trihexidyl)	2 mg	$4.65/1000
	5 mg	$6.25/1000
Veratex	2 mg	$6.40/1000
	5 mg	$8.80/1000
Wolins (Parcotane)	2 mg	$6.95/1000
	5 mg	$9.90/1000

TRI-HIST
See Schein under Triaminic®.

TRI-HYDROSERPINE
See Darby and Modern under Ser-Ap-Es®.

TRILION
See IDE under Triaminic®.

TRIPHENYL
See Modern under Triaminic®.

TRIPLE SULFAS TABLETS, N.F. AND/OR U.S.P.

Contains 2½ grains of sulfamethazine, 2½ grains of sulfadiazine, and 2½ grains of sulfamerazine—for *N.F.*

Squibb (Terfonyl®)*	7½ gr tabs	$22.50/1000
Darby	7½ gr	$13.50/1000
IDE	7½ gr	$10.40/1000
Modern	7½ gr	$13.25/1000
Moore	7½ gr	$13.50/1000
Schein	7½ gr	$12.95/1000
Veratex	7½ gr	$13.70/1000
Wolins	7½ gr	$13.50/1000

TRISULFAPYRIMIDINES TABLETS, U.S.P.
See Triple Sulfas Tablets.

TRIWOL
See Wolins under Triaminic®.

TUINAL®

Lilly (Tuinal®)

capsules { 45 mg secobarbital / 45 mg amobarbital } $27.74/1000

capsules { 100 mg secobarbital / 100 mg amobarbital } $36.92/1000

Darby	capsules	$10.50/1000
IDE	capsules	$8.50/1000
Modern	capsules	$10.50/1000

Schein

capsules { 45 mg amobarbital / 45 mg secobarbital } $10.50/1000

capsules { 100 mg amobarbital / 100 mg secobarbital } $10.95/1000

Wolins

capsules { 45 mg amobarbital / 45 mg secobarbital } $8.50/1000

capsules { 100 mg amobarbital / 100 mg secobarbital } $9.80/1000

* This is the *U.S.P.* version. It is entirely comparable to the *N.F.* versions.

TUSS-ADE
See Schein and Veratex under Tuss-Ornade®.

TUSSADON
See Modern under Tuss-Ornade®.

TUSS-CHLORPHENADE
See Wolins under Tuss-Ornade®.

TUSS-ORNADE®
Smith Kline & French

(Tuss-Ornade®)	liquid	$6.50/pint	
	Spansules®	$58.50/500	($6.15/50)
Modern (Tussadon)	T.D. capsules	$15.65/1000	
Schein		$6.75/pint	
(Tuss-Ade)		$18.95/1000	
Veratex (Tuss-Ade)		$19.80/1000	
Wolins (Tuss-Chlorphenade)		$18.95/1000	

TYLENOL® (Acetaminophen, N.F.)
Brand names:

Eaton (NEBS®)	325 mg tabs	$12.00/1000
McNeil (Tylenol®)	325 mg	$17.90/1000
Mead Johnson		
(Tempra®)	300 mg	$33.90/1000
Smith Kline & French		
(SK-APAP®)	325 mg	$14.50/1000
Squibb (Valadol®)	325 mg	$16.78/1000

Generics:

Darby (5 gr acetaminophen)	tablets	$7.50/1000
IDE	325 mg tabs	$7.50/1000
Modern (Apap)	325 mg	$7.50/1000
Moore	325 mg	$7.75/1000
Schein (Apap)	325 mg	$2.50/1000
Veratex (Apap)	325 mg	$7.20/1000
Wolins (5 gr acetaminophen)	tablets	$7.50/1000

TYLENOL® (Acetaminophen, N.F.) WITH CODEINE
McNeil (Tylenol®

with Codeine)	¼ gr (15 mg) tabs	$20.65/500	($4.35/100)
	½ gr (30 mg)	$58.90/1000	($6.55/100)

Darby	¼ gr	$21.30/1000 ($10.65/500)
	½ gr	$36.50/1000 ($18.25/500)
IDE	¼ gr	$27.50/1000 ($2.75/100)
	½ gr	$45.00/1000 ($4.50/100)
Modern	¼ gr	$21.30/1000 ($10.65/500)
	½ gr	$36.50/1000 ($18.25/500)
Schein	¼ gr	$18.50/1000
	½ gr	$29.50/1000
Veratex (Apap with codeine phosphate)	¼ gr	$22.90/1000
	½ gr	$39.90/1000
Wolins	¼ gr	$29.50/1000
	½ gr	$51.00/1000 ($25.50/500)

VALISONE® (Betamethasone Valerate, N.F.)
Schering	creams 0.01% $1.22/15 g	$2.81/60 g
	0.1% $2.13/15 g	$4.12/45 g
	ointment 0.1% $2.13/15 g	$4.12/45 g
	lotion 0.1% $5.14/60 cc	

VALIUM® (diazepam)
Roche	2 mg tabs $28.75/500
	5 mg $35.00/500
	10 mg $48.50/500

VASODILAN® (isoxsuprine hydrochloride)
Mead Johnson (Vasodilan®)	10 mg tabs $64.26/1000	
	20 mg $114.12/1000	
Darby	10 mg $31.20/1000	
Modern	10 mg $31.20/1000	
	20 mg $56.40/1000	($28.20/500)
Moore	10 mg $27.90/1000	
	20 mg $49.20/1000	
Schein	10 mg $27.50/1000	
	20 mg $47.50/1000	

V-CILLIN K® (Potassium Phenoxymethyl Penicillin, U.S.P.)
Brand names:
Lilly (V-Cillin K®)

125 mg tabs (200,000 Units)	$5.48/100	
250 mg (400,000 Units)	$43.09/500	($9.13/100)

Wyeth (Pen-Vee® K)

       125 mg tabs (200,000 Units) $35.60/1000 ($2.12/36)

Generics:

Darby (Penicillin V)

       125 mg tabs (200,000 Units) $15.90/1000
       250 mg   (400,000 Units) $16.85/1000

IDE (Penicillin V)

       125 mg tabs (200,000 Units) $16.00/1000 ($1.60/100)
       250 mg   (400,000 Units) $19.00/1000

Modern (Penicillin VK)

       125 mg tabs (200,000 Units) $16.50/1000
       250 mg   (400,000 Units) $16.70/1000

Moore (Penicillin VK)

       250 mg tabs (400,000 Units) $19.90/1000

Schein (Penicillin VK)

       125 mg tabs (200,000 Units) $14.50/1000
       250 mg   (400,000 Units) $14.90/1000

Veratex (Penicillin VK)

       250 mg tabs (400,000 Units) $20.70/1000

Wolins (Penicillin V)

       125 mg tabs (200,000 Units) $16.50/1000
       250 mg   (400,000 Units) $18.45/1000

V-CILLIN K® (Potassium Phenoxymethyl Penicillin, U.S.P.) ORAL LIQUID

Lilly (V-Cillin K® Oral Liquid)

       125 mg/5 cc $2.13/150 cc ($1.53/100 cc)
       250 mg/5 cc $3.18/150 cc ($2.08/100 cc)

Darby (Penicillin V)

       125 mg (200,000 Units) $1.27/150 cc ($.85/100 cc)
       250 mg (400,000 Units) $1.72/150 cc ($1.15/100 cc)

IDE (Penicillin V)

       125 mg (200,000 Units) $9.00/150 cc

Modern (Penicillin VK)

       125 mg (200,000 Units) $1.12/150 cc ($1.00/100 cc)
       250 mg (400,000 Units) $1.50/150 cc ($1.00/100 cc)

Moore (Penicillin VK)

       125 mg (200,000 Units) $1.10/200 cc ($.95/150 cc)
                                              $.80/100 cc)
       250 mg (400,000 Units) $1.50/200 cc ($1.25/150 cc)
                                                $.99/100 cc)

Schein (Penicillin VK)
  125 mg (200,000 Units) $1.15/200 cc ($.75/100 cc)
  250 mg (400,000 Units) $1.65/200 cc ($1.00/100 cc)
Veratex (Penicillin VK)
  125 mg (200,000 Units) $1.30/200 cc ($.80/100 cc)
  250 mg (400,000 Units) $1.80/200 cc ($1.10/100 cc)
Wolins (Penicillin V)
  125 mg (200,000 Units) $1.35/150 cc
  250 mg (400,000 Units) $1.65/150 cc

VIBRAMYCIN® (doxycycline hyclate) *

Pfizer (Vibramycin®)	50 mg caps $36.60/100 ($18.10/50)	
	100 mg	$21.40/50
Darby	100 mg	$21.40/50
IDE	50 mg	$14.75/50
	100 mg	$21.75/50
Modern	100 mg	$19.95/50
Moore	50 mg	$14.50/50
	100 mg	$212.00/500
Schein	50 mg	$13.50/50
	100 mg	$19.95/50
Wolins	50 mg	$15.00/50
	100 mg	$22.30/50

VIOFORM®-HYDROCORTISONE

CIBA (Vioform®-Hydrocortisone)	cream	$3.65/20 g	
IDE (iodochlor w/hydrocortisone)		$1.00/20 g	$10.50/lb
			$30.50/3 lb
Modern (iodochlorhydroxyquin 3% w/hydrocortisone)		$.90/20 g	
Moore (iodochlorhydroxyquin w/hydrocortisone)		$.48/5 g	
		$.96/20 g	$10.50/lb
Schein		$3.65/20 g	
Veratex (Iodo-HC)		$1.00/20 g	$13.20/lb
Wolins (Iodo-HC)		$.50/5 g	$.99/20 g
			$10.95/lb

* See also Pfizer under Tetracycline and Tetracycline-Like Products.

VISTARIL® (hydroxyzine pamoate)

Pfizer	25 mg caps	$42.65/500
	50 mg	$51.99/500
	100 mg	$60.34/500
	25 mg/5 cc oral suspension	$13.77/pint

VITAMIN B$_{12}$ INJECTION, U.S.P.

Brand names:

Lilly (Betalin 12®)
    10 cc vial, 1000 micrograms/cc $2.07/vial
Merck, Sharp & Dohme (Redisol®)
    10 cc vial, 1000 micrograms/cc $1.58/vial
Parke, Davis (Sytobex®)
    10 cc vial, 1000 micrograms/cc $1.89/vial
Upjohn (Berubigen®)
    10 cc vial, 1000 micrograms/cc $2.37/vial

Generics:

Darby
    10 cc vial, 1000 micrograms/cc $.36/vial ($3.45/10 vials)
    30 cc vial, 1000 micrograms/cc $.60/vial ($5.60/10 vials)
Modern
    10 cc vial, 1000 micrograms/cc $.36/vial ($3.45/10 vials)
    30 cc vial, 1000 micrograms/cc $.59/vial ($5.50/10 vials)
Moore
    10 cc vial, 1000 micrograms/cc $.43/vial ($3.95/10 vials)
    30 cc vial, 1000 micrograms/cc $.82/vial ($7.65/10 vials)
Schein
    10 cc vial, 1000 micrograms/cc $3.50/10 vials
Wolins
    10 cc vial, 1000 micrograms/cc $.49/vial ($4.50/10 vials)
    30 cc vial, 1000 micrograms/cc $.79/vial ($7.50/10 vials)

WARFARIN (Sodium Warfarin, U.S.P.)
See Coumadin®.

ZYLOPRIM® (allopurinol)

Burroughs Wellcome	100 mg tabs	$6.60/100
	300 mg	$17.30/100

Appendices

APPENDIX A
Prescribing for Children

The doctor who cares for children is concerned primarily with preventive medicine; *i.e.,* administration of vaccines and early discovery of correctable abnormalities. A large number of common childhood illnesses need no therapy and may be made worse by unnecessary drugs. However, a number of the diseases the doctor has to manage do need therapy. Prescribing can generally be kept simple, safe, and inexpensive. Here are some of the "pediatric basic drugs," listed by categories, about which the *Handbook* offers commentary.

I. Anti-Infection Drugs

A. PENICILLIN PRODUCTS

These are for oral use; there is currently little reason to give injections of penicillin in office practice.

---

* This appendix was prepared with the close collaboration of Dr. Hyman Shrand, a pediatrician who is Director of Pediatrics, Mount Auburn Hospital, Cambridge, Massachusetts, and with another eminent pediatrician in private practice near Boston who prefers not to be identified.

1. Penicillin G Tablets (Potassium Penicillin G Tablets, U.S.P.)

The least expensive way for the doctor to prescribe penicillin G is as "Penicillin G Tablets, *U.S.P.* (Soluble), 200,000 units." The tablet can be dissolved in anything that will mask its taste, preferably something very sweet, such as strawberry jam. To be certain the tablet goes into solution, it should be crushed into powder between two spoons. (It is easier to crush it between a teaspoon and a tablespoon than between two equal-sized spoons.) Should a soluble tablet not be available, the more commonly dispensed buffered penicillin G tablet can be used. Penicillin tablets are stable indefinitely, if kept dry. One hundred soluble tablets, each containing 200,000 units, can be bought very cheaply.

Another way to prescribe penicillin G is as flavored penicillin G powder in a 16- or 30-dose bottle. Tap water is added to the neck of the bottle to put the material into solution. One teaspoonful will contain 200,000 or 400,000 units. A disadvantage of the syrup is gradual deterioration of the penicillin in solution over a period of 2 to 3 weeks. However, this is of minor or no importance, because the entire contents should have been used in this time. The following price information might be useful:

16 tsps (400,000 units/tsp)	$ .90	Interstate Drug Exchange
16 " " "	1.10	Wolins
20 " " "	1.68	Squibb (Pentids® for Syrup)

2. Penicillin V (Potassium Phenoxymethyl Penicillin, U.S.P)

Many doctors currently prescribe penicillin V products (Penn-Vee® K, V-Cillin K®, Compocillin-V®, and Compocillin-VK®). They are more expensive than penicillin G, unless the latter is bought as Pentids® for Syrup, and have but a single theoretical advantage: if they are taken when there is food in the stomach, significantly more penicillin will find its way into the bloodstream than when penicillin G is used. Since the doctor nearly always prescribes penicillin to treat infections caused by either the hemolytic streptococcus or the pneumococcus—organisms exquisitely susceptible to penicillin—any such higher blood level is usually of little or no clinical importance. However, should a doctor feel that the blood level is clinically important, he can tell the mother to administer penicillin G when the child's stomach is empty and then wait about 30 minutes before giving food. (Physicians and patients might like to know that flavored penicillin V powder for syrup is now available generically from nearly all suppliers of generic drugs. Enough to provide 100 cc—20 teaspoonfuls containing 200,000 units each—sells at a wholesale cost of $0.75. This is not more expensive than flavored penicillin G for syrup.) When a doctor treats a child with streptococcus infection, he is advised by the American Heart Association and other authorities to prescribe penicillin 3 times a day for 10 days. Many doctors believe it is wise to treat other members of the family, including parents, even if they are without symptoms. In many cases, it is economically feasible to do this only if one uses penicillins bought at the lowest possible price.

3. Ampicillin Syrup (Amcill®, Polycillin®, Omnipen®, Penbritin®, Principen®)

Nearly all anti-infection drugs given to children in office and home practice are for upper respiratory infections due to hemolytic streptococcus, pneumococcus, and/or *Hemophilus influenzae*. Penicillin G and a sulfonamide will nearly always do the therapeutic trick.

Ampicillin covers essentially the same spectrum of activity as penicillin G plus a sulfonamide—but at much higher cost. Prices of three competing brands of ampicillin are much alike:

Ampicillin for Oral Suspension
(16 tsps = 80 cc)

16 tsps (400,000 units/tsp)			$2.20	Squibb (Principen®)
16 "	"	"	2.63	Bristol (Polycillin®)
20 "	"	"	2.26	Ayerst (Penbritin®)
20 "	"	"	1.65	Modern (Ampicillin, U.S.P.)
20 "	"	"	1.90	Wolins (Ampicillin, U.S.P.)

B. SULFONAMIDES

Triple sulfas (Trisulfapyrimidines Tablets, U.S.P.) is universally available and cheap. It is commonly given for urinary tract infections. Sometimes the doctor will wish to prescribe it along with penicillin G.

C. TETRACYLINE HYDROCHLORIDE, U.S.P.

Although tetracycline was once widely used in pediatric practice, most authorities now believe it is contraindicated for children under five (and for a woman in the last half of pregnancy) because the child's teeth, both first and second sets, may be permanently discolored. Even one course of tetracycline can cause developing teeth to become discolored, and the more it is used, the worse the discoloration. As a matter of interest, many of the organisms once sensitive to tetracycline (pneumococcus, streptococcus, and staphylococcus) are now resistant.

Therefore, this appendix does not bother to list prices and sources of tetracycline.

D. METHENAMINE MANDELATE, U.S.P.

This drug is useful only in treating chronic pyelonephritis and therefore may have to be given for months or even years. Hence, cost is always an important consideration. Tablets are prescribed. (For young children a portion of a tablet may be crushed and dissolved in jam.) For further comments see Mandelamine® in the Addenda.

E. ERYTHROMYCIN, U.S.P.

This has the same spectrum of antibacterial action as penicillin G, and its only indication for use is where there is known allergy to penicillin G (which is unusual in children). At present, erythromycin is more expensive than penicillin G or V.

The prevailing wholesale costs for granules of erythromycin ethylsuccinate for suspension should be looked up in the Price Lists.

Note that one erythromycin, Ilosone®, is not recommended for use since it may have a toxic effect on the liver, causing jaundice.

II. Sedative and Anti-Epilepsy Drugs

A. CHLORAL HYDRATE SYRUP, U.S.P.

For the occasional child who is too excited to sleep, chloral hydrate syrup is the safest sedative. See Chloral Hydrate Syrup, U.S.P., in the Price Lists.

B. PHENOBARBITAL ELIXIR, U.S.P. (PHENOBARBITAL TABLET, U.S.P.)

This is still the cornerstone of treatment for epilepsy. As the duration of treatment is at least 2 years, cost is an important consideration. An expensive way to prescribe phenobarbital is as Luminal®.

This drug should always be dispensed in a bottle that is difficult for children to open, and it should be kept out of their reach.

III. Drugs for Treating Stuffy Nose (as in the Common Cold)

A. PHENYLEPHRINE HYDROCHLORIDE, U.S.P.

As a ⅛ or ¼ percent solution, this is the most effective way to open a stuffy nose. The child should be held with nostrils pointed to the ceiling. Four drops should be put into each nostril and the child held in this position for a minute. Then he should be turned over with nostrils pointed to the floor; any secretions can be wiped away. Never use nose drops repeatedly for more than 3 days. Phenylephrine nose drops can be bought without a prescription for $1 or less.

"Decongestants," advertised for children who will

not take nose drops, are not recommended. These substances are vasoconstrictors; it is not sensible to give anyone a systemic vasoconstrictor in the hope of constricting the blood vessels in the nose, since there is no evidence that these blood vessels are more sensitive to the action of vasoconstrictors than blood vessels elsewhere. The administration of enough systemic vasoconstrictor to affect the nose might well cause the blood pressure to rise. Most decongestant drugs are really mixtures of items, including an antihistamine with the same actions as diphenhydramine. It is strongly suspected that the vasoconstrictor decongestant agent in such mixtures is present in amounts too small to have a pharmacological effect, and that any benefit is derived from the drying action of the antihistamine on nasal secretions. It is questionable whether it is always beneficial to dry up secretions in a child with a respiratory infection.

The *Handbook* recommends the use of phenylephrine nose drops as first choice for relief of a stuffy nose.

B. DIPHENHYDRAMINE ELIXIR, U.S.P.

This is an antihistamine drug whose side effects—sedation and drying up of nasal secretions—may be useful. However, phenylephrine drops, because they are not given systemically, are much to be preferred. The usual prescription for diphenhydramine elixir is for 4 ounces. As Benadryl® Elixir the wholesale cost is 83 cents; it is hardly worthwhile shopping around.

IX. Drugs for Cough

Many children cough a great deal when they have common colds. Often, the cause is postnasal drip from a runny nose. The correct use of phenylephrine nose drops will decrease the drip and the need to cough. Keeping the child in a steamy bathroom for 10 minutes is often helpful, as is a warm drink of a solution of honey.

Many pediatricians prefer not to treat simple cough lest the suppressive action should cause secretions to enter the lungs. If such treatment does become necessary, the following drugs might be useful:

A. DEXTROMETHORPHAN HYDROBROMIDE, N.F.

This is an excellent cough suppressant and is available at low cost, but as a matter of fact it is not commonly needed. Companies always seem to include it in mixtures with minor and mongrel items in order to sell a polypharmacal at a high price. General advice is to avoid non-prescription cough syrup containing dextromethorphan, because any child with cough that severe needs consultation with a doctor, not suppression of his symptom.

Dextromethorphan is available without a prescription in proprietary mixtures. One should ask the pharmacist.

B. CODEINE SULFATE, N.F.

This is a narcotic. It should be used only as a last resort in children.

V. Drugs for Gastrointestinal Disorders

A. Most simple diarrheas are self-limiting and will be helped by stopping all milk and solid food for 24 hours. Water *must* be given, small sips at a time. In older children a popsicle serves this purpose emiently well. If diarrhea should persist severely for more than 24 hours on this regimen, or should blood appear in the stools, a doctor should be consulted. Some pediatricians say that they prescribe kaolin-containing preparations "in order to treat the anxious parents," but a little advice and reassurance would often serve as well.

B. Most vomiting is self-limiting, but persistence (as with diarrhea) may require hospitalization for diagnosis and treatment. The *Handbook* is reluctant to suggest the use of antinausea and antivomiting drugs in children.

VI. Drug for Eczema and Eczematoid Conditions

A. HYDROCORTISONE CREAM 1%, U.S.P.

See Hydrocortisone Cream, U.S.P., in the adult Prescription Drug List. In pediatric practice the most common need is for treating eczematoid skin conditions. In many cases, no treatment is necessary at all because the condition is localized and self-limiting.

VII. Drug for Hay Fever (and Possibly for Hives)

A. DIPHENHYDRAMINE ELIXIR, U.S.P.

This antihistamine may be usefuly in hay fever. Its effectiveness for hives is less certain, but its sedative side effect can help the "itchy" child with hives who cannot sleep.

VIII. Drugs for Asthma and/or Acute Wheezing

A. EPHEDRINE SULFATE, U.S.P.

This is a relatively safe and effective drug for treating a child with wheezing. Since it is often taken regularly over long periods of time, it should be prescribed and purchased as written above. Writing for Tedral®, a tablet containing ephedrine along with small doses of two other drugs, theophylline and phenobarbital, leads to unnecessary expense. See Ephedrine Sulfate, U.S.P., in the adult Prescription Drug List, and in the Price Lists.

B. PREDNISONE, U.S.P.

Occasionally an acute wheezing attack or other acute allergic condition requires a short course of prednisone. A useful system is to prescribe thirty-six 5 milligram tablets with directions to take 8, 7, 6, 5, 4, 3, 2, and 1 tablet on 8 successive days.

Less commonly, chronic allergic conditions will

necessitate a very small daily or every-other-day dose of prednisone on a maintenance basis. At a dose level of 5 milligrams per day, growth and development are unlikely to be affected.

See Prednisone, U.S.P., in the adult Prescription Drug List and also in the Price Lists.

IX. Vitamins and Diet Supplements

It is traditional, as well as generally recommended practice, to give dietary supplements of vitamins C and D to children until age two, and of D and sometimes A to older children who for whatever reason have a poor diet. A convenient but expensive way to take vitamin C is as fresh orange juice. It is not easy to find a simple pediatric vitamin mixture containing only A, D, and C. However, one is Tri-Vi-Sol® Drops (Mead Johnson); a 50 cc bottle costs the druggist $2.05. A preparation with the same vitamins, Tri-Vite® Drops, is sold to druggists by Wolins Pharmacal Corp., which asks only 89 cents for 60 cc. Either preparation, 0.6 cc, provides 3000 U.S.P. units of A, 400 U.S.P. units of D, and 60 milligrams of vitamin C. The daily dose should not exceed this in otherwise normal children.

Where drinking water is not naturally rich enough in fluoride, or where communities have not supplemented drinking water with this chemical, it is generally recommended that children be given 1 milligram of sodium fluoride daily. For infants and small children, dropper bottles of sodium fluoride solution containing 2 milligrams/cc are available inexpensively, although it is possible to pay extra if it is bought by the name Luride®. The standard dose is 10 drops daily. For older children, many drugstores sell unbranded sodium fluoride tablets, each containing 2.2 milligrams. A tablet every other day is a sufficient dose. The wholesale cost of 1000 such tablets is approximately $1.75.

Neither cod-liver oil nor any other vitamin supplement serves as a tonic to promote appetite. Cod-liver oil is still an official *N.F.* preparation. It is a good source of vitamins A and D and is inexpensive. A pint (480 cc) can retail for as little as $2.50. The dose is 1 teaspoonful (5 cc) a day. Its disadvantage is its taste, although many children can take it without batting an eyelash.

X. Analgesics

When an infant or child has a condition associated with pain, the correct dose of aspirin is still the safest analgesic. However, if ingested in excess, aspirin is a common poison. *Because much commercial aspirin resembles candy, it should be kept out of children's reach.*

XI. Iron

Iron-deficiency anemia from inadequate diet is the most common nutritional deficiency among the poor. The best-absorbed specific treatment is the cheapest: ferrous sulfate pediatric drops, which have inexplicably been dropped from both the *United States Pharmacopeia* and the *National Formulary* in recent editions. In a previous edition of the *U.S.P.*, ferrous sulfate syrup containing 40 milligrams (8 milligrams iron) per cc was official. One teaspoonful (5 cc), therefore, contained 40 milligrams of iron. The recommended dose is 2 milligrams of elemental iron per pound of body weight per day. For the average one-year-old who needs iron, 60 milligrams daily is adequate.

Very few companies sell ferrous sulfate pediatric drops, an oversight that demands correction in view of the widespread need. Feosol® Elixir is commonly available. The cost for enough to treat a one-year-old for 2 months will be close to $5. For a poor family with several iron-deficient children, this could be a burden. Surely other manufacturers could move into this area of the market with palatable elixirs that might be even lower-priced. (See Addenda.)

Syrups and elixirs containing anything in addition to iron are nearly always more expensive, serve no additional purpose, and therefore need not be used.

As with all other medications, *is is imperative that iron preparations of any kind be kept out of the reach of children.* Iron poisoning is easily produced in children, and can be fatal without immediate treatment.

N.B.

1. A common cause of death in the home is ingestion of drugs. All drugs should be kept in a safe place out of the reach of inquisitive hands. If a child does swallow a drug, a good treatment is immediate administration of Ipecac Syrup, U.S.P., to induce vomiting. Drugstores dispense it without a prescription, often free. The usual dose is 1 tablespoonful, no matter what the child's age. It usually acts within 20 minutes. If not, the dose should be repeated once. The parent can help to induce vomiting by putting a finger firmly down the child's throat. If this treatment fails to bring about vomiting, the child should be taken to the nearest hospital.

2. Local anesthetic and antihistamine ointments should never be applied to the skin indiscriminately, because of the high incidence of sensitivity. Only certain antibiotic ointments should be used for superficial infections—and then only on a doctor's advice.

APPENDIX B
The Top 200 Drugs Prescribed in 1974*

Drug	Rank†	Drug	Rank
Achromycin® V	26	Butazolidin® Alka®	23
Actifed®	16	Butisol Sodium®	75
Actifed-C® Expectorant	131	Chlor-Trimeton®	51
Afrin®	59	Cleocin®	52
Aldactazide®	57	Combid®	94
Aldactone®	175	Compazine®	85
Aldomet®	17	Cordran®	151
Aldoril®	39	Cortisporin®	89
Ambenyl® Expectorant	144	Coumadin®	102
Amcill®	142	Cyclospasmol®	162
Ampicillin	2	Dalmane®	21
Antivert®	48	Darvocet-N®	24
Apresoline®	192	Darvon®	68
Aristocort®	84	Darvon® Compound-65	3
Artane®	178	Darvon-N®	199
Atarax®	135	Darvon-N®/A.S.A.	195
Atromid-S®	93	DBI-TD®	83
Azo Gantrisin®	123	Decadron®	137
Bellergal®	198	Declomycin®	173
Benadryl®	18	Demerol®	159
Bendectin®	110	Demulen®-21	124
Bentyl®	149	Diabinese®	54
Bentyl®/Phenobarbital	174	Digoxin	61
Benylin® Expectorant	62	Dilantin Sodium®	36
Butazolidin®	140	Dimetane®	145

* Information supplied by the Food and Drug Administration.

† Drugs ranked among the first 50 accounted for slightly more than thirty-five percent of new and refill prescriptions; those among the second 50 accounted for about fifteen percent; the last 100 drugs make up approximately fifteen percent of new and refill prescriptions.

Drug	Rank	Drug	Rank
Dimetapp®	13	Medrol®	148
Diupres®	121	Mellaril®	30
Diuril®	25	Meprobamate	70
Donnagel-PG®	200	Minocin®	143
Donnatal®	15	Mycolog®	58
Doriden®	104	Mycostatin®	71
Dramamine®	196	Mylanta®	161
Drixoral®	67	Mysteclin-F®	130
Dyazide®	22	Naldecon®	113
Elavil®	29	Nembutal®	125
Empirin® Compound/		NeoDecadron®	188
Codeine	8	Neosporin®	87
E-Mycin®	184	Nicotinic Acid	136
Equagesic®	82	Nitroglycerin	105
Equanil®	73	Noludar®	177
Erythrocin®	19	Norgesic®	101
Erythromycin	56	Norlestrin®-21	88
Esidrix®	107	Norlestrin® FE 28	166
Etrafon®	170	Novahistine®-DH	157
Feosol®	153	Novahistine® Expectorant	179
Fiorinal®	34	Novahistine® Singlets	183
Fiorinal®/Codeine	189	Omnipen®	112
Flagyl® Oral	158	Oracon®-21	164
Gantanol®	118	Orinase®	47
Gantrisin®	64	Ornade®	40
Garamycin®	185	Ortho-Novum®	122
Hydergine®	160	Ortho-Novum® 1/50-21	44
Hydrodiuril®	12	Ortho-Novum® 1/80-21	49
Hydropres®	65	Ovral®	9
Hygroton®	63	Ovulen® 21	33
Ilosone®	27	Parafon Forte®	117
Inderal®	50	Paregoric	150
Indocin®	11	Pavabid®	53
Ionamin®	127	Pediamycin®	134
Isopto Carpine®	155	Penbritin®	194
Isordil®	66	Penicillin G Potassium	95
Kaon®	176	Penicillin VK	79
Keflex®	35	Pentids®	69
Kenalog®	97	Pen-Vee® K	74
Lanoxin®	14	Percodan®	55
Lasix®	7	Periactin®	109
Librax®	32	Peri-Colace®	182
Librium®	4	Peritrate® SA	181
Lomotil®	28	Phenaphen®/Codeine	46
Macrodantin®	90	Phenergan®	154
Marax®	115	Phenergan® Expectorant	129

Drug	Rank	Drug	Rank
Phenergan® Exp./		Synalar®	132
Codeine	77	Synthroid®	81
Phenergan® VC		Talwin®	60
Expectorant	187	Tandearil®	120
Phenergan® VC Exp./		Tedral®	133
Codeine	108	Teldrin®	116
Phenobarbital	20	Tenuate®	76
Placidyl®	128	Terramycin®	147
Polaramine®	168	Tetracycline HCl	6
Polycillin®	78	Tetrex®	169
Poly-Vi-Flor® Chewable	193	Thorazine®	37
Prednisone	41	Thyroid	42
Premarin®	5	Tigan®	165
Principen®	111	Tofranil®	92
Pro-Banthine®	146	Tolinase®	167
Proloid®	152	Tranxene®	86
Provera®	171	Triaminic®	197
Pyridium®	190	Triavil®	38
Quinidine Sulfate	126	Tuinal®	191
Rauzide®	186	Tuss-Ornade®	96
Regroton®	119	Tylenol®	99
Reserpine	163	Tylenol®/Codeine	45
Ritalin®	141	Valisone®	72
Salutensin®	114	Valium®	1
Seconal®	138	Vasodilan®	106
Ser-Ap-Es®	43	V-Cillin K®	10
Serax®	103	Vibramycin®	80
Sinequan®	100	Vioform®-	
Stelazine®	91	Hydrocortisone	156
Sterazolidin®	180	Vistaril®	172
Sudafed®	139	Zyloprim®	98
Sumycin®	31		

APPENDIX C

Some Distributors of Generic Drugs

Darby Drug Co., Inc
100 Banks Ave.
Rockville Centre
L.I., New York 11570

Interstate Drug Exchange, Inc.
Engineers Hill
Plainview, New York 11803

Modern Wholesale Drug Co., Inc.
1 Randall Ave.
Rockville Centre
L.I., New York 11570

H. L. Moore Drug Exchange
370 John Downey Drive
P.O. Box 1296
New Britain, Conn. 06050

Henry Schein, Inc.
39-01 - 170th Street
Flushing, New York 11358

Veratex Corporation
18610 Fitzpatrick
Detroit, Michigan 48228

Wolins Pharmacal Corp.
75 Marcus Drive
Melville, New York 11746

Index

Index

A

Abbott Laboratories, 48, 246, 264, 270
Abortion, 189n, 206, 255, 292
  See also Pregnancy
Abuse, drug (addiction, dependence, habituation, overdose, suicide), 163, 167, 172, 176-77, 178, 183-84, 197, 231, 232, 237, 246, 252, 263, 274, 275, 283, 292, 297
Acetaminophen, N.F., 153, 166, 167, 177-78, 202, 221, 262-63
  See also Tylenol®
Achromycin-V®. *See* Tetracycline Hydrochloride, U.S.P.
Acne, drugs for, 265
Actifed®, 139-40
Actifed-C®, Expectorant, 140
  See also Actifed®
Addiction, drug. *See* Abuse, drug
Adrenalin®, 184
Adrenaline, 184, 195, 204, 248
Afrin®, 140-41
Agranulocytosis, 148
Akineton®, 151
Alcohol, U.S.P., 202, 237, 250, 253, 279-80
Alcoholism, 149
Aldactazide®, 141-42, 143, 284
Aldactone®, 142-43, 284
Aldomet®, 143-44
Aldoril®, 144
Aldosterone, 142-43
Alka-Seltzer®, 152
Allergic reactions, and drugs for, 147, 157, 248, 275
Aludrox®, 145
Aluminum hydroxide. *See* Magnesium and aluminum hydroxides mixtures
AMA *Drug Evaluations*, 176, 263
Ambenyl® Expectorant, 145

Amcill®, 147, 266
  See also Ampicillin, U.S.P.
Amenorrhea. *See* Menstrual disorders
Aminophylline, U.S.P. (theophylline ethylenediamine), 145-46
Aminosalicylic Acid, U.S.P. (PAS), 240
Amitriptyline Hydrochloride, U.S.P., 201-2, 208-9
Ammonium Chloride, U.S.P., 145, 160
Amphetamines, 204, 296, 297
  See also Dextroamphetamine Sulfate, U.S.P.
Amphotericin B, 243-45
Ampicillin, U.S.P., 146-47, 213, 227-28, 235, 265-66, 283, 287
Amyl nitrite, 251
Angina pectoris (heart pain), 218, 220, 225-26, 251, 264, 277-78
Ankylosing spondylitis, 221
  See also Arthritis
Ansolysen®, 223
Antacids and antacid mixtures, 232-34, 243, 288
Antibiotics, 146, 240, 241, 242, 243, 244, 245, 247, 260, 263, 265
  See also Cephalexin monohydrate; Chloramphenicol (Chloromycetin®); Erythromycin estolate (Ilosone®); Erythromycin ethylsuccinate; Erythromycin Stearate, U.S.P.
Anticholinergics, 288
Antiflatulants, 243
Antihistamines, 147-49
Antipsychotic and antidepressant drugs, BDI. *See* Amitriptyline Hydrochloride, U.S.P.; Benzodiazepine drugs; Chlorpromazine Hydrochloride, U.S.P.
Antivert®, 148, 149-50, 250

433

APC and APC-like drugs, 166, 167, 179 and n, 202-3, 211, 252, 273
Appendicitis, 279
Appetite suppressants (anorexiants), 223
Aristocort®, 151
Artane®, 151
Arthritis, drugs for, 65, 120-21, 153, 161
Ascriptin®, 153
Aspirin, U.S.P., 148, 152-53, 166, 167, 177-79, 202-3, 205, 211, 220-21, 246, 252, 262, 273-75, 278, 289
Asthma and drugs prescribed for, 219
    Aminophylline, U.S.P., 202
    Antihistamines, 147
    Ephedrine Sulfate, U.S.P., 204, 235-36
    Theophylline, N.F., 205, 235-36
Atarax®, 149, 153, 235, 276
Atromid-S®, 154, 175, 250
Atropine Sulfate, U.S.P. and atropinelike drugs, 139, 151, 154-55, 157, 158-59, 169, 194-95, 230, 232, 288
Azo Gantanol®, 292
Azo Gantrisin®, 155, 292
Azulfidine, 155-56

B

Bactocill®, 201
Banthine®, 288
Banting, Frederick Grant, 222
Barbital, 281 and n
Belladonna Tincture, U.S.P., 156. *See* Tincture of Belladonna
Benadryl®, 148-49, 150, 153, 156, 157, 164, 170, 197, 198, 276, 285
Bendectin®, 157-58
Bendroflumethiazide, 294-95
Benemid®, 169, 221
Ben Gaffin & Associates, 26
Bentyl®, 154, 157, 158-59
Bentyl® with Phenobarbital, 159
Benylin® Expectorant, 159-60
Benzalkonium Chloride, U.S.P., 141
Benzodiazepine drugs, 230
Best, Charles Herbert, 222
Betamethasone Valerate, N.F., 216
Biogenic amines, 275
Biperiden, 151
Birth Control. *See* Contraception
Bladder infections. *See* Urinary tract infections
Blood pressure disorders. *See* Hypertension; Hypotension

Blood-sugar-lowering drugs. *See* Oral blood-sugar-lowering drugs
Blood vessel dilators (vasodilators), 227
Bretylium, 223
Bristol Laboratories, 200
Bromodiphenhydramine hydrochloride, 145
Brompheniramine Maleate, N.F., 164, 190-92
Bronchitis, 146, 147, 165, 265
    See also Upper respiratory tract infections
Bronchospasm. *See* Asthma
Brooklyn Eagle, 30
Brunton, Lauder, 251
Bufferin®, 152
Burns, and drugs prescribed for, 241, 247, 248
Butabarbital. *See* Sodium Butabarbital, U.S.P.
Butalbital, N.F., 211
Butazolidin®, 161, 162, 167, 175, 221 and n
Butazolidin® Alka, 161-62
Butisol® (Butisol Sodium®), 162, 283

C

Cafergot®, 207
Caffeine, U.S.P., 177, 179, 202-3, 207, 211, 252
Calcium carbonate, 233
Campbell, E.J.M., 261, 262
Candicidin, 243
Candida albicans. See Yeast infections
Canker sores. *See* Silver Nitrate, Toughened, *in* Addenda
Carbenicillin, 213
Casanthrol, 276-77
Cascara anthraquinones, 276
Casden, E.J., 29
Cephalexin monohydrate, 213, 227-28
Chicken pox, 275
Chloral Hydrate, U.S.P., 162-63, 175, 176-77, 197, 237, 246, 252, 281
Chloramphenicol, 16, 40, 50-51, 199
    See also Chloromycetin®
Chloriazepoxide Hydrochloride, N.F., 14, 48, 176, 230-32
Chloroform, N.F., 160, 253, 279-80
Chloromycetin®, 16, 40-41, 147, 180n, 258
Chlorothiazide, N.F., 192-94
Chlorpheniramine Maleate, U.S.P., 149, 153, 164, 191, 198, 245-46, 253, 258, 275, 276, 283

Chlorpromazine Hydrochloride, U.S.P., 279
See also Thorazine ®
Chlorpropamide, U.S.P., 187-88
See also Diabinese ®
Chlorthalidone, U.S.P., 217-18, 295
Chlor-Trimeton ®, 149, 153, 164, 191, 198, 246, 275, 276, 283
See also Chlorpheniramine Maleate
Chlor-Trimeton ® Repetabs ®, 164
Chlorzoxazone, 262-63
Cholesterol, 154, 250, 285
Cinchona, 293-94
Cirrhosis, 233
Citric Acid, U.S.P., 279-80
Cleocin ®, 164-65
Clidinium bromide, 230
Clindamycin hydrochloride, 164
Clofibrate, 154, 175, 250
Clorazepate dipotassium, 313
See also Tranxene ®
Cloxacillin, 200, 201
Cobenemide ®, 289
Cocaine, 289
Codeine Phosphate, U.S.P. and/or Codeine Sulfate, N.F., 140, 145, 160, 166-67, 172-73, 179, 183, 202-3, 205, 232, 252-53, 273, 275, 278, 279-80
Cogentin ®, 151
Colace ®, 276
Colchicine, U.S.P., 167-69, 221, 289
Colds. *See* Common colds
Colitis, ulcerative, and drugs prescribed for, 155, 165, 230
Combid ® Spansules ®, 169
Common colds, and drugs prescribed for, 139, 140, 148, 198, 245, 246, 248, 253, 258, 279-80
See also Cough remedies
Compazine ®, 169-70, 279
Competitive Problems in the Drug Industry, 150n
Compoz ®, 148
Congestive heart failure, 284
Conjugated Estrogens, U.S.P., 189n, 286-87
Constipation, and drugs for, 233, 234
Contraceptives. *See* Intrauterine devices (IUD's); Oral contraceptives
Cordran ®, 170-71, 216
Cortisporin ® Ointment, 171-72, 240, 248
Cough remedies (antitussives), 172-74, 253, 258, 279-80
Coumadin ®, 163, 174-75

Cyclandelate, 175-76
Cyclospasmol ®, 175-76, 264
Cyproheptadine, 149, 275-76

D

Dalmane ®, 163, 176-77, 246
Darvon ® and Darvon ® formulations, 168, 177-79
"Day-after" pill, 189, 255
DBI-TD ®, 179-80 and n
Decadron ®, 180-81, 286
Decavitamin Capsules, U.S.P. (or Tablets), 157, 181-82, 215, 239
See also Hexavitamin; Vitamins
Declomycin ®, 182-83, 238
Demeclocycline Hydrochloride, N.F., 182, 238
Demerol ®, 166, 167, 183-84, 273, 274
Demethylchlortetracycline Hydrochloride, N.F., 182-83
See also Demeclocycline Hydrochloride, N.F.
Demulen-28 ®, 256
Dependence, drug. *See* Abuse, drug
Depression. *See* Mental disorders
DES. *See* Diethylstilbestrol
Desiccated thyroid, 290
Dexamethasone Sodium Phosphate, N.F., 180-81, 247
Dexbrompheniramine Maleate, N.F., 198
Dexchlorpheniramine Maleate, N.F., 149, 283
Dexedrine ®, 14-15, 185
Dextroamphetamine Sulfate, U.S.P., 14-15n, 184-86
Dextromethorphan Hydrobromide, N.F., 160, 186-87, 253, 280
Diabetes, and drugs prescribed for, 9, 179-80 and n, 187-88, 193-94, 219, 220, 222, 242, 250, 257-58
Diabinese ®, 179, 187-88
Diarrhea, and drugs for, 147, 155, 165, 167, 169, 232, 233, 234, 245, 263
Diazepam, 176
See also Valium ®
Dicloxacillin. *See* Sodium dicloxacillin
Dicumerol ®, 174-75
Dicyclomine Hydrochloride, N.F., 157, 158, 159
Diethylstilbestrol, U.S.P. (Stilbestrol) (DES), 188-89 and n, 255
Diet pills. *See* Appetite suppressants
Digitalis, 168
Digoxin, 30, 189-90

Dihydroergocornine methane sulfonate, 215
Dihydroergocristine methane sulfonate, 215
Dihydroergokryptine methane sulfonate, 215
Dihydromorphinone, 183
Dihydroxyphenylalanine. *See* Dopa
Dilantin®️ Sodium, 175, 190
Dilaudid®️, 183
Dimenhydrinate, U.S.P., 31, 148, 197
Dimetane®️, 164, 190-91, 198
Dimetapp®️, 191-92
Dioctyl Sodium Sulfosuccinate, N.F., 276-77
Diphenhydramine Hydrochloride, U.S.P., 145, 147-49, 150, 153, 156, 159, 164, 170, 197, 198, 276
Diphenoxylate hydrochloride, 232
Diphenylhydantoin, 175
d-Isoephedrine sulfate, 198
Diupres®️, 192-93, 217, 226, 284
Diuril®️, 193-94, 226, 228, 284, 295
Dizziness. *See* Vertigo
Donnatal®️, 194-95
Dopa (L-Dopa [Levodopa]; Dihydroxyphenylalanine), 151, 195-96 and n
Dopamine, 195-96
Doriden®️, 196-97, 283, 292
Dormethan®️, 187
Doxycycline hyclate, 238
Doxylamine succinate, 157
Dramamine®️, 148-49, 156-57, 197
Dried Aluminum Hydroxide Gel, U.S.P., 161
Drixoral®️, 198
Dyazide®️, 198-99, 284
Dymelor®️, 180n, 188
Dynapen®️, 199-201, 227
Dyrenium®️, 198-99

E

Ear infections, and drugs for, 265, 272
Ecolid®️, 223
Elavil®️, 201-2, 209, 296
Eli Lilly, 177, 178, 205, 207, 270, 297
Elixophyllin®️, 202
Emotional disorders. *See* Mental disorders
Emphysema, 173-74, 161, 262
Empirin®️ Compound with Codeine Phosphate, 166, 202-3
E-Mycin®️, 203
Endocarditis, 271n
Enduron®️, 203-4, 229, 284, 295
Entero-Vioform®️, 263

Ephedrine Sulfate, U.S.P. and Ephedrine-like drugs, 204-5, 235-36, 258
    See also Pseudoephedrine
Epilepsy, and drugs for, 190, 281
Epinephrine, 184
    See also Adrenaline
Equagesic®️, 205
Equanil®️, 24, 206, 237
Ergomar®️, 207
Ergonovine Maleate, U.S.P., 206-7
Ergot, 168, 206
Ergotamine Tartrate, N.F., 206-7
Ergotrate®️, 207
Erythrocin®️ Stearate, 207-8, 218, 264, 265
Erythromycin Estolate, N.F., 218
    See also Ilosone®️
Erythromycin ethylsuccinate, 264-65
Erythromycin Stearate, U.S.P., 165, 199, 203, 207-8, 218, 227
Esidrix®️, 208, 216, 226, 229, 284, 295
Estrogen, 253, 255, 256
    See also Conjugated Estrogens
Ethambutol, 240
Ethchlorvynol, 283
    See also Placidyl®️
Ethinyl estradiol, 256
Ethoheptazine Citrate, N.F., 205
Ethynodiol diacetate, 256
Etrafon®️, 208-9
Excedrin®️-PM, 148
Extentabs®️, 191, 192, 195
Eye disorders, and drugs for, 225

F

FDA. *See* Food and Drug Administration
Feosol®️, 209 and n
Fergon®️, 257
Ferrous Gluconate, N.F., 358
Ferrous Sulfate, U.S.P., 209-10 and n
Fever-reducing drugs. *See* Antipyretics
Fiorinal®️, 211
5-HT, 275
Flagyl®️, 211
Fluocinolone acetonide, 216
    See also Synalar®️
Flurandrenolide, N.F., 170, 216
Flurazepam hydrochloride, 163, 176-77
    See also Dalmane®️
Food and Drug Administration (FDA), 149, 156, 176, 180n
Franklin, Benjamin, 168

Fungus infections, 214, 240, 241, 242, 244
   See also Yeast infections
Furadantin®, 234
Furosemide, 228-29
   See also Lasix®

G

Gangrene, 206
Gantanol®, 212-13
Gantrisin®, 146, 212-14, 265
   See also Azo Gantrisin®
Gardner, John W., 54
Glaucoma, 225
Glutethimide, N.F., 196-97
   See also Doriden®
Glyceryl guaiacolate, 140, 173, 253
Glyceryl trinitrate. *See* Nitroglycerin, U.S.P.
Glycine, 140
Gonorrhea, 266, 271
Gout, and drugs for, 9, 161, 167-69, 221, 250, 288-89
Gramicidin, 240-42
Griseofulvin, N.F., 214
Guanethidine Sulfate, U.S.P., 223-24

H

Habituation. *See* Abuse, drug
Hay fever, and drugs prescribed for, 139, 147
Headaches, and drugs for, 183
   See also Migraine headache
Hepatic dysfunction. *See* Liver disorders; Jaundice
Hexavitamin Capsules, N.F. (or Tablets), 214-15, 239
High blood pressure. *See* Hypertension
Histamine, 147, 275
"Hives" (urticaria), and drugs for, 147, 275
Hoffmann-LaRoche, Inc. *See* Roche Laboratories
Hydergine®, 215
Hydrochlorothiazide, U.S.P., 141-42, 143, 144, 193, 198-99, 204, 208, 216-17, 295
Hydrocortisone, 161, 171, 216, 285-86
Hydrocortisone Cream, U.S.P., 170-71, 216, 228, 242, 247, 271, 276, 286
Hydrocortisone cream, 151
Hydrodiuril®, 144, 193, 199, 204, 208, 216-17, 226, 229, 284, 295
Hydropres®, 217, 226, 284

Hydroxyzine Hydrochloride, N.F., 149, 153, 235-36
   See also Atarax®
Hygroton®, 217-18, 226, 229, 284, 295
Hyoscine hydrobromide, 194-95
Hyoscyamine Sulfate, N.F., 194-95
Hyperactive ("hyperkinetic") children, drugs for, 297
Hypertension (high blood pressure), and drugs prescribed for, 192-94, 204, 216, 217-20, 223, 248, 249, 254, 284, 295, 296
Hypotension (low blood pressure), 196, 279

I

Ilosone®, 208, 218, 265
Immunosuppressives, 24
Inderal®, 118-20
Indocin®, 167, 220-21
Indomethacin, N.F., 220-21
   See also Indocin®
INH. *See* Isoniazid, U.S.P.
Insulin Injection, U.S.P., 179, 188, 219, 222-23, 257, 258
Intrauterine devices (IUD's), 255
Inversine®, 223
Ionamin®, 223
Ipecac, fluid extract of, 279-80
Iron Sulfate. *See* Ferrous Sulfate, U.S.P.
Irritable bowel syndrome ("nervous" stomach), 154, 158, 162, 169, 194, 230, 233
Ischemia, drugs prescribed for, 264
Ismelin®, 223-24
Isoniazid, U.S.P. (INH, Isonicotinic Acid Hydrazide), 224-25, 240
Isopropamide iodide, 169, 258
Isopto Carpine®, 225
Isordil®, 225-26, 251, 277
Isosorbide dinitrate, 225-26
   See also Isordil®
Itching. *See* Pruritis
IUD's. *See* Intrauterine devices

J

Jaundice, 218, 279
   See also Liver disorders
Johnson, Lyndon B., 54, 55
Joint disorders. *See* Arthritis
Journal of the American Medical Association (JAMA), 172

K

Kaochlor®, 284

Kaolin mixture with pectin, 263
Kaon ®, 226-27, 284
Kaopectate ®, 263
Keflex ®, 213, 227-28
K-Lor ®, 284
K-Lyte ®, 284
Kemadrin ®, 151
Kenalog ®, 151, 216, 228

L

Labels, warning. *See* Warning labels
Lasix ®, 228-29, 284, 295
Laxatives and stool softeners, 276-77
L-Dopa. *See* Dopa
Leritine ®, 183
Levodopa. *See* Dopa
Librax ®, 230
Librium ®, 14, 48, 176, 177, 230-32, 264, 281
Ligament injuries. *See* Sprains
Lincocin ® (lincomycin hydrochloride). *See* Addenda
Lipids. *See* Cholesterol
Liver disorders, 250, 264, 281
   See also Jaundice
Local anesthetics, 289
Lomotil ®, 232, 263
Low blood pressure. *See* Hypotension
Lung disease, 147

M

Maalox ®, 145, 153, 232-34, 243
Macrodantin ®, 234-35
Magnesium and aluminum hydroxides mixtures, 11, 232-34, 243
   See also Maalox ®
Magnesium trisilicate, U.S.P., 161
Mahuang, 204
Mandelamine ®, 235. *See also* Addenda
Marax ®, 235-36
Mecamylamine, 223
Meclizine Hydrochloride, U.S.P., 148, 149-50
Medical Letter, 152n, 165n, 172, 272
Medrol ®, 236, 286
Medroxyprogesterone Acetate, U.S.P., 291-92
Mellaril ®, 236, 281
Meningitis, drugs for, 265
Menopausal symptoms, drugs for, 189n, 286-87, 291
Menstrual disorders (amenorrhea), 254
Mental disorders (anxiety, depression, nervousness, neurosis, psychosis, schizophrenia, senility, etc.), and drugs for, 282, 296

Menthol, 160
Meperidine Hydrochloride, U.S.P., 183-84, 274
   See also Demerol ®
Meprobamate, N.F., 24, 205, 206, 237
Merck, Sharp & Dohme, 36, 270, 275, 289
Mestranol, 256
Metahydrin ®, 204, 226, 284, 295
Methadone, 183-84, 273, 274
Methantheline, 288
Methaqualone, 292
Methenamine hippurate, 234
Methenamine Mandelate, U.S.P., 234.
   See also Addenda
Methicillin, 200
Methyclothiazide, 203-4
   See also Enduron ®
Methyldopa, U.S.P., 143-44
Methylphenidate Hydrochloride, N.F., 296-97
Methylprednisolone, N.F., 236
   See also Medrol ®
Methyprylon, N.F., 251-52
   See also Noludar ®
Metronidazole, U.S.P., 211
Michigan State Board of Pharmacy, 29
Micronor ®, 254, 256
Migraine headache, 206-7
Milk of magnesia, 277
Miltown ®, 24, 237
Minocin ®, 238-39
Minocycline hydrochloride, 238-39
Miscarriage. *See* Abortion
Morning sickness, and drugs prescribed for, 157-58, 254
Morphine, 274
Motion sickness (seasickness), and drugs for, 148-49, 150, 153, 156, 229, 279
Multiple vitamins, 239
Muscle pains (spasm), and drugs prescribed for, 262
Myambutol ®, 240
Mycolog ®, 171, 240-42, 248
Mycostatin ®, 242-43, 244
Mylanta ®, 243
Mysteclin-F ®, 243-45 and n

N

Nafcillin, 201
Naldecon ®, 245-46
National Academy of Sciences—National Research Council (NAS-NRC), 139, 149, 156

National Formulary (N.F.), 169
National Research Council. *See* National Academy of Sciences
Nausea and vomiting, and drugs prescribed for, 148, 150, 153, 156, 169-70, 196, 234, 239, 240, 279, 280
Nelson, Gaylord, 257
Nembutal®, 49, 176, 246, 282, 283
NeoDecadron®, 247
Neomycin Sulfate, U.S.P., 171, 240-42, 247-48
Neosporin®, 247-48
Neo-Synephrine®, 4, 198, 246, 248-49, 269, 280
Nephrotic syndrome, and drugs prescribed for, 143
"Nervous stomach." *See* Irritable bowel syndrome
Nicotinamide (niacinamide), 224
Nicotinic acid (niacin), 149-50, 249-50, 264
Nilstat®, 243
Nitrofurantoin, U.S.P., 234-35
Nitroglycerin, U.S.P. (Glyceryl Trinitrate), 226, 277-78
Nixon, Richard M., 57
Noludar®, 251-52, 283
Norethindrone, 256
Norgesic®, 252
Norgestrel, 256
Norinyl®, 256
Norlestrin®, 256
Nor-Q.D.®, 254
Novahistine® DH, 252-53
Novahistine® Expectorant, 253
Nystatin, U.S.P., 240-43
Nytol®, 148

O

Obesity, 258
See also Appetite suppressants
Omnipen®, 147, 266
Opium, 168, 264
See also Paregoric, U.S.P.
Opium-like synthetic narcotics, 232
Oral blood-sugar-lowering drugs, 179-80 and n, 187-88, 193-94, 222, 257
Oral contraceptives ("the pill"), 90, 242, 243, 254-57
Oral steroids, 276
Orinase®, 179, 180n, 187-88, 257-58
Ornade®, 258
Orphenadrine citrate, 252
Ortho-Novum®, 256
Osteoarthritis, 140
Osteoporosis, 281

Overdose, drug. *See* Abuse, drug
Ovral®, 256
Ovrette®, 254
Ovulen®, 256
Oxacillin, 200, 201
Oxycodone hydrochloride, 273-75
See also Percodan®
Oxycodone terephthalate, 273-75
See also Percodan®
Oxygen, U.S.P. (100 percent oxygen), 259-62
Oxymetazoline Hydrochloride, N.F., 140
Oxyphenbutazone, N.F., 175
See also Tandearil®

P

Pagitane®, 151
Pancreatitis, 194
Panmycin®, 262
Papaverine Hydrochloride, N.F., 263-64
Parafon Forte®, 262-63
Paraldehyde, 281
Paregoric, U.S.P. (Camphorated Tincture of Opium), 167, 232, 263
Parke, Davis & Company, 16, 40
Parkinsonism, and drugs for, 151, 196
PAS. *See* Aminosalicylic Acid, U.S.P.
Pathocil®, 200
Pavabid®, 263-64
Pectin, kaolin mixture with, 263
Pediamycin®, 264-65
Pellagra, and drugs for, 249
Penbritin®, 147, 265-66
Penicillin, 380
Pentaerythritol tetranitrate, 277-78
See also Peritrate®
Pentids®, 271, 272-73
Pentobarbital. *See* Sodium Pentobarbital, U.S.P.
Pentolinium, 223
Pen-Vee® K, 272, 273
Peptic ulcer, 153, 154, 158, 161-62, 169, 194, 230, 233, 250, 288
See also Irritable bowel syndrome; Stomach disorders
Percodan®, 166, 167, 183, 273-75
Periactin®, 149, 275-76
Peri-Colace®, 276-77
Peristim®, 276
Peritrate®, 225, 251, 277-78
Peritrate® SA, 225, 277-78
Perphenazine Hydrochloride, N.F., 208-9, 281

Pfizer, Inc., 36, 187, 270
Pharmacopeia of the United States of America (U.S.P.), 52, 56 and n, 169, 181-82, 190, 191, 192, 195, 202, 239, 245, 258
Phenacetin, U.S.P., 177, 179, 202-3, 211, 252, 273-75, 278
 See also APC
Phenaphen ®, 278
Phenaphen ® with Codeine, 278
Phenazopyridine hydrochloride, 155, 292
 See also Salicylazosulfapyridine
Phenergan ®, 278-79, 309
Phenergan ® Expectorant, 279
Phenergan ® Expectorant with Codeine, 279
Phenergan ® VC Expectorant, 280
Phenergan ® VC Expectorant with Codeine, 280
Phenformin hydrochloride, 179-80
Phenobarbital, U.S.P., 153, 159, 162, 169, 190, 194-95, 204, 205, 211, 230, 231, 235, 237, 276, 278, 280-82, 283
Phenothiazine drugs, 169-70, 279
 See also Compazine ®; Phenergan ®; Thorazine ®
Phentermine resin, 223
Phenylbutazone, U.S.P., 161, 175
 See also Butazolidin ®
Phenylephrine Hydrochloride, U.S.P., 141, 148, 191-92, 198, 245-46, 248-49, 252-53, 280
Phenylmercuric acetate, 141
Phenylpropanolamine hydrochloride, 191-92, 245-46, 258
Phenyltoloxamine citrate, 245-46
Photosensitivity, 183
Physicians' Desk Reference (PDR), 141
Pilocarpine Hydrochloride, U.S.P., 225
Pipanol ®, 151
Placidyl ®, 283, 292
Plateau CAPS ®, 264
Pneumonia, 165, 207, 265, 271
Poison ivy, drugs for, 276
Polaramine ®, 149, 164, 283
Polycillin ®, 147, 266, 283
Polymixin B Sulfate, U.S.P., 171, 247-48
Potassium Chloride, U.S.P., 198, 199, 227, 229, 284
Potassium depletion, and drugs for, 142, 193, 198-99, 217, 226-27, 229, 277, 284, 295
Potassium gluconate, 226-27
 See also Kaon ®

Potassium guaiacolsulfonate, N.F., 145
Potassium Guaiacolsulfonate, U.S.P., 279-80
Potassium Penicillin G Tablets, U.S.P., 165, 200, 207, 221, 227, 265, 266, 269-73
Potassium Phenoxymethyl Penicillin, U.S.P. (Penicillin V), 165, 200, 207, 266, 270, 271-72, 273
 see also Penicillin
Potassium retention, 198, 284
Prednisolone, U.S.P., 74, 151, 236, 285
Prednisone, U.S.P., 74, 151, 236, 260, 285-86
Pregnancy, 157-58, 189 and n, 242, 285
 See also Abortion; Intrauterine devices (IUD's); Oral Contraceptives
Premarin ®, 189n, 286-87
Principen ®, 147, 266, 287
Pro-Banthine ®, 154, 287-88
Probenecid, U.S.P., 169, 221, 288-89
Procainamide Hydrochloride, U.S.P., 289-90, 293, 294
Procaine, 289
Prochlorperazine Maleate, U.S.P., 169, 279
Procyclidine, 151
Progesterone, 251, 254
Progestin, 255, 256
Progestogens, 254
Proloid ®, 272, 290-91
Promethazine Hydrochloride, U.S.P., 170, 278-80
Pronestyl ®, 290
Propantheline Bromide, U.S.P., 287-88
 See also Pro-Banthine ®
Propranolol Hydrochloride, U.S.P., 218-20
Prostaphlin ®, 201
Provera ®, 290-92
Pruritis (itching), 149, 153, 275-76
Pseudoephedrine hydrochloride, 139, 140
Psychiatric disorders. *See* Mental Illnesses
Pulvules ®, 178, 297
Pyridium ®, 155, 292
 See also Salicylazosulfapyridine
Pyridoxine Hydrochloride, U.S.P., 157

Q

Quaalude ®, 292
Quinaglute ®, 293

Quinidine gluconate, 293
Quinidine Sulfate, U.S.P., 289, 293
Quinine, 293-94

R

Rapid-eye-movement (REM) sleep, 163
Rauwolfia Serpentina, N.F., 294-95, 296
  See also Rauzide ®
Rauzide ®, 284, 294-95
Raynaud's phenomenon, and drugs prescribed for, 175-76
Regroton ®, 284, 295
REM sleep. *See* Rapid-eye-movement sleep
Reserpine, U.S.P., 144, 168, 192-93, 217, 218, 223, 295, 296
Rheumatic fever, and drugs for, 270-71, 272
Ringworm infections. *See* Fungus infections
Ritalin ®, 296-97
Robitussin ®, 173
Roche Laboratories (Hoffmann-La Roche Inc.), 176, 177, 212, 230
Romilar ®, 187

S

Salicylazosulfapyridine, 155
  See also Phenazopyridine hydrochloride
Salt retention. *See* Sodium retention
Sandoz Pharmaceuticals, 207
Seasickness. *See* Motion sickness
Secobarbital. *See* Sodium Secobarbital, U.S.P.
Seconal ® Sodium, 176, 282, 283, 297-98
Ser-Ap-Es ®, 284
Serax ®, 230, 281
Serpasil ®, 27
Silver Nitrate, Toughened. *See* Addenda
Simethicone, 243
Smith Kline & French Laboratories, 14-15, 36, 184-85, 198
Sodium bicarbonate, 152, 233
Sodium Butabarbital, U.S.P., 162, 237, 283
Sodium Citrate, U.S.P., 160, 279-80
Sodium dicloxacillin, 165, 199-201, 227
Sodium Diphenylhydantoin, U.S.P., 63, 190
Sodium Pentobarbital, U.S.P., 48-49, 176, 197, 246, 252, 282, 283, 297

Sodium retention, 142, 152, 161
Sodium Secobarbital, U.S.P., 176, 197, 246, 252, 282, 283, 297-98
Sodium Warfarin, U.S.P., 163, 174-75, 177, 246
Sominex ®, 148
Sorbitol, 140
Spansules ®, 169n, 258, 275
Spironolactone, U.S.P., 141-43
  See also Aldactazide ® ; Aldactone ®
Sprains, 161
Squibb & Sons, E.R., 243, 244, 245n, 270, 271, 272
St. Anthony's Fire, 206
Staphylococcus infections, and drugs prescribed for, 165, 199-201, 227, 239, 265, 267-68
Stomach disorders, 243
  See also Irritable bowel syndrome; Peptic ulcer
Stool softeners. *See* Laxatives and stool softeners
Subcommittee on Monopoly, 257
Suicide. *See* Abuse, drug
Sulfamethoxazole, 212-13
Sulfisoxazole, U.S.P., 146, 155, 212-14, 227
  See also Gantrisin ®
"Sustained action" preparations, 209, 245-46
  See also Extentabs ® ; Spansules ®
Synalar ®, 216, 228

T

Talwin ®, 273, 274
Tandearil ®, 175, 221 and n
Tedral ®, 205, 235
Tegopen ®, 200
Telangiectasis, 216
Terpin hydrate and codeine elixir, 172
Thalidomide, 157
Theophylline, N.F., 202, 205, 235-36
Thiazides, 223, 224, 228-29, 284, 295, 296
Thioridazine, 236, 281
Thorazine ®, 169, 279
Throat infections, and drugs prescribed for, 227, 265, 270, 272
Thrombophlebitis, and drugs prescribed for, 174-75, 291-92
"Thrush." *See* Vaginal disorders
Thyroglobulin, 290-91
  See also Proloid ®
Tinactin ®. *See* Addenda
Tincture of Belladonna (Belladonna Tincture. U.S.P.) and Belladonnalike drugs, 154-55, 156,

Tincture of Belladonna (cont.)
158-59, 195, 230, 252, 288
See also Atropine Sulfate, U.S.P.
Tincture of opium. *See* Paregoric,
U.S.P.
Tinea. *See* Fungus infections
Tofranil ®, 296
Tolbutamide, U.S.P., 187-88, 257-58
See also Orinase ®
Tolinase ®, 179, 180n, 188
Tolnaftate, U.S.P. *See* Addenda
Topical antibiotics, 247-48
Topical steroids, 170-72, 216, 228,
247-48, 276, 285, 286
Toughened Silver Nitrate, U.S.P.
See Addenda
Trademark law, 246
Trantoin ®, 234
Tranxene ®, 231, 281, 313
Tremin ®, 151
Triamcinolone Acetonide, U.S.P.,
151, 216, 228, 240-42
Triamterene, 198-99
Triavil ®, 406
Trichlormethiazide drugs, 193, 199,
204, 208, 224, 229, 295, 296
See also Thiazides
Trichomonads, drugs for, 211, 242
Tricyclic antidepressants, 296
See also Elavil ®
Triglycerides, 250
Trihexyphenidyl Hydrochloride,
U.S.P., 151
Trilafon ®, 209
Tripelennamine Hydrochloride,
U.S.P., 149
Triple antibiotic ointment. *See* Neo-
sporin ®
Triple Sulfas Tablets (Trisulfapy-
rimidine Tablets, U.S.P.), (Sul-
facetamide, Sulfadiazine, and
Sulfamerazine Tablets, N.F.),
146, 212, 213, 214
Triprolidine hydrochloride, 139, 140
Trisulfapyrimidine Tablets, U.S.P.
See Triple Sulfas Tablets
Tuberculosis, and drugs for, 173, 240
Tums ®, 233
See also Ornade ®
Tylenol ®, 70, 166, 167, 202, 273
See also Acetaminophen, N.F.
Typhoid fever, 147
Tyrosine, 195

U

Ulcerative colitis. *See* Colitis
Ulcer, stomach. *See* Peptic ulcer;
stomach disorders
Unipen ®, 201
Upjohn Company, The, 17, 36, 164,
187, 203, 257, 262, 270
Upper respiratory tract infections,
147, 165, 172-74, 227, 245, 246
Urethan, 281
Urinary tract infections, and drugs
prescribed for, 146, 155, 212, 213,
227, 234-35, 239, 265
Urticaria. *See* "Hives"

V

Vaginal disorders, and drugs for, 211,
240-42, 254, 286
Valisone ®, 216
Valium ®, 176, 177, 230, 281
V-Cillin K ®, 272
Venereal disease. *See* Gonorrhea
Ventimask ®, 261
"Venturi mask," 261
Veracillin ®, 200
Veronal ®, 281
Vertigo (dizziness), 148-50, 239
Vibramycin ®, 238
Vick's "Cough Silencers ®," 187
Vistaril ®, 149, 276
Vitamins, 325
Vomiting. *See* Nausea and vomiting

W

Wallace Pharmaceuticals, 36
Warfarin. *See* Sodium Warfarin
Warner/Chilcott Laboratories, 205,
277, 290
Whiskey, 251
Wound healing, and drugs prescribed
for, 171, 240, 241, 247-48
Wyeth Laboratories, 200, 205, 237

Y

Yeast infections. *See* Vaginal disorders

Z

Zinc Bacitracin, U.S.P., 171, 247-48
Zyloprim ®, 289

Addenda

Addenda

Addendum to Chapter 3, I: The Character of the Onslaught Against Us, page 89

During the late 1950s and through the 1960s, for example, one of the most profitable and heavily prescribed items was a product, Panalba®, marketed by the Upjohn Company. Panalba® was a capsule containing two antibiotics: tetracycline and novobiocin. The rationale for including the novobiocin, according to Upjohn promotion, was to discourage superinfection with toxic staphylococcus germs. These germs are not harmed, in many cases, by tetracycline. Thus, when tetracycline knocks out many other species of germs in the gastrointestinal tract, there is always the latent possibility that these toxic staphylococcus germs will overgrow abundantly in the absence of competing organisms. In debilitated people, this kind of staphylococcus can enter and has entered the bloodstream and caused death from septicemia.

When the National Academy of Sciences–National Research Council study of drug efficacy was undertaken in the mid-1960s, Panalba® was studied and declared to be ineffective as a fixed-dose combination. The mixing of two or more drugs in one tablet or capsule is poor medical practice—as has been pointed out again and again in the *Handbook*. Infectious-disease experts consider it an especially poor practice with antibiotics. In the case of Panalba®, it was decided that better drugs existed than novobiocin to treat tetracycline-resistant staphylococcus infections, anyway. The NAS-NRC therefore advised the FDA to take Panalba® off the market.

There ensued a gigantic brouhaha, with Upjohn sending letters to doctors informing them of the company's intention to fight the FDA. Upjohn spoke of the tried-and-true nature of Panalba® and hinted of government encroachment on doctors' rights to prescribe as they see fit.

In the end, Upjohn lost its case; but before the story was closed, an FDA inspector discovered, on March 7, 1969, that Upjohn had substantial evidence in its files, at least prior to 1966 and possibly as early as 1960, that when tetracycline and novobiocin are taken together each inhibits the absorption of the other into the bloodstream. The very item that Upjohn was touting as good for possible overwhelming staphylococcus infections was found, in some clinical trials, to have its absorption into the blood so badly interfered with that hardly any of it could be found in the bloodstream!

This vital information concerning Panalba®, which had been in the Upjohn files for years, had never been made known until the FDA inspector discovered it. As a properly constituted federal regulatory agency, the FDA had a right to know about these data, and Upjohn had a responsibility to provide them.

The story in all its detail appears in *Present Status of Competition in the Pharmaceutical Industry*, Part 12, pages 5147 *et seq.*

Addenda to Chapter 3, II: Derogatory Euphemism, page 91, footnote 15

DOCUMENTATIONS:

"Nosocomial Bacteremias Associated with Intravenous Fluid Therapy—U.S.A.," *Morbidity and Mortality Weekly Reports of the Center for Disease Control,*

Suppl. Vol. 20, No. 9 (released March 12, 1971). The article alludes to 150 bacteremias ("septicemias") and 9 deaths.

"Follow-up on Septicemias Associated with Contaminated Intravenous Fluids—United States," *Morbidity and Mortality Weekly Reports of the Center for Disease Control*, Vol. 20, No. 11 (released March 26, 1971). The article alludes to 350 septicemias known to have been reported as of March 22, 1971. The bacteria recovered from the blood of the septicemia victims included *Enterobacter cloacae*, a sewer organism, and another, *Enterobacter agglomerans* (also known as *Herbicula lathyri*).

Addendum to the Basic Drug List, pages 133, 134

Decavitamin, U.S.P., and Hexavitamin, N.F., are listed primarily for educational purposes. Doctors and students of medicine should be aware of their existence: great care has gone into their composition. Yet, from a practical standpoint, there are such an overwhelming number of relatively inexpensive over-the-counter multivitamin preparations facing the prospective buyer that trying to find either of these official preparations would be like trying to find the proverbial needle in a haystack. Also, to ensure that a patient received either of the official vitamin mixtures would almost surely require specific instructions—*i.e.*, a prescription—from doctor to pharmacist. This would increase the cost to the patient.

Addendum to the Prescription Drug List, Antivert®, page 150

On June 1, 1975, the FDA annual updated report on final decisions on drug efficacy declared Antivert® to be "ineffective" for all the conditions for which it

had been promoted. The manufacturers of Antivert®
then quietly removed the nicotinic acid component.

Addendum to the Prescription Drug List, Cleocin®, page 164

FDA witnesses told Senator Nelson's subcommittee
on July 9, 1975, that in their opinion Cleocin® is probably indicated for use in only about 5 percent of the
instances where it is currently being prescribed. Bearing
in mind that Cleocin® was the 52nd most-prescribed
drug in the United States in 1974, the testimony of the
FDA witnesses, if correct, makes a mockery of the
oft-repeated slogan "Doctors should be free to prescribe
as they wish without government interference in the
doctor-patient relationship." The testimony, if correct,
points up again the need for much of the medical profession to learn how to prescribe drugs rationally.

Addendum to the Prescription Drug List, DBI-TD®, page 179

On July 9, 1975, FDA experts reported to the United
States Senate Subcommittee on Monopoly that, in their
opinion, there is no justification for continuing to use
phenformin (sold as DBI® and DBI-TD®) as a prescription drug. The University Group Diabetes Program
(UGDP) study found it to be causing excessive mortality from heart disease at an even faster clip than
Orinase®. No evidence exists to show that phenformin
retards progression of disease in the small blood vessels. It is the latter that is the important killer of real
diabetes patients; the elevated blood sugar is of com-
paratively minor importance.

Addendum to the Prescription Drug List, page 232

LINCOCIN®   lincomycin hydrochloride

In hearings (July 1975 before the Nelson subcommittee, a substantial amount of testimony was provided by experts who supported the contention that Lincocin's® toxicity (severe diarrhea, bloody ulcerative colitis, and deaths attributable to its use) outweighs its usefulness. These experts contended that Lincocin® should be removed from the market.

Addendum to the Prescription Drug List, page 235

MANDELAMINE® Methenamine Mandelate, U.S.P.

This is a good drug, which should be more widely used than it is. It is recommended by many experts for "suppressive" treatment of urinary tract infection in persons prone to recurrences. Its more important component is the part of the molecule which is derived from mandelic acid. Mandelic acid in the un-ionized form can kill bacteria. As with most organic molecules, it is only the un-ionized (hence, fat-soluble) form that can enter into cells (bacteria are single cells). The trick to changing mandelic acid into the un-ionized form is to put it in a fairly acidic environment. For this purpose it is sometimes necessary for patients to take 4 to 8 grams a day of ascorbic acid (vitamin C), which is harmlessly excreted in the urine and usually acidifies it nicely.

Two points about the use of methenamine mandelate:

1. Prescribed and bought as "methenamine mandelate" it can be inexpensive (0.5 gram tablets at $7.50 per 1000). Economy is usually an important consideration because the drug is meant to be taken regularly for long periods of time. Writing Mandelamine® on the prescription makes economy impossible. The "suppressive" dose is 1 gram three or four times a day.

2. The patient should check the urine occasionally with indicator paper to be sure that the pH is 5.0 or less. If pH is higher than this, the patient will have to take 4 to 8 grams a day of ascorbic acid, which many

pharmacists will sell in large quantities cheaply (0.5 gram tablets wholesale for $7–$10 per 1000). If ascorbic acid fails to lower the pH, the chronic infection is probably with *Proteus mirabilis*, an organism which alkalinizes the urine by "splitting" urea into ammonia. In such cases methenamine mandelate is useless treatment.

Addendum to the Prescription Drug List, Orinase®, page 257

In September 1975 a hearing was held in which the FDA made known its proposal to require that all advertisements for Orinase® contain information concerning its potential lethal effects. The FDA decided to take this action after the Biometric Society, a highly respected international organization of biostatisticians, had made a detailed review of the data collected by the University Group Diabetes Program (UGDP), an American multi-university study program. In a ten-year study, the UGDP had shown that Orinase® not only is ineffective in preventing long-term vascular complications of diabetes but that it probably accelerates the development of blood-vessel disease. The Biometric Society's conclusion, after scrutinizing the UGDP's study, was this: "We consider that in the light of the UGDP findings, it remains with the proponents of the oral hypoglycemics to conduct scientifically adequate studies to justify the continued use of such agents."

The complete report by the Biometric Society appears in *Competitive Problems in the Drug Industry*, Part 28, pp. 13,337–13,377.

Addendum to the Prescription Drug List, page 300

SILVER NITRATE, TOUGHENED (TOUGHENED SILVER NITRATE, U.S.P.)

Painful "canker sores" in the mouth are a common reason for visiting the doctor. A good method of treatment—fast and reliable—is with silver nitrate on applicator sticks, available to the doctor for about 2 cents apiece. The hard, crystalline tip of the applicator is moistened with a drop or two of tap water and touched for a moment to the "canker." A residue of nitric acid is left on the lesion, which turns whitish-gray and, after an initial stinging sensation, becomes painless. When there are multiple "canker sores," no more than four should be treated at a single visit.

A less common use of the drug is to apply it to the surface of warts, including plantar warts. Often, if one is persistent and patient, the wart turns black to its "roots," separates itself from the healthy surrounding skin, and is easily "shelled out."

Addendum to the Prescription Drug List, page 310

TINACTIN®   Tolnaftate, U.S.P.

This is the single brand name for tolnaftate, a drug for athlete's foot and certain other Trichophyton infections. It is a good drug, and as a little bit goes a long way, it is reasonably economical. It does not work against fungus infections of nails or hair, and cannot affect monilia infections ("thrush," or candidiasis).

Addendum to Appendix A: Prescribing for Children, page 424

Since this section was written, generic manufacturers have marketed ferrous sulfate elixir, and comparison of their prices with that of Feosol® Elixir shows a little price-saving. For example, while 12 ounces (¾ pint) of Smith Kline & French's Feosol® Elixir wholesales for $1.45, Wolins sells 16 ounces (1 pint) for $1.65. Moore's price is $1.60 per pint.

Dr. Richard Burack, first chairman of the Massachusetts Drug Formulary Commission, served on the Harvard Medical School staff and faculty for 23 years. In 1974 he became a Medical Director of a major industrial concern. Dr. Fred J. Fox is currently completing training in internal medicine at the University of Washington Affiliated Hospitals in Seattle, Washington, and is interested in clinical pharmacology as a career.